WOMENOPAUSE:
STOP PAUSING AND START LIVING

FEELING FIT, FEMININE, AND FABULOUS IN FOUR WEEKS

ক৵ড়

THE MENOPAUSE MAKEOVER

ক৵ড়

WOMENOPAUSE:
STOP PAUSING AND START LIVING

FEELING FIT, FEMININE, AND FABULOUS IN FOUR WEEKS

❧

THE MENOPAUSE MAKEOVER

❧

Lovera Wolf Miller, M.D., F.A.C.O.G., N.C.M.P.

and

David C. Miller, M.D., M.A., D.A.B.P.M., N.C.M.P.

BOOKS

Winchester, UK
Washington, USA

First published by O-Books, 2010
O Books is an imprint of John Hunt Publishing Ltd., The Bothy, Deershot Lodge, Park Lane, Ropley,
Hants, SO24 0BE, UK
office1@o-books.net
www.o-books.com

Distribution in:

UK and Europe
Orca Book Services Ltd

Home trade orders
tradeorders@orcabookservices.co.uk
Tel: 01235 465521 Fax: 01235 465555

Export orders
exportorders@orcabookservices.co.uk
Tel: 01235 465516 or 01235 465517
Fax: 01235 465555

USA and Canada
NBN
custserv@nbnbooks.com
Tel: 1 800 462 6420 Fax: 1 800 338 4550

Australia and New Zealand
Brumby Books
sales@brumbybooks.com.au
Tel: 61 3 9761 5535 Fax: 61 3 9761 7095

Far East (offices in Singapore, Thailand,
Hong Kong, Taiwan)
Pansing Distribution Pte Ltd
kemal@pansing.com
Tel: 65 6319 9939 Fax: 65 6462 5761

South Africa
Stephan Phillips (pty) Ltd
Email: orders@stephanphillips.com
Tel: 27 21 4489839 Telefax: 27 21 4479879

Text copyright Lovera Wolf Miller &
David C. Miller 2009

Design: Stuart Davies

ISBN: 978 1 84694 321 8

A CIP catalogue record for this book is
available from the British Library.

Printed in the UK by CPI Antony Rowe
Printed in the USA by Offset Paperback Mfrs,
Inc

We operate a distinctive and ethical publishing philosophy in all
areas of its business, from its global network of authors to
production and worldwide distribution.

CONTENTS

"...it's a fabulous book. Womenopause is a very well-rounded, comprehensive compendium on the female transition commonly termed menopause. Lovera and David Miller offer a refreshing look at a natural process that affects every aspect of the midlife woman's health and well-being. They challenge standard social concepts of menopause as well as provide a new paradigm that focuses on vitality and wellness. The book offers a clear and understandable, yet thorough and scientifically sound explanation of the physiology of menopause and the anticipated physical, psychological and mental changes. The authors offer a well-balanced view of available remedies for symptoms including hormonal, nonhormonal-pharmaceutical, and alternative treatments. Also, they nicely discuss behavioral and lifestyle approaches. This book is tremendous resource for any woman seeking to employ an intelligent and multifaceted approach to the Womenopause transition."

Sharon J. Parish, M.D.

Associate Clinical Professor of Medicine, Albert Einstein School of Medicine Board of Directors: The International Society for the Study of Women's Sexual Health

"...wonderfully knowledgeable while tastefully entertaining. Womenopause: Stop Pausing and Start Living is an insightful guide for women explaining in a light-hearted manner premenopause, the transition, and postmenopause. Women of all ages would benefit from the knowledge provided in this book written to take away the fear of menopause and provide empowerment in its stead."

Irwin Goldstein, MD

Clinical Professor of Surgery, University of California at San Diego Editor-in-Chief, The Journal of Sexual Medicine

Book Reviews for WOMENOPAUSE: STOP PAUSING AND START LIVING

Nothing plays havoc with marital intimacy like misunderstood menopause. Couples struggle individually and together--- often in all-out conflict attempting to make sense of the changes. Frequently, women embrace self-blame, ridicule, and a sense of being less than they are. And when husbands are insensitive or *simply clueless, women can begin to feel downright crazy. Even in 'best case menopause' with a strong partnership, a couple's relationship is stressed in ways previously not experienced.*

For decades in my work as a licensed marital therapist, I have been seeking a resource to assist my clients to gain understanding, acceptance, and active management of this normal life cycle transition. Confused couples, especially those in their late 30s-early 40s, have frequently come to me for therapy wondering whether their marital problems and decline in sexual intimacy could be related to menopause.

In Womenopause: Stop Pausing and Start Living Lovera Wolf Miller, MD and David C. Miller, M.D. provide remarkable insight into the menopause transition for women and the men who love them. With frequent spoonfuls of sugar, the Millers, who are certified menopause specialists, translate the mystery using everyday metaphors and analogies. The authors supply frequent, unexpected spurts of humor to break up the dryness of necessary medical terminology. Readers seeking detailed explanations of the menopause process will not be disappointed. At the same time, the format is friendly for those who prefer to skim for main points.

No discussion of menopause would be complete without a full review of the impact of perimenopause and post-menopause on sexual and emotional intimacy. In straightforward, no-nonsense language, the Millers describe the specific body and mood changes triggered by hormonal shifts. Chapter 18, Sexercise is likely to be the section that women assign as required reading to their partners. Written with clarity and wit, men will benefit from this insider's view of how menopause affects a woman's sexual desire and arousal. And while they have the book in hand, men may just be drawn to read chapter 25, Manopause to help them make sense of their own hormonal transition.

Womenopause propels readers beyond understanding to a commitment for action through challenges and behavioral assignments at the close of each chapter. Simple to do, these challenges are designed with specific direction and goals for becoming healthier and strengthening intimate partnerships during menopause.

Womenopause demonstrates that there is no "one size menopause fits all". Each woman's experience is her own, yet there is a set of familiar symptoms. The book provides useful charts for you to evaluate based on symptoms, your position in what the authors refer to as "a naturally evolving transformation of life". Being clear about what is happening to you is the first step to decision making about available remedies.

The authors also take a fresh look at the findings from the Women's Health Initiative (WHI) 2002.The initial published results threw a scare into women taking or considering hormones. This study of 6,000 women yielded early findings that were incomplete--- since less than 1000 of the participants were in early post-menopause, under the age of 60. The Millers report on facts reached through the subsequent analysis of the WHI data; which yield a more optimistic look at Menopause Hormone Therapy (MHT) as a solution to be considered--- after weighing all the individual risks and benefits.

This book can be your go-to guide for menopause information for years to come. Through its positive and proactive tone, you and your partner will be encouraged and guided to journey through this transition united in understanding, support, harmony, and action.

Patt Hollinger Pickett, PhD

Licensed Marriage and Family Therapist Licensed Professional Counselor

Certified Professional Coach Clinical Member of the

American Association for Marriage and Family Therapists (AAMFT)

Author of *Dr. Coach Love's Life Coaching Tips* at

www.DrCoachLove.com

Where was this great informative, humorous and uplifting book ten years ago when I needed it? Well, fortunately it is here now and for those of you that want to take your life back and bring some pizzazz into it read my review of Womenopause and get the low down on Menopause and more. In order to understand the rationale behind this informative book I decided to take the Womenopause challenge...

Fran Lewis of Bookpleasures.com

Dr. Lovera Wolf Miller and Dr. David C. Miller, are the personification of the couple all us women over 50 want to be a part of! They wanted to share what worked for their life with all us women out there that face the same challenges brought on by menopause. It offers real life solutions that are designed to make menopause the wonderful new chapter of life and "relationship enhancer" it can be. I highly recommend this insightful, articulate, fresh take on menopause from a unique couple living the dream!

Roberta Speyer, Publisher

www.OBGYN.net The Universe of Women's Health

#1 women's health and ob/gyn destination website.

"Womenopause: Stop Pausing and Start Living" is the perfect book for a woman approaching or in the early stages of menopause — or, as the book's authors like to term it: "womenopause." "Womenopause" encourages women to be proactive about taking control of health problems — from specific symptoms associated with menopause to bigger issues such as obesity — that can cut short or reduce the quality of a person's life. For those who planned their pregnancies, why not also plan this phase of your life? And to others, who "go with the flow," you will also benefit from acquiring the knowledge to actually recognize what's going on, because there's a lot more to know about perimenopause than hot flashes and mood swings.

Jana Peterson, Duluth Budgeteer News

"What I liked best about Womenopause is that it takes the fear and dread out of menopause by providing so many down-to-earth actionable ideas for living well before, during and after this important life passage."

Christine Crosby, Editorial Director, GRAND Magazine

Through changes in diet, exercise, use of supplements, and informed decisions made in partnership with one's doctor, readers will experience a new and better state of being, perhaps finding themselves more fit and feminine in later life than ever before. Womenopause is the definitive guide to the second half of life, and no woman should be without it.

Dawn Williams Managing Editor Chicagoland Senior News – 50 and Better!

In Womenopause: Stop Pausing and Start Living, the authors explain how to make the "post-menopause" years the best of a woman's life. I encourage all women to take the Womenopause Challenge! The authors' appreciation for the way a woman's body works shines through this well written and accessible book. Womenopause takes all the negative stereotypes associated with menopause and turns them on their head! A must read for women of all ages!
Andrea I. Weinstein, Esq. Co-founder and President
CommitmentNow.com

The years a woman goes through "the changes" come with several unique challenges. We may feel our bodies have betrayed us, as what has always seemed normal suddenly goes off-kilter. So it's understandable that we reach for support during these turbulent years. In Womenopause, authors Lovera Wolf Miller, M.D. and David C. Miller, M.D. explore some of these changes, and offer their suggestions in how to handle them.
Alice Berger bergerbookreviews.wordpress.com

I highly recommend menopausal women to read this book! Very educational! It gives you the information that the doctors do not!
Sandy Draelos, Publisher
Boomers! Newspaper Milwaukee, WI

DEDICATION

To our daughters,
Sasha Fay Miller Franger
And Brienna Ginelle Miller,
Your love makes our life complete.

ACKNOWLEDGEMENTS

One rarely gets the chance to publicly thank family and friends for their love and support, so we savor this opportunity. For our parents Dr William E. and Armina Carter Wolf, and John Robert and the late Marjorie Calvert Miller, we have no words that could ever come close to expressing our love and appreciation. Our children Sasha Fay Miller Franger and Brienna Ginelle Miller, you make life FUN.

Our appreciation goes to our new son Kash Franger for legal advice (frangerlaw.com). To our brothers and sisters, we say thanks for the years of love and patience: John, Victoria, Mina, Lana, Mark, Randy, Susan, Bill, Renee, Lisa, and Scott. We want to honor our friends who have laughed and cried with us , who keep us honest, and who no doubt, would drop everything to come bail us out of a Bangkok prison: Bob and Cindy Cutler, Ben and Dar Mannix, Chris and Jenny Hawkins, Mike and Debbie McDermott, Kai and Starr Nyby, Joe Finelli, and Mr. Duck. We give many thanks to Karen Ellison for the yoga lessons and inspirations (karensyoga.com).

We are grateful to our co-workers who have given us so much slack while we wrote this book: Tammy, Nikki, Melissa, Jackie, and Jenny thank you all. Thanks also to our partners and the staff at Woodland HealthCare and our hospital partners: St. Anthony's Memorial Hospital of Michigan City, IN and LaPorte Regional Health Center in LaPorte, IN.

We give a special thanks to Timothy J. Winski for graphic design and encouragement (574-210-2334).

A huge thank you goes to our literary agent Laura Strachan (strachanlit.com), who believed in us and the book from the beginning and helped us fulfill our hope of bringing *Womenopause* to print.

To our proof-readers: Yolanda Craft, Sasha, and Brienna, we

value your opinions and expertise, and you helped make this book mouer b;ed"d-r..

We also send our thanks to John Hunt, publisher of O-Books. We appreciate his vision and innovations.

Chapter 1

Feeling Fit, Feminine, and Fabulous
in Four Weeks

Part I:
Menopause Makeover

Many women dread menopause. As a symbolic dividing line, the prospect of menopause may unnecessarily conjure visions of decline and demise. This book turns that notion around. There are robust reasons why menopause and beyond should be the best years of a woman's life.

The menopause opinion makeover begins right now. Menopause is a woman's last menstrual period, the pausing of menstruation. Of course, the word menopause is ironic since "men" do not get menopause (they really don't get it). The term "womenopause" suits the situation better because it's about women, and it's about NOT pausing. Many use the term menopause, loosely, to describe the later years of life after the cessation of regular periods. It's okay to refer to it that way, but we recommend dividing the time surrounding menopause into two parts. First, "perimenopause" refers to the interval of irregular periods and hot flashes that may occur for a decade before periods officially cease. Second, all the time following the last menstrual period is "postmenopause".

While menopause is an important milestone, it does not signal finality. A good analogy for menopause is High School graduation "commencement exercises". The end of formal schooling points toward beginning (commencing) the next phase of life with a fresh, bold confidence and hope. The same is true for menopause.

It is possible for you to be healthier at age 60 than you were at age 40. It is possible for you to be stronger, leaner, keener, and happier. It is possible. How do you get there? You will not get there by chance. You will not get there by wishful thinking. Unfortunately, you will not get there by just reading this book. There are steps you can take, beginning today, to help you manage your menopause that will have tremendous long-term health consequences. Learning about menopause is useful only when that information is put to work. Nothing changes without action.

This menopause book is not like reading a romance novel; it is more like trekking the Andes and discovering Machu Picchu. Reading about Machu Picchu is one thing, seeing the video is another, but hiking to the place is something altogether more rewarding. Womenopause is an invitation to action.

Menopause is not an isolated medical incident. Menopause is a naturally evolving transformation of life that progresses within a woman's pivotal years. General health, fitness, diet, marriage, ethnicity, children, church, job, parents, finances, friends, social life, and community involvement, all factor in to how menopause may become expressed. It is important to consider that menopause does not occur within a no-strings-attached void; it transforms women within the context of an already convoluted life and within the complexities of a marriage and/or other dynamic relationships. Every woman will go through menopause, but none will experience it in exactly the same way.

Have you ever shopped for jeans? There must be about a million shapes, colors, styles, and sizes. Everyone expects their jeans to have the best possible fit. Fortunately, today, women have about as many choices to help them manage their midlife change. Just as you would insist on the right jeans, you should expect a perfect designer healthcare fit for your menopause.

Part II:
You Are Not Alone

Every single day, 6000 American women reach menopause. That's a big number. This means over two million women kiss their periods goodbye each year. The average age of menopause at 51 does not appear to be changing over time. What *has* changed is women's life expectancy. A hundred years ago few women lived past their menopause. Today, however, if a woman is healthy at age 50, she most likely will live long into her eighties (Figure 1-1).

The decisions a woman makes regarding how she manages the midlife changes of her perimenopause and beyond have enormous consequences. These decisions will determine her health and well-being for the second half of her life.

If this excites you, you are in good company. Many women are confused about what they have heard regarding menopause and, particularly, the role of menopausal hormone therapy (MHT). MHT replaces the term with which you may be more familiar: hormone replacement therapy (HRT). This book will help you set

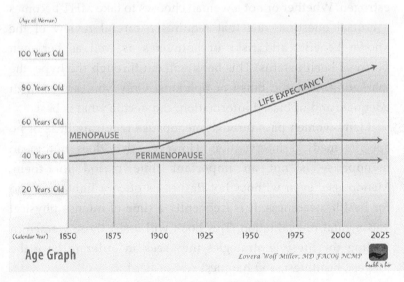

Figure 1-1 Age Graph

in motion a medical plan that suits your specific needs.

It is hard to find a more controversial medical topic than the use of menopausal hormone therapy (MHT). Never has there been a more over-hyped or more maligned medical treatment option. Proponents and opponents publicly disparage each other, and menopausal women are the ones who end up suffering the most from the dispute. The controversy has been brewing for the past century, and it is not likely to go away any time soon. It seems like everyone has an opinion about hormone therapy, and those opinions seem to change every month. This book will help you separate the truths from the trends. Many women have a love/hate relationship with the notion of hormone therapy. If you are one of them, you are definitely not alone.

Before any discussion about menopausal hormone therapy may proceed, a certain point has to be made. There is one scientific fact, the proverbial elephant in the room; menopause is linked to a drastic decline of circulating estrogen. Certainly, many physical, social, and emotional events factor into the change, but none compare to the direct consequences of very low estrogen. Whether or not a woman chooses to take MHT becomes a crucial question, one that requires a careful review of the known benefits and risks of hormones as well as her own personal health status. This book will cut through the hype, the marketing, and the noise of opinions. Only you, armed with adequate and unbiased information, can decide what is best.

Many women pass through menopause requiring little or no specific medical intervention. However, that does not mean menopause is not an important time period for them. Menopause, even without hot flashes, is often a lightening rod for health awareness. It is frequently a time of intense physical and mental re-evaluation. This book will assist those women in finding the lifestyle strategies they seek in order to have the longest, healthiest, and happiest rest-of-her-life.

Part III:
The Womenopause Challenge:
Feeling Fit, Feminine, and Fabulous in Four Weeks

Magic wand! Isn't that what we all want to use to get something we really crave? Hey Presto! Abrakadabra! If we were kids, we might cling to that notion, but we are not children. We have lived long enough to know how this universe is constructed. It goes something like this, "Everything worthwhile is hard to get." We can wish the world to be different, but it's not going to change. For example, a trip to Hawaii would be great. It's not going to be easy to get there. We have to get a good job, we show up and work everyday for years, we save the money, we make the arrangements, and finally catch the rays on Waikiki (remembering to pack the sunscreen). It's not going to be easy, but it is so worth it.

We cannot pretend that health and well-being are easy to attain, but they are absolutely worth it. If you have been pausing a little, maybe coasting, letting life do the spinning while you do the resting, letting your relationships slide; if that is you, then now is the time to stop pausing and start living. The sun will come up tomorrow. There is no jumping forward; there is no going back. Why would you when there is infinitely more interesting things to do today.

Take the WOMENOPAUSE Challenge. Make a decision to live life fully, every moment of every day. The Womenopause Challenge can help by organizing the process into small achievable steps. Here they are:

- Step #1 *w*Score and *w*Chart: Establish your baseline and track your cycle
- Step #2 Womenopause *w*TimeLine: Pinpoint your day
- Step #3 Hot Flashes: Cool it
- Step #4 Vaginal Health: Discover your balance

- Step #5 Sleep Hygiene: Control your context
- Step #6 Real Food: Eat real food not fake food-like substances
- Step #7 Supplements: Take vitamins, minerals, and complementary remedies
- Step #8 Vitamin-X: Exercise like you mean it
- Step #9 Sexercise: Work-outs for intercourse and outercourse
- Step #10 Relaxation: Practice your method
- Step #11 Designer Therapy: Select the perfect prescription fit
- Step #12 Skin Care: Assess your skin and pick your products
- Step #13 Boning Up: Build stronger bones
- Step #14 Breast Cancer: Reduce your risk
- Step #15 Heart Health: Reduce your risk
- Step #16 Smoke Free: Stop in one week
- Step #17 Memory Exercises: Build-up your brain
- Step #18 wScore: Nothing compares to you

First, we recommend rehabilitating your opinions about yourself and your body. Start here by saying: "I am an amazing unique creation. My life has meaning and purpose. I am just one being — not a spirit trapped inside a physical form — I am this one-wonderful thing."

How we feel emotionally affects how our body physically works. How our body works affects how we feel. That's because it's all united into one. If someone eats right, exercises right, but lets her marriage slide, she will not be optimal. Conversely, if someone totally commits to her relationship but lets her health erode, she will not be optimal either. When the body and soul are joined for a common goal, then amazing things can happen. And the best part is, you can choose to make it happen.

WOMENOPAUSE is an interactive program because knowing

all about menopause is useful only when that knowledge prompts action. Here are three important definitions:

- **Feeling Fit:** Physical and emotional fitness describes how well we function within the duties and challenges of our life. From mundane things like climbing the basement stairs with a laundry basket of wet towels to handling the emotional outbursts of a co-worker, we must strive to become powerfully fit.
- **Feeling Feminine:** How well a woman matches up to her internal self-image defines her femininity. External standards are often destructive. Knowing who you are, where you came from, and where you are going are the essential statements you need answers to. Incorporating the answers to these questions into your worldview is as important as lacing up your boots before starting a hike.
- **Feeling Fabulous:** A fabulous woman is at peace with her fitness and femininity. From the endeavor of a purposeful plan emerges matchless well-being.

Here is the four week plan.

Part IV:
Introduction to the wScore Worksheet

When all is said and done, it only matters what was done. This book recommends steps you can **do** to upgrade your health and well-being. The fun part is keeping track of the progress. If you have ever seen *Extreme Makeover Home Edition*, it's the before and after scenes that are the killer moments. When the family comes back after being at Disney, they can see what the Makeover crew has done. Before and after pictures are powerful reinforcements that all the trouble and effort are worth it. As you begin the Womenopause Challenge take your first step and fill-out a *w*Score (Figure 1-2).

wSCORE	Lovera Wolf Miller, MD FACOG (219) 879-5143

Name:_____ Date:_____ Age:_____ Email:_____

Current Treatement:_____

FIT, FEMININE, AND FABULOUS IN FOUR WEEKS

Circle: ☺ Not a Problem One **W**-Mild Problem Two **WW**-Moderate Problem Three **WWW**-Severe Problem

HOT FLASH FEVER

•Hot Flash	☺	W	W	W
•Hot Dread (Stressful)	☺	W	W	W
•Warm Flush	☺	W	W	W
•Night Sweats	☺	W	W	W
•Wet Nightgown	☺	W	W	W
•Cold Crash	☺	W	W	W
•# Per Day <3 <9 >9	☺	W	W	W

Total_____

MOOD MATTERS

•Not Feeling Myself	☺	W	W	W
•Mood Swings	☺	W	W	W
•Crying Spells	☺	W	W	W
•Meno-Fog	☺	W	W	W
•Anxiety	☺	W	W	W
•Incomplete Tasks	☺	W	W	W
•Not Socializing	☺	W	W	W

Total_____

SEXERCIZE

•Lack of Desire	☺	W	W	W
•Lack of Comfort	☺	W	W	W
•Lack of Orgasm	☺	W	W	W
•Pain	☺	W	W	W

Total_____

BMI_____   TOTAL W [   ]

VAGINA SAHARA

•Sahara (Dry)	☺	W	W	W
•Burning	☺	W	W	W
•Itching	☺	W	W	W

Total_____

SKINNY ON SKIN

•Dry	☺	W	W	W
•Wrinkles	☺	W	W	W
•Oily / Pimply	☺	W	W	W
•Dry Thin Hair	☺	W	W	W
•Facial Hair	☺	W	W	W

Total_____

INSOMNIA QUEEN

•Going to Sleep	☺	W	W	W
•Staying Asleep	☺	W	W	W
•Daytime Fatigue	☺	W	W	W

Total_____

PLUMBING & PAIN

•Urinary Problems	☺	W	W	W
•Joint Pain	☺	W	W	W
•Headaches	☺	W	W	W
•Breast Tenderness	☺	W	W	W

Total_____

PLAN:_____

Figure 1-2 *w*Score

The *w*Score serves as a before and after measure of the changes you might expect to make after four weeks on the Womenopause Challenge. The *w*Score helps identify potential midlife health problems women commonly notice, and some problems women commonly try to ignore. This book contains the account of thirty real women who participated in the Womenopause Challenge. You will no doubt find that some of their stories hit close to home.

Filling out the wScore is simple and quick. Seven boxed categories gather commonly associated problems together. For instance, the *Hot Flash Fever* box lists seven symptoms related to vasomotor disturbances seen in perimenopause and beyond. Each item has a separate score.

The first listed symptom is *Hot Flash*. It can be scored by circling one "W" to indicate mild hot flashes, circle two "W W" to indicate moderate hot flashes, or circle three "W W W" to indicate severe hot flashes. If hot flashes are not a problem, then circle the smiley face "☺".

The second item in the Hot Flash Fever box is called *Hot Dread*. A Hot Dread adds the emotional component to a hot flash and refers to the aura and anxiety some women experience when they flash. *Mood Matters* refer to emotional changes that sometimes interfere with family and social relationships. *Vagina Sahara* keeps track of vaginal dryness (as you probably know, the Sahara desert is a dreadfully dry expanse across northern Africa), a commonly overlooked and embarrassing menopausal problem. The *Skinny on Skin* focuses on skin and hair issues, which may concern many menopausal women. *Insomnia Queen* helps track sleep disturbances. *Plumbing and Pain* brings together some wide-ranging problems like urinary problems, joint pain, breast tenderness, and headaches.

Finally, the *Sexercise* group examines sexual function in several ways. Sexual desire is frequently referred to as libido. If you have a little less desire for sex, circle one "W". If you have a lot less desire for sex than you used to have, circle two "W W". If you have no interest in sex, circle three "W W W". If your interest in sex is good and there has been no appreciable change lately, then circle the smiley face "☺". Some women who are single, divorced, or widowed have difficulty knowing how best to fill-out this section. It might be helpful to consider the desire for sex is not exactly the same thing as having sex, but the issue is certainly complicated.

The answer is not a grade school arithmetic test you have to show your mom. Since the responses are purely subjective, whatever answer you give is the only correct answer. The total wScore is like your golf game; you are always trying to lower your score and improve your game.

When it comes to filling out the wScore, it is interesting to note that some women have a cluster of problems in one area, and none in other areas. For instance, one woman may have no problems with hot flashes, but her vagina is dry, making sex painful. Hormone changes during perimenopause and postmenopause do not affect everyone in the same way. Identifying the most conspicuous problem may lead to a better-targeted individual designer treatment.

Near the bottom of the wScore notice the BMI line. BMI stands for Body Mass Index. The BMI is a yardstick to measure the progress made in the areas of food and exercise. Food is discussed in Chapter 14, and Vitamin-X, exercise, is covered in Chapter 16. Remember, before and after pictures are your greatest reinforcement for the efforts you are about to make. Where you stand right now is only the beginning. Do not get discouraged before you have a chance to make things better. The BMI chart, (Figure 1-3) looks a little complicated, but it's not. Find your height on the far left column. For example, if you are five feet five inches tall (5 X 12" = 60", 60" + 5" = 65") track down the column until you find "65". Move to the right along the line to find your weight. Let's say you weigh 144 pounds. Stop at the 144 and follow that column up to the top to find your BMI = 24. Great, you are what we call "fine figured", congratulations.

Determination of the BMI should be used as a motivational tool and not the be-all and end-all of success. God made people

wBODY MASS INDEX

Body Weight (pounds)

Height (inches)	SLIM FIGURED						FINE FIGURED					FULL FIGURED										FULLSOME FIGURED														
BMI	19	20	21	22	23	24	25	26	27	28	29	30	31	32	33	34	35	36	37	38	39	40	41	42	43	44	45	46	47	48	49	50	51	52	53	54
58	91	96	100	105	110	115	119	124	129	134	138	143	148	153	158	162	167	172	177	181	186	191	196	201	205	210	215	220	224	229	234	239	244	248	253	258
59	94	99	104	109	114	119	124	128	133	138	143	148	153	158	163	168	173	178	183	188	193	198	203	208	212	217	222	227	232	237	242	247	252	257	262	267
60	97	102	107	112	118	123	128	133	138	143	148	153	158	163	168	174	179	184	189	194	199	204	209	215	220	225	230	235	240	245	250	255	261	266	271	276
61	100	106	111	116	122	127	132	137	143	148	153	158	164	169	174	180	185	190	195	201	206	211	217	222	227	232	238	243	248	254	259	264	269	275	280	285
62	104	109	115	120	126	131	136	142	147	153	158	164	169	175	180	186	191	196	202	207	213	218	224	229	235	240	246	251	256	262	267	273	278	284	289	295
63	107	113	118	124	130	135	141	146	152	158	163	169	175	180	186	191	197	203	208	214	220	225	231	237	242	248	254	259	265	270	278	282	287	293	299	304
64	110	116	122	128	134	140	145	151	157	163	169	174	180	186	192	197	204	209	215	221	227	232	238	244	250	256	262	267	273	279	285	291	296	302	308	314
65	114	120	126	132	138	144	150	156	162	168	174	180	186	192	198	204	210	216	222	228	234	240	246	252	258	264	270	276	282	288	294	300	306	312	318	324
66	118	124	130	136	142	148	155	161	167	173	179	186	192	198	204	210	216	223	229	235	241	247	253	260	266	272	278	284	291	297	303	309	315	322	328	334
67	121	127	134	140	146	153	159	166	172	178	185	191	198	204	211	217	223	230	236	242	249	255	261	268	274	280	287	293	299	306	312	319	325	331	338	344
68	125	131	138	144	151	158	164	171	177	184	190	197	203	210	216	223	230	236	243	249	256	262	269	276	282	289	295	302	308	315	322	328	335	341	348	354
69	128	135	142	149	155	162	169	176	182	189	196	203	209	216	223	230	236	243	250	257	263	270	277	284	291	297	304	311	318	324	331	338	345	351	358	365
70	132	139	146	153	160	167	174	181	188	195	202	209	216	222	229	236	243	250	257	264	271	278	285	292	299	306	313	320	327	334	341	348	355	362	369	376
71	136	143	150	157	165	172	179	186	193	200	208	215	222	229	236	243	250	257	265	272	279	286	293	301	308	315	322	329	338	343	351	358	365	372	379	386
72	140	147	154	162	169	177	184	191	199	206	213	221	228	235	242	250	258	265	272	279	287	294	302	309	316	324	331	338	346	353	361	368	375	383	390	397
73	144	151	159	166	174	182	189	197	204	212	219	227	235	242	250	257	265	272	280	288	295	302	310	318	325	333	340	348	355	363	371	378	386	393	401	408
74	148	155	163	171	179	186	194	202	210	218	225	233	241	249	256	264	272	280	287	295	303	311	319	326	334	342	350	358	365	373	381	389	396	404	412	420
75	152	160	168	176	184	192	200	208	216	224	232	240	248	256	264	272	279	287	295	303	311	319	327	335	343	351	359	367	375	383	391	399	407	415	423	431
76	156	164	172	180	189	197	205	213	221	230	238	246	254	263	271	279	287	295	304	312	320	328	336	344	353	361	369	377	385	394	402	410	418	426	435	443

Figure 1-3 *w*Body Mass Index

in all shapes and sizes, and they are all perfect. We are all works in progress. Trying to get yourself into what your vision of yourself looks like is the object. Also notice the usual terms at the top of the BMI chart identifying "normal", "overweight", "obese", and "extreme obesity" have been changed. Most people find those terms offensive, and Womenopause recommends the terms: slim figured (BMI 19 – 24), fine figured (BMI 25 – 29), full figured (BMI 30 – 40), and fulsome figured (BMI 41 – 54). As an example, a person 5'4" (64") weighing 122 pounds has a BMI of 21 and is slim figured. If a 5'4" person weighs 157 pounds her BMI is 27, and she is fine figured. A person 5'4" weighing 192 pounds has a BMI of 33 and is full figured. A 5'4" person weighing 256 Pounds has a BMI of 44 and is fulsome figured. Being fulsome figured or full figured would have no significance, except there is solid evidence that women in those categories have significantly more serious health problems and a shorter life span.

Scoring the wScore is easy. Simply add the number of "W" in each box, then total all the boxes for the Total "W" score at the bottom. The wScore should be filled out at the beginning of the Womenopause Challenge, then once more at the end of the four weeks. The wScore often helps women identify problems they had barely recognized as part of their transition or have been trying to ignore. Everyone has the opportunity to decide which problems are of significant magnitude to warrant discussion with their healthcare provider.

Part V:
The Womenopause Challenge:
Feel Fit, Feminine, and Fabulous in Four Weeks

1. Determine your life expectancy on the Age Graph Figure 1-1.
2. Calculate your initial wScore Figure 1-2.
3. Determine your initial Body Mass Index Figure 1-3.
4. Now is the time to stop pausing and start living.

Chapter 2

Ovaries R Us

Part I:
Y Women Love Genes (XX)

Ovaries are God's gift to women. These white, almond-sized organs nestled in the rim of the pelvis, perform amazing work. The products of the ovaries: estrogen, progesterone, and testosterone define what we call female, the sound and shape of a woman. Women have ovaries, men don't. It's all in the genes. Of the 46 chromosomes, almost everything about women and men is the same, except that women have an "XX", and men have an "XY". A woman's "X" factor makes all the difference. Some say the extra "X" gene explains why women look so good in their jeans.

Part II:
Reproductive Endocrinology 101

Of all the cycles found in nature, none are more beautifully conceived than the female menstrual cycle (Figure 2-1). Every month, the brain area called the hypothalamus releases a hormone named GNRH (gonadotropin releasing hormone, for those of you who must have all the details). GNRH instructs another part of the brain, the pituitary, to release a pair of hormone messengers, FSH (follicle stimulating hormone) and LH (luteinizing hormone). These messengers travel a great distance through the bloodstream to be received by cells within the ovary. The ovary responds with enlarging eggs that freely pour out estrogen, progesterone, and inhibin A and B, (follicular phase). In mid-cycle, the ovary releases an egg (ovulation). When the hypothalamus senses enough estrogen, and especially enough inhibin B, it stops telling the pituitary to release FSH and LH. The declining FSH and LH signal the ovary to curb

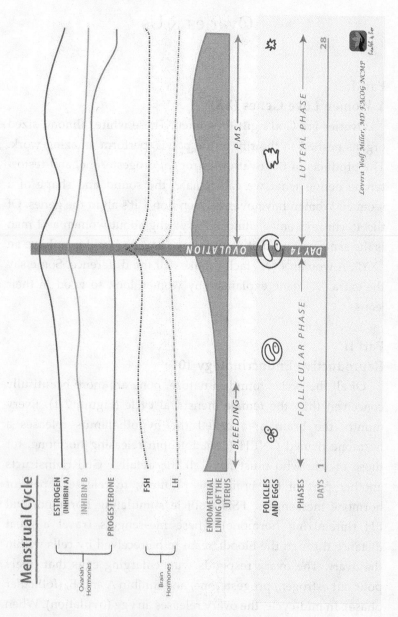

Figure 2-1 Menstrual Cycle

14

production of estrogen (luteal phase), permitting the cells within the ovary to calm down. The surge of estrogen, progesterone, and inhibin fall back to baseline. All is quiet until the next month, only to be reborn (Figure 2-1). Such are the wonders of the female hormone cycle, the ebb and flow of signals, switches, and system responses.

Part III:
Menstrual Music: Estrogen and Progesterone Know How to Play the Organs

During the monthly menstrual cycle, the rise and fall of hormones, especially estrogen and progesterone, produce dramatic changes in many organs. The primary organs include the brain, uterus, ovary, breasts, and skin; however, the heart, blood vessels, intestines, kidney, liver, and muscle are all influenced by the reproductive hormones. The lining of the uterus, the endometrium, responds loudly to the ovarian stimulation. When the endometrium is under the influence of estrogen and progesterone during a normal monthly menstrual cycle, there is growth of the glandular tissue of the uterus. This thickens the uterine lining and prepares the uterus for an implantation of a fertilized egg, allowing for possible pregnancy. When the estrogen and progesterone decline in the second half of the menstrual cycle, the endometrial lining sheds. The shedding of the uterine lining is affectionately known as a menstrual period. There is more happening behind the scenes.

When FSH and LH stimulate the ovaries, several eggs initially begin to mature, but only one usually becomes the dominant egg for that month (when there are two eggs that mature simultaneously, that's when it's possible for "fraternal twins"). Around the dominant egg, there develops a ring of cells called the follicle. The follicle rapidly expands during the first half of the monthly cycle. At mid-cycle, there is s dramatic surge of FSH and LH that results in the egg being released from the follicle. The release of the dominant egg from its follicle is termed ovulation. The follicle remaining within the ovary produces high quantities of progesterone that continues as the source of stimulation for the uterus. The ejected egg becomes captured by the tendril ends of the fallopian tubes and gets transported down the tube into the uterus. If a pregnancy occurs, the early developing embryo sends a signal back to the follicle to keep up the production of progesterone. Most of the time there is no pregnancy, and the ovarian follicle winds down and then stops production of progesterone. All of the remaining ovarian eggs slow down their production of estrogen; the uterus gives up (for this month) and sheds the endometrial lining (the period).

Much like the way estrogen and progesterone stimulate the uterus to prepare for pregnancy, estrogen and progesterone also stimulate and prepare the breasts. The glandular tissue in the breasts is necessary for milk production in the event that ovulation leads to pregnancy. For many women, at the time of menstrual bleeding there is an accompanying soreness of the breasts.

Sweat glands get the same treatment from estrogen and progesterone. They clog with debris, get infected, irritable, and may erupt into a pimply protest upon withdrawal of estrogen and progesterone.

Withdrawal of these hormones may manifest itself in a variety of mood changes, which may vary widely from woman to woman. Many areas of the brain are influenced by these reproductive hormones. It is not unusual to hear sighs of relief when the period begins, and estrogen and progesterone settle down. Premenstrual Syndrome (PMS) is a cyclically recurring physical and mood change that appears in the last two weeks of the menstrual cycle during the decline of estrogen and progesterone. Some women may notice any combination of the following:

• Moodiness

- Pimples
- Breast tenderness
- Bloating
- Headaches
- Insomnia
- Joint Pains
- Constipation or diarrhea

Part IV:
A Trio of Estrogens

When most people hear the term "steroid hormone", they think of professional ball players getting into trouble. That is partially true. Anabolic hormones like testosterone, the primary sex hormone in men, stimulate muscles and are chemically a steroid structure. Technically, estrogen, the female sex hormone, is a steroid too. Estrogen does not have the same properties as testosterone. Our bodies make dozens of "steroid" hormones, each with its unique function.

General Motors (GM) is a big American car company. Under their business, they manufacture several different brands: Chevrolet, Buick, and Cadillac. Estrogen is like the name of a hormone company. The trio of brand-named estrogens: estradiol (pronounced: estra-dye-all), estriol (es-tree-all), and estrone (es-trone). As there are significant differences between a Chevy and a Caddy, there are even more differences between estrogens. Estradiol, also known as 17 beta-estradiol or E2, is the Corvette convertible of estrogens. Estradiol comprises the most active sex hormone in young menstruating women and is primarily synthesized in the ovaries. Estriol (E3) is the predominant estrogen of pregnancy, a mini van if you will. E3 is manufactured by the placenta and has 95 percent less activity than estradiol (E2). Estrone (E1) has approximately 80 percent less activity than 17 beta-estradiol (E2), and it is this less active estrogen (E1) that is present during postmenopause, more like a golf cart.

Figure 2-2 Estrogen Potency

E1 20% potent	Estrone	After menopause	Golf Cart
E2 100% potent	Estradiol	Before menopause	Corvette Convertible
E3 5% potent	Estriol	Pregnancy	Mini Van

Figure 2-2 Estrogen Potency

Postmenopausal estrone is made by the conversion of other precursors in fat and muscle tissue after the ovaries have shut down production. The primary source of estrogen in postmenopausal women comes from the adrenal gland whose steroid precursors are acted upon by the important enzyme aromatase. Testosterone, the primary male sex hormone, is produced in small but pivotal quantities in women by the support cells within the ovaries and by conversion of other precursors.

Part V:
Nothing Lasts Forever

A woman is born with over two million eggs; each one, a possible new being, waits for the call to ovulation. Incredibly, only about four hundred of those eggs are released during a woman's fertile years; the rest shrivel up and die, a process termed atresia. By the time of menopause there remain fewer than two thousand eggs; none of which can hear the FSH call. Young ovaries, with their multitude of eggs, reliably respond to FHS and LH to produce an exceptional quantity and variety of estrogen and progesterone. Hundreds of cycles later, the ovaries are exhausted. The FSH level goes up and up (ten to fifteen times premenopausal levels), but the eggs do not respond. Estrogen production becomes erratic, declines, then all but stops. The familiar monthly periods may become unfamiliar and unfriendly. Irregular periods, hot flashes, and erratic PMS are harbingers of perimenopause and may begin before age forty. The ovaries cease being the center of the female endocrine universe at an average age of 51.

Part VI:
Ovarian Cancer

Cancer of the ovary, frequently referred to as "the silent killer", is rare (Figure 30-1). Many young women worry about cancer because there is confusion about what a cyst in the ovary means. As discussed earlier in this chapter, the ovaries develop follicles with eggs, every month. There are usually several follicles in various stages of development within the ovary at any one time. Follicles are cystic structures. It is perfectly normal for menstruating women to have "cysts" in their ovary. Once in a blue moon, one of the follicles enlarges to the point of discomfort and can be seen on an ultrasound. Those cysts are not in any way related to cancer and usually go away with two months of treatment with cycle control pills or the vaginal NuvaRing (also known as birth control). Uncommonly, ovarian cysts in young women persist and may require further investigation, treatment, and occasionally surgery.

Of importance is the recent reassuring research that finds women who have used birth control pills have a 50 percent reduction of ovarian cancer. The risks of ovarian cancer are covered in Chapter 31: Death Prevention.

Part VII:
Charting the Course: The wChart

The best way to begin understanding your unique menstrual pattern is to chart your periods on the wChart (Figure 2-3). The wChart is designed to be a special calendar for keeping track of all the relevant events related to hormone changes as they progress through a monthly menstrual cycle. When all the information about the menstrual cycle is condensed onto one sheet, as is illustrated in the wChart, it is easier to spot certain trends and problems, which in turn, leads to individualizing each woman's management according to her own unique situation.

The column on the left of the chart identifies the months of the year, and the numbers across the top of the chart are the days of the month. You may start graphing your periods today, and you do not need to wait for the beginning of the month. If, for instance, today is June 15th, go down the left column to JUN, then follow over the line to the box under 15 and make your first mark.

The "key" below the chart on the right gives some suggestions about how to signal certain events on the chart for consistency and comparison purposes. If, for example, on June 15th you were starting your period, menstrual bleeding, put a small "X" in the corresponding box for that day. If it is only spotting instead of a normal flow, place an "O" in the box instead. Use a back slash "/" to indicate light flow and a small dark box "■" to indicate heavy flow. Associated symptoms should be included when present such as "C" for cramping, "P" for premenstrual symptoms like grouchy mood, pimples, or breast tenderness, and "Sx" for any perimenopausal symptoms like hot flashes, vaginal dryness, insomnia, mood swings, and meno-fog. Meno-fog is a minor memory malfunction noticed during perimenopause.

Over time, regular periods march out across the chart like clockwork. Women experiencing perimenopause may, initially, notice menstrual irregularity, followed later by randomness of periods. Knowing the exact pattern of menstrual periods is critical in helping women determine where they stand on the wTimeLine (Figure 3-1). During the reproductive years, women might come to expect minor irregularities in the timing of their menstrual periods and predictable PMS as part of what defines their "normal". Beginning in perimenopause, most women notice progressive menstrual irregularities. Unpredictable bleeding

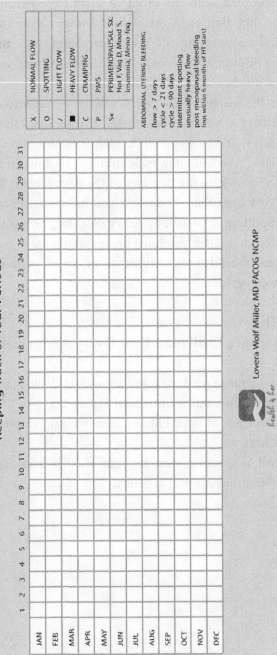

Figure 2-3 wChart

may be coupled with the onset of distinctive perimenopausal problems: hot flashes, night sweats, insomnia, and/or vaginal dryness. Incorporating all the information into the *w*Chart simplifies finding your place on the *w*TimeLine and, if necessary, leads to a quicker targeted treatment.

Below the *w*Chart on the left, is a series of menstrual bleeding abnormalities, which may be serious. These exceed the "normal" irregularities. If you experience menstrual bleeding that lasts longer than 7 days, if your cycle (number of days from the first day of one period to the first day of the next period) is less than 21 days or longer than 90 days, if you have intermittent unpredictable spotting or unusually heavy bleeding, or if you have any vaginal bleeding after you have presumably passed menopause; then, you should seek advice from your gynecologist or healthcare provider.

Part VIII:
Womenopause Challenge: Four Ovary Assignments

1. Find your exact day on the Menstrual Cycle Figure 2-1.
2. Begin filling out your *w*Chart Figure 2-3.
3. Keep track of your PMS or menopausal symptoms on the *w*Chart.
4. Send a greeting card to your mother and father (God willing they are still around).

Chapter 3

wTimeLine: The Life Cycle of
Menstrual Cycles

Part I:
Beyond the Monthly Cycle

The monthly menstrual cycle dominates a woman's health attention throughout her reproductive years. Fewer than 10 percent of women believe they are "regular". Normal variations in the timing of menstruation puzzle nearly everyone. That is why it is hard for women to know when the normal irregularity becomes an abnormal irregularity. Sometime during their forties, most women begin to notice distinctive changes in the pattern of their menstrual cycles. Periods usually stop completely around age 51 (plus or minus ten years).

Menopause is a single day in the life of all women. It is neither an epoch nor a season; it is a woman's final bloody flow. The catch is, one can only know the final menstrual period (FMP) in retrospect. Exactly one year after the FMP, menopause can be identified as the moment of that last red drop; but by then, it's already a year too late to throw a goodbye party. **Perimenopause** is the four-year to ten-year time span preceding menopause and persisting for one additional year after menopause. "Peri" means around; therefore, perimenopause surrounds the day of menopause, much of it before and for exactly one year after menopause.

Premenopause is a confusing term. A toddler, a teenager, or a young mother of three could all be called premenopausal. In each of those young women, very different endocrine activities are taking place.

Part II:
The Confusing Part

One terminology scheme divides women's menstrual cycles into three groups: reproductive, menopausal transition, and postmenopause, (*Stages of Reproductive Aging Workshop (STRAW), Menopause 2001*). The reproductive stage is subdivided into early, peak, and late. Menopausal transition and postmenopause are subdivided into early and late, with perimenopause overlapping both. When menstrual cycles are superimposed, the STRAW partitions into five categories. In the early reproductive phase, menstrual cycles are variable, becoming more regular during the peak and late reproductive time. In the menstrual transition of perimenopause, menstrual periods are highly variable. There may be short cycles, followed by longer cycles, and in some months, the period may be skipped completely. Flow volumes are erratic. Throughout postmenopause, menstrual bleeding completely stops. The postmenopause stage lasts for the rest of a woman's life, hopefully a long, long time. A total of seven stages are categorized from the STRAW schema ranging from "minus five" to "plus two" with the FMP defining the zero mark. To say the least, it can be a little confusing.

Part III:
The Simpler Part

The endocrine *w*TimeLine (Figure 3-1) helps women identify their present hormone status and gives them a perspective on where they are headed. Figure 3-1 consolidates all this information into a single, simple chart. In this figure, the seven stages on the *w*TimeLine outlined above are projected onto a calendar depicting the seven days of one week, Sunday through Saturday. The days of the week are labeled with a preceding "*w*" to designate that it is a *w*omenopause category.

The left side of the chart begins with puberty at 12:01 AM *w*Sunday morning. For most females, puberty, the first period, usually occurs between the ages of twelve to fourteen. Teenage periods may arrive at unexpected times. With maturity, FSH coordinates with the ovary to release predictable amounts of estrogen. At ovulation in midcycle, an egg is released switching on the production of progesterone. Near the end of the cycle, declining estrogen and progesterone may trigger PMS. The beginning of the next cycle starts with the onset of menstrual flow. Yes, it has always seemed counterintuitive to begin counting the days of a new cycle by the bleeding from the endometrium stimulated in the last cycle. However, the first spot is the only reliable reference point in the cycle so it makes sense to start the clock there.

Moving toward the right along figure 3-1, wMonday and wTuesday constitute a woman's most fertile years, her twenties and thirties. During this time, menstrual cycles are the most predictable: estrogen rises and falls like waves on the sea, FSH peaks in midcycle, egg releases, progesterone kicks in, PMS wakes up, then the menstruation flows, just like clock work (at least on paper). Of course there are important sidebars to this scheme. Many women take cycle control pills, (formerly known as birth control pills) during their fertile years. Some women interrupt the cycles and take a nine-month hiatus for pregnancy. Cycle control pills and pregnancy create a protective hormonal environment. Cycle control is covered in more detail in Chapters 5 & 22.

After the age of 40, many women notice menstrual irregularities corresponding to wWednesday, on Figure 3-1. **Perimenopause** constitutes all day wWednesday and wThursday until early wFriday morning. Periods usually become increasingly erratic. FSH rises subtly trying to stimulate the ovary to make more reliable quantities of estrogen, and estrogen levels begin fluctuating unpredictably. Periods may be short, long, heavy or light. PMS may be usual, as on wTuesday, or more severe and almost continuous. PMS rarely gets better at this stage. Some women may notice the gradual onset of what is termed "mood swings" as something different from their usual PMS. Hot flashes and insomnia may make their first appearances on *w*Wednesday.

By the time *w*Thursday, arrives, there is little doubt about the presence of significant changes. As figure 3-1 graphically demonstrates, estrogen levels go bonkers. FSH and the ovaries lose their linkage, and menstrual periods lose their periodicity.

For many women, *w*Thursday is the most difficult time. Hot flashes may progress from annoying to debilitating, disrupting an already disturbed sleep. PMS may be experienced any time of the month. At about this same time, many women complain of "not quite feeling like themselves". Sometimes women notice that problem as a memory malfunction or a vague mental cloud, referred to as "meno-fog". Vaginal dryness may be an increasing problem during *w*Thursday. In addition to the constant irritation, vaginal dryness may present an obstacle to intimacy.

The final menstrual period, **menopause**, occurs *w*Thursday at midnight. It would be cause for celebration if all the problems would go away at the same time. They don't. Because periods can be so irregular prior to the final period, it is almost impossible to know for sure when the last one happens. By convention, you wait for a full year of no bleeding before declaring that menopause has officially happened. That means you know the date of menopause only in retrospect, one year after the fact. Perimenopause is considered to be finished when you hit that magical one-year mark. Perimenopause ends at sunrise on *w*Friday morning on Figure 3-1. Rarely, a woman who has had no periods for more than a year may resume menstruating. More than a few families have been blessed with children whose mother had conceived after she believed her menopause to have taken place.

Osteoporosis, a reduction in the quantity of strong bone, is primarily a disease of postmenopausal women. Estrogen and testosterone produced in the ovary stimulate normal bone growth. When a woman's hormone system cycles normally through wWednesday, bone strength is high and risk of fracture is low because of the protection afforded by high estrogen and testosterone. During the two or three years immediately surrounding menopause, dramatic declines in bone density may occur in concert with declining estrogen and testosterone. It is critical for women to take steps during this time to insure the conservation of bone strength for the later years (Chapter 26: Boning Up 4 Osteoporosis).

Postmenopause usually is a time of gradually receding menopausal symptoms. Meno-fog and memory lapses that were annoying in perimenopause, usually improve within a year of the final menstrual period. Similarly, mood swings that drove you (and everyone around you) a little nutty, gradually remit, and most women say they feel more like themselves with time. Likewise, insomnia problems dissipate, and normal sleep patterns can be expected.

For some women, certain menopausal symptoms last indefinitely. Vaginal dryness is a particularly progressive problem over the long run (Chapter 10: Vagina Sahara). Because vaginal dryness interferes with comfort during sexual intercourse, it may have significance in complicated matters of well-being beyond what a simple dryness might be expected to cause (Chapter 18: Sexercise). More than 20 percent of women continue to complain of persistent hot flashes throughout postmenopause. Hot Dreads may not be quite so debilitating for women in their seventies, but they may remain a significant annoyance for many women. A Hot Dread is a shot of hot flash with a twist of anxiety (Chapter 9: Hot Flash Fever). Osteoporosis marches forward through the postmenopause time and may result in major disabilities and mortality for elderly women.

Now, take a few moments and locate yourself on the wTimeLine Figure 3-1. It is not difficult to locate which day of the wWeek you are. Which of the problems depicted on the chart

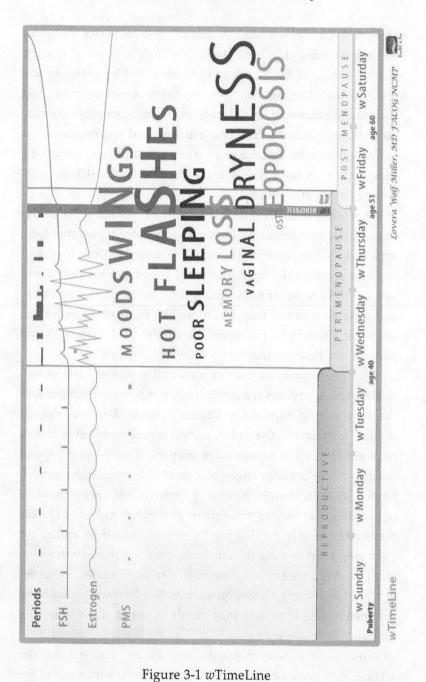

Figure 3-1 wTimeLine

Part IV:
The Fun Stuff

Estrogen joins a bike club and begins cycling wSunday afternoon and travels on some very nice eco tours all wMonday. On wTuesday afternoon estrogen loses some of its enthusiasm for the cycle routine and looks around for a new challenge. This leads estrogen to begin a bungie-jumping hobby on wWednesday, and on wThursday tries skydiving. At midnight wThursday, estrogen leaves the plane, for the last time, without a parachute. Early wFriday morning, estrogen is found laying on a desert floor somewhere. It's not underground, but it's close. Very low estrogen occurs all day wSaturday.

Part V:
The Serious Part

Even though hot flashes are recognized as the most unmistakable feature of menopause, there are other serious health matters brewing under the surface. Menopausal women are, on average, age 51. In many aspects of life, professionally and personally, 51 can be a woman's personal peak, yet 51 might also signal the commencement of decline and demise. Or, seen differently, 51 just might be the launching pad for unexxxpected fulfillment.

The health strategies that are set into motion around menopause will shepherd you to a place of *your* choosing. The symptoms of menopause often compel women to step back for a moment and consider how their lifestyle choices affect their well-being, both physically and mentally. It comes as a surprise to most women that the steps taken to control menopause problems have far-reaching effects. This book recommends lifestyle choices that solve both the transition problems, as well as, the terminal ones.

Is it aging or is it menopause? Midlife is the time when serious chronic diseases get a foothold. Cardiovascular disease, cancer, diabetes, osteoporosis, dementia, and lung disease express themselves with aging. These diseases kill women prematurely. These diseases are optional not inevitable. Womenopause helps channel your menopause options toward solutions that have broad health benefits (Chapter 30: Death Prevention).

Part VI:
What Figure 3-1 Does Not Show You

Figure 3-1 maps out the typical "life-cycle of the menstrual cycle" and includes the predominate symptoms accompanying the changes in hormones for the average woman. We've never actually met an "average" woman and do not know anyone who aspires to be one. There are huge variations among "normal" women. Even in the same woman, there may be stretches of time where her periods go off on a binger, only to return somewhat normal later on. This can be normal. Abnormal uterine bleeding may signify that something is wrong (Figure 2-3). Do not hesitate to ask your doctor if you are concerned.

Part VII:
The Womenopause Challenge: Three Steps on the wTimeLine

1. Find "your wDay" on the wTimeLine Figure 3-1.
2. Discover if you are experiencing any of the common perimenopausal symptoms.
3. Begin osteoporosis prevention: vitamin D 4000 IU, calcium 1500 mg, and walking 10,000 steps a day.
4. Put some flowers in the kitchen.

Chapter 4

Uterus News: Film at Eleven

Part I:
The Uterus is the Katie Couric of Feminine Endocrinology

The uterus is amazing. It starts out smaller than a pear and expands bigger than the biggest baby, if only they could put that kind of spandex into jeans. Of course, the uterus is appreciated because it's a womb for children. Perhaps just as importantly, the uterus constantly "broadcasts" the news pertaining to the condition of the entire female hormone system. The lining of the uterus, the endometrium, is stimulated to grow each month first by estrogen, then by estrogen and progesterone. When those hormones are withdrawn, the uterus sheds its lining and a period, menstrual bleeding, takes place. The health of a woman's hormone system is not hard to monitor because the uterus grows, cramps, and bleeds each month, only if all the components are working in sync. When a woman's hormones change, the uterus lets her know. For instance, if pregnancy occurs, progesterone does not decline as usual, and there is no menstrual period.

In perimenopause, erratic estrogen levels may trigger the uterus to bleed erratically. Throughout the course of a women's life, the uterus sends out signals announcing what day of the *w*Week it is. (Figure 3-1) Like a Katie Couric announcement on the CBS Evening News, the uterus informs and updates women about the state of affairs of their hormones.

31

Part II:
More Serious Stuff

For the first three days of the wWeek: wSunday, wMonday, and wTuesday (roughly, puberty to age 40ish), the uterus announces, "all is well" with the hormones by providing regular monthly periods. Although some variations occur, most women recognize this usual news pattern. Although a 28 day cycle is considered the norm, it is acceptable for the monthly cycle to range anywhere from 21 to 45 days in length and for the period to last from four to seven days. When women arrive on wWednesday, and certainly by wThursday, the uterus announces a disturbance of the hormones by producing periods at unpredictable intervals. Instead of the six o'clock news, Katie Couric might come on at 3:15 in the afternoon, or skip a whole news cycle. On wFriday the uterus stops all regular broadcasts. The one year silence of the uterus yells menopause.

When the uterus sends out confusing messages and bleeds irregularly, there are several important clues women may need to investigate. A woman should seek medical advice for abnormal uterine bleeding for the following reasons:

- There is absence of bleeding or irregular bleeding (may represent pregnancy).
- Bleeding is lasting longer than seven days.
- The menstrual cycle is less than 21 days long.
- The menstrual cycle is more than three months long.
- Bleeding is too heavy.

Abnormal uterine bleeding may require one or more of the following tests: pregnancy test, cultures for sexually transmitted infection tests (STI), complete blood count (CBC), thyroid hormone test (TSH), prolactin hormone test, follicle-stimulating hormone (FSH), luteinizing hormone (LH), biopsy of the uterine lining (pipelle), and/or an ultrasound of the uterus.

Pipelle biopsy of the uterus is an easy and convenient way to sample cells of the uterus to find out exactly how it feels about its hormones. Getting a pipelle for the uterus is much like getting a Pap test for the cervix. For a pipelle, a small tube, much like a coffee stirrer, is inserted through the cervix and into the uterus. A miniscule sample of tissue from the endometrium can be examined under a microscope to definitively classify the state of the uterus and reassure women that all is clear – or not. Sometimes, abnormal uterine bleeding means pre-cancerous cell changes or cancer of the uterus; therefore, getting an accurate evaluation matters.

An ultrasound of the uterus can measure the thickness of the endometrium if the pipelle is unobtainable or inconclusive. An endometrial "stripe" is measured. If the endometrial stripe is less than 5mm thick, it is considered normal. Anything thicker than that may indicate a problem and may need a follow-up ultrasound or a D & C, dilatation and curettage (scraping and cleaning) of the lining of the uterus.

Part III:
Back to the Fun Stuff

After menopause, the uterus retires from broadcasting and moves to Arizona. Sometimes, even in retirement, the uterus makes guest appearances, and those announcements must be carefully considered with the woman's healthcare provider. Uterus news from the retirement community in Arizona usually represents a minor problem but not always. The uterus remains our best early news source for uterine cancer.

Unlike the uterus, the cervix is tight-lipped and has taken a vow of silence about the condition of its health. The cervix, which is the opening of the uterus into the vagina, must be coaxed into the conversation by acquiring a regularly scheduled Pap test; otherwise, she respectfully declines all interviews. Human Papilloma Virus (HPV), transmitted through sexual contact, causes almost all cancers of the cervix, and while 80 percent of women will become positive for HPV during their reproductive years, 90 percent of those infections will spontaneously convert to negative within two years. The Pap test is a reliable screen for pre-cancerous abnormalities and cancer of the cervix.

Birth control pills, also known as cycle control pills, put the ovaries and uterus down for a nap allowing the endometrial lining to have a rest. The endometrial lining ceases the continual, reproductive cycle of thin-thick-shed. It is not synonymous with simply turning off the TV. With cycle control, the TV is still on, there is just less news to report from the hormone world. This hormone rest is not only safe, but some research indicates it actually protects the uterus from multiple diseases, including endometriosis and cancer.

Part IV:
Good News

Deaths from cancer of the uterus and cervix are on the decline. That's good news. Reducing the risk for contracting cancer of the uterus and cervix still has room for improvement. Uterine cancer affects 3 percent of women and over 95 percent of those survive with today's early diagnosis and treatments. The following list identifies the most important risk factors for cancer of the uterus.

- Age over 50 years
- Family history positive for uterine cancer
- BMI over 30, full figured and fulsome figured (Figure 1-3)
- High fat diet
- Diabetes and hypertension
- Early first period and/or late menopause
- Nulliparity (no pregnancies) and/or no breastfeeding
- Estrogen therapy alone without progesterone
- Tamoxifen chemotherapy (a hormonal treatment for breast cancer)

34

Here are two things you can do to reduce your risk even further:

1. You can lower your Body Mass Index (BMI) with diet and exercise. These are big-ticket items, and we devote a whole chapter to each of these topics, (Chapter 14: Real Food), and (Chapter 16: Vitamin-X, Exercise)

2. You can take cycle control pills (birth control pills, CCPs). They reduce uterine cancer risk. Women who take them have 75 percent less uterine cancer and 50 percent less ovarian cancer, eliminate their PMS, control their menstrual cycles, and avoid unplanned pregnancies. The protection from uterine cancer persists for 20 years or more after stopping CCP, protecting them on wThursday and into wFriday. Cycle control pills and vaginal birth control rings usually contain both estrogen (E) and progesterone (P). After menopause, menopausal hormone therapy (MHT), for women with a uterus, also contains both E and P but at much lower doses (one-fourth the dose). Estrogen treatment alone increases the risk of uterine cancer, but adding progesterone therapy to estrogen therapy will return the uterine cancer risk to below the level of women not on hormones.

Human papillomavirus (HPV) causes 95 percent of cancers of the cervix. HPV is contracted through sexual contact. Fortunately, most infections of HPV do not lead to cancer, and most of them resolve spontaneously by the action of our own immune system within two years. HPV infections leading to dysplasia of the cervix may denote a pre-cancerous change. In the United States, twenty-five million women are currently infected with HPV. The following list identifies the major risk factors for cancer of the cervix.

- Sex at a young age

- Multiple sexual partners
- Unsafe sex (condoms do not give complete protection)
- Smoking (another reason to quit)
- Lack of regular gynecologic examination

Here are five things you can do to reduce your risk of cervical cancer even further:

1. Know your sexual partner and stay in a committed relationship, forever (that is good advice for a lot of reasons).
2. Young women should seriously consider getting the HPV vaccine (Gardasil). In a perfect world, a woman would meet, fall in love, and marry the person who was "meant" for her. Well, this isn't a perfect world. It is possible for a virgin woman to fall in love with someone who is (unknowingly) not a virgin. She may innocently contract a deadly sexually transmitted cancer. Gardasil provides protection from 75 percent of the HPV viruses and is recommended for all young women, and especially, for teens before they are sexually active or before they even think of being sexually active.
3. There is no substitute for getting regular Pap tests. Pre-cancer and cancer of the cervix can be cured if caught early. It is important to remember, cancer of the cervix is a sexually transmitted disease and getting cultures for other possible infections is not part of the standard Pap test. Cultures should be obtained at the time of the annual exam to evaluate other possible infections such as herpes, gonorrhea, chlamydia, trichomonas vaginalis, syphilis, hepatitis B, HPV, and HIV. Vaginal atrophy, caused from low estrogen, increases the risk for all of these infections.
4. If you are still smoking, this is another reason for stopping; it reduces your risk of cancer of the cervix (and many other

cancers).

5. Take vitamin C and vitamin D. Vitamins are covered in more detail in Chapter 17.

Part V:
The Womenopause Challenge: Three Uterus Assignments

1. Determine if your bleeding pattern is abnormal.
2. If you have not done so this year, schedule an appointment with your healthcare provider (physician, nurse practitioner, or physician's assistant) for a pelvic exam and Pap test.
3. Ask your healthcare provider about vaccination with Gardasil.
4. Get a date and take time to go out to a movie.

Chapter 5

Perimenopause: A Euphemism for Chaos

Part I:

Let the Show Begin

Before the curtain rises on a Broadway musical, the orchestra plays an overture. The overture gets everyone's attention and previews the up-coming show. It compacts the production's melodies, tenderness, comedy, and drama into a sonic version of a fast-paced movie trailer. Brief runs of the horns, majestic strings, and pulsating percussions get woven into a mini art form. PMS is the overture for perimenopause.

When the menstrual cycle hums along regularly in a woman's teens, twenties, and thirties (wSunday, wMonday, and wTuesday), women learn to expect some minor physical and emotional patterns that keep pace with their periods. Things like headaches, cramping, bloating, breast tenderness, pimples, and trivial alter-ations of their otherwise sunny disposition, come and go in sync with their internal calendar. PMS, premenstrual syndrome, is seen during the last one to two weeks of the cycle but disappears as the blood flow comes to its peak.

During perimenopause, many of the annoying things of PMS morph into something different. Ninety percent of women in their forties begin to notice irregularities in their menstrual periods' interval and flow if they are not on cycle control pills or vaginal ring (birth control) or other hormones. It begins so gradually many do not give it any attention for years. Those period irregularities are a backdrop to the next wave of change – —hot flashes, the hallmark of perimenopause. Hot flashes, similarly, creep up over time. Initially, they are feelings of warmth and no big deal; then gradually, they can develop into full-blown Hot Dreads. They are called Hot Dreads because the term hot flash does not do them justice. Many women report a trapped feeling like, "I gotta get out of my skin," and no amount of wardrobe creativity can solve that problem. Hot Dreads may be punctuated with cold crashes and drenched nightgowns.

At this time, the usual two or three days of restlessness with monthly PMS mushrooms into a continuous problem. Mood swings that used to be a bother for a few days before each period start cropping up unpredictably any time of the month. For some women, the only new problem is a foggy brain (Meno-Fog). For others, there might be an annoying vaginal itch that was never present before. Some women experience everything, all the time. Irregular periods, vaginal dryness, mood-swings, insomnia, and cognitive impairment are common problems noticed by perimenopausal women. If you have noticed any of these annoyances: good morning. Welcome to the beginning of wWednesday.

The customary problems of PMS may intensify during perimenopause, but that does not explain the new features. Like a musical overture that leaves out the showstoppers, hot flashes, vaginal dryness, and insomnia may have little PMS equivalent. These are mostly new problems unique to the hormone changes of wWednesday and wThursday.

Perimenopause is wWednesday and wThursday through sunrise Friday morning found on the wTimeLine Figure 3-1 (Chapter 3). Perimenopause is not a disease; it is the next day of the wWeek.

It's important to remember, Wednesday is not an *illness* of having been Tuesday; six is not an *imbalance* of having been five; sixth grade is not a *disorder* for having passed through fifth grade. wWednesday is simply the anticipated next day.

Part II:
Defining Moments

Perimenopause is defined by changes in menstrual cycles; however, it is an imprecise science. Women who have predictable periods can usually spot a cycle change within a few months and presume that perimenopause has commenced. The other 90 percent of women are left guessing, sometimes for years: short periods, long periods, and heavy or light flow. wWednesday officially starts when periods become irregular.

Underlying the outward signs of menstrual irregularities are the interior changes in the reproductive hormones. Chapters 2 & 3 examined the hormone changes that occur over time. The number of eggs and follicles decline with age, and they respond less reliably to FSH and LH stimulation (the hormones from the brain that stimulate the ovaries to develop eggs and to release estrogen and progesterone). Estrogen production by the ovary becomes erratic.

In some women, estrogen levels may swing wildly up and down many times a day. Estrogen fluctuations trigger hot flashes, cold crashes, night sweats, insomnia, forgetfulness (Meno-Fog) and moodiness. There is no reliable way of measuring estrogen in the blood to predict which symptoms a woman will get or how severe they may be. Mood swings and insomnia commonly begin around the same time as hot flashes, but not always. Some women never get hot flashes even though they may suffer from memory malfunction or insomnia. And the good news is that 20 percent of (lucky) women notice nothing except minor menstrual irregularities. Fertility rapidly declines during the time of irregular periods as a consequence of ovarian failure; however, pregnancy is still possible up until the final menstrual period: menopause.

Menstrual cycles may become shorter or longer. If a woman skips a period altogether, 60 days of no bleeding, wThursday, late perimenopause, has officially begun. For many women *w*Thursday is a lot like *w*Wednesday, only magnified. Hot flashes, mood swings, memory lapses, insomnia, and vaginal dryness all usually crescendo through *w*Thursday on their way toward menopause. The duration of perimenopause, *w*Wednesday and *w*Thursday, is all over the map. Two to ten years is commonly used as a guesstimate for how long perimenopause will last, but nobody takes much solace in that. For sure, perimenopause does not last forever, even though it may seem like it at certain times. Menopause is the final menstrual period (FMP). Perimenopause lasts from the beginning of menstrual irregularities until one full year after the final menstrual period. Women on cycle control pills (birth control) do not experience the symptoms of perimenopause because the estrogen in their pills prevents their symptoms.

When a woman in her forties begins noticing irregular periods, it is a sure bet that menopause is on the horizon. Get a head start on perimenopause: Stop Pausing and Start Living today.

Part III:
Take a Deep Breath

A woman's life is a dangerous and exciting high-wire act. The trick is learning to balance whatever comes your way. Women approaching 50 benefit from all the experiences that enrich life. Days of splendor, joy, and amazement make their marks on the soul. Youthfulness has nothing to compare to a wedding day, the births of children, special vacations, richness of a mature marriage, or the peace that spiritual progress provides. Food tastes better; wine is more complex; bed sheets are crisper; and fires radiate more warmth. These are some of the appreciated blessings of maturity. Perimenopause is a temporary yin of that yang. Nothing is gained without giving something else back. Fertility is one of the givebacks, but with maturity what you gain is worth it. Perimenopause heralds the opening of the curtain and the start of a new musical play. Perimenopause is sometimes called the menopause transition. The hormone upheaval accompanying perimenopause can sometimes cause chaos. Fortunately, most perimenopausal problems can be safely and effectively managed.

Part IV:
Cycle Control for Perimenopause

The dominant driver of perimenopausal problems is erratic ovarian function. The ovaries can no longer be counted on to produce reliable waves of estrogen and progesterone. Like a wind coming across the water, perimenopause can convert the regular quiet hormones lapping against the beach into a category V storm that rips boats off the pier then tries to wash-out the entire beach. Of course, it is not like that for everyone, but the perimenopause storm can catch women off guard and can be quite brutal. Good news, hushing the perimenopause storm can be achieved through simple steps.

Have you ever been in a piazza in Rome on a sunny summer afternoon? There are streets going in every direction, and each one can take you to an interesting place: a monument, ruin, church, café. There are lots of choices. Like most big cities, however, there are some places in Rome you should stay away from.

The following personal studies should be read like examples of walking tours in a travel book. The cases steer away from the danger areas and make some suggestions about points of interest most women find particularly worthwhile. Everyone's trip is unique, and sometimes going off the beaten path is the most fun part.

Connie J.

Connie J. is a healthy and happily married mother of two teenage daughters. She is an extraordinarily active and fulfilled, stay-at-home mom. At 46 with a BMI of 20, she looks and acts younger than her years. She credits her health to good genes because, as she admits, she certainly does not put any effort into eating right or exercising.

At her annual gynecology check-up, her wChart revealed considerable menstrual irregularities. She reported several embarrassing episodes of being caught unprepared for her period. Her PMS, cramps, and bloating seemed to be getting worse and worse. Her children complained to her that she didn't act herself any more, and she attributed it to her recent sleep problem.

Connie confided she and her husband are at an impasse in their marriage. Despite loving him dearly, she simply has had less desire for sex than when she was younger. She thought getting a tubal ligation last year might help, but it didn't. She uses Vaseline to relieve some of the vaginal discomfort during sex, but she has come to dread intercourse.

Connie's physical exam was normal except for a significant dryness of the vaginal mucosa. A Pap test was done and vaginal cultures were obtained. Because of the abnormal uterine bleeding, Connie was advised to have a pipelle test. A pipelle is a sampling of the cells inside the uterus performed by inserting a small tube, like a coffee stirrer, through the cervix and into the inside of the uterus. A pipelle is a minor procedure done to exclude the unlikely possibility that her abnormal uterine bleeding was caused by any abnormality of the uterus cells, including endometrial cancer. Mammogram, thyroid, and hemoglobin tests were ordered.

Fortunately, all of the tests came back normal.

The Womenopause wTimeLine (figure 3-1) helped Connie recognize her seemingly diverse problems may all be related to hormone changes. Connie determined that she was living a wWednesday life with irregular periods, mood swings, memory loss, dry vagina, and a loss of sex drive. Connie had not experienced anything she felt could be called a hot flash or night sweat. She was relieved to know she was not losing her mind but concerned about how to get feeling better. Connie accepted the Womenopause Challenge.

Connie filled out a wScore (Figure 1-2) and her group totals were as follows:

1. Hot Flash Fever: all☺
2. Mood Matters: 11 W
3. Sexercise: 10 W
4. Vagina Sahara: 6 W
5. Skinny on Skin: 5 W
6. Insomnia Queen: 9 W
7. Plumbing and Pain: 2 W

Connie had a total wScore of 43 W with most problems centered on sleep, vaginal dryness, and sex.

The first step toward health for Connie was undertaking some lifestyle changes she had been putting off. She began by agreeing to:

1. eat only "real food" (Chapter 14: Real Food)
2. exercise regularly (Chapter 16: Vitamin-X: Exercise)
3. take appropriate supplements (Chapter 17: Vitamins)
4. initiate a relaxation program (Chapter 12: Mood Matters)

In Connie's case this was starting a yoga class taught by a friend who had been trying to get her to do it for several years.

To control her out-of-control periods, Connie chose to start taking Yaz, a cycle control hormone pill. Yaz is a prescription medication containing estrogen (ethinyl estradiol) and proges-terone (drospirenone). She was to take the active pill for 24 days then go off for four days to resemble a regular monthly cycle. Because Yaz is such a low dose, Connie was advised she might experience some irregular bleeding for the first three months but not to be alarmed by it. Because of Connie's severe vaginal dryness and loss of sex drive, she used a vaginal testosterone cream for a short time to jump-start the recovery of vaginal health and libido. Testosterone cream may be used off-label for women with sexual arousal disorder (Chapter 18: Sexercise). She started by applying the testosterone cream three times a day for a month and would then evaluate the effects before beginning to taper the next month.

The health risks of cycle control hormones were important considerations for Connie, and she was understandably worried because of what she had read. For Connie, cycle control hormones:

1. reduce her risk of uterine cancer by 75 percent
2. reduce her risk of ovarian cancer by 50 percent
3. reduce her risk of colon cancer
4. have no known effect on breast cancer
5. have a minimal and debatable risk of blood clots in healthy non-smoking individuals

The combination of lifestyle changes coupled with Yaz cycle control hormone pills resulted in significant health improvements for Connie by the time of her follow-up appointment four weeks later. She remarked that everything seemed to improve after she left the office, before she even implemented any changes. She found it reassuring just knowing where she was on the wWeek. She had no problems with irregular periods, cramping, or bloating since starting the Yaz. She slept better, and her kids noticed the return of their familiar mom. Most importantly to Connie, she believed that sex had been better this month than it had been in years. It was comfortable and fun for Connie. She enjoyed exercising and especially valued the yoga class. Her children missed their familiar comfort foods, but her husband had lost five pounds on the family's new real food plan. She also found that appealing.

The wScore after four weeks changed from 43 W to 10 W. Connie felt that seeing her score change like that was a big encouragement to keep up the program.

The next month Connie tapered down on the use of testosterone cream, and the Yaz pills were adjusted for her to have a three-month cycle instead of having a period every month. This is a personal, safe choice and even more reliable as birth control. A woman on cycle control pills or vaginal ring (NuvaRing) may choose if and when she wants to have a few days of bleeding, similar to a period, as long as she has had at least 21 days of hormone control in a row. It's not a real period due to ovulation, but an induced bleeding from withdrawing the hormones. She may take the active pill every day, straight through for as long as she desires without increasing any known risks. For the long term, Connie could choose to stay on Yaz until menopause, skipping all of the perimenopausal problems. After menopause, Connie can consider what she wants to do during postmenopause (Chapters 22 & 23).

Brenda Z.

Brenda Z. at age 39 is an immaculately dressed bundle of intensity. She and her husband are partner-tracked lawyers in a big firm. They have no children. Brenda is a highly structured person who eats only organic foods and exercises religiously. She believes her gynecologist is the only person in the world who knows that she is a closet cigarette smoker.

Brenda immediately lets down her guard and says that in the past year, her body and mind have started a rebellion against her. She states she is constantly tired; she sneaks away to cry "over nothing"; she has a headache almost all the time; and her periods are just plain crazy. She has had frequent heavy periods recently, but six months ago she skipped several periods. Brenda complains that in the worst possible moments, usually at work, she feels trapped with a hot pressure around her neck, like she is going to choke unless she gets outside. She has been waking up three times a night to change her wet nightgown; now she just sleeps in t-shirts.

She is afraid that people at work will think she is "losing her edge".

Brenda's physical exam was normal. Her pregnancy test was negative; and Pap test, blood tests, mammogram, and vaginal cultures were obtained. A quick hemoglobin check showed anemia at 10.2 grams. A pipelle endometrial sample was taken and later showed disordered endometrial cells, which is a benign typical finding during wWednesday and wThursday when estrogen is erratic.

After studying the Womenopause wTimeLine, Brenda surmised she was perimenopausal. The real question was had she already reached menopause because of the long intervals of no periods, or was she still a wThursday woman with irregular periods? The point is important because wWednesday and wThursday women frequently have irregular periods, but if a wFriday woman bleeds it may be a sign of endometrial cancer. The pipelle test was reassuring as it showed benign, but it was not definitive evidence of where she was on the wTimeLine. In Brenda's situation, a lab check of her FSH level would be helpful. Brenda's FSH was 11, indicating she was probably not postmenopausal and still in wThursday. Three FSH levels above 30 implies probable menopause. The definitive diagnosis is one year with no periods in a woman who has a uterus. An ultrasound of her uterus showed a normal endometrium.

The wScore results for Brenda were as follows:

1. Hot Flash Fever: 17 W
2. Mood Matters: 19 W
3. Sexercise: 2W

4. Vagina Sahara: 1 W
5. Skinny on Skin: 3 W
6. Insomnia Queen: 6 W
7. Plumbing and Pain: 1 W

Her total was 49 W, and her problems clustered around hot flashes, mood, and sleep. Brenda undertook the Womenopause challenge. She was motivated to make changes to regain her previous level of performance and to exceed it.

She already had exemplary eating and exercise habits. She began taking the recommended supplements (Chapter 17) with three extra doses of iron. She tracked her menstrual cycles on a wChart and tried to anticipate her periods. She took 600 mg of ibuprofen four times a day for one to two days prior to and throughout the time of her bleeding. This helps prevent menstrual cramps and cuts the amount of blood flow in half. Brenda accepted counseling for smoking cessation and a prescription for Chantix to help her quit. Brenda's menopausal symptoms have commenced earlier than average possibly due to cigarette smoking. Brenda was not a candidate for simple cycle control hormone pills or ring because she was a smoker and over age 35. Her risk of blood clots would be too high. After carefully weighing the risks and benefits, Brenda decided to try a low dose transdermal estrogen, Vivelle-Dot 0.05 (17beta-estradiol), coupled with oral progesterone, Prometrium. Both of these are wBodyIdentical hormones (Chapter 21), identical to the ones naturally made within our body. The Prometrium would be cycled 24 days on, and four days off to resemble a monthly menstrual cycle. The estrogen was prescribed for the purpose of slowing down the incapacitating hot flashes/night sweats. Menopausal hormone therapy such as this is not effective as a contraceptive, but her husband had had a vasectomy years ago.

After one week on Chantix, Brenda successfully quit smoking; but, unfortunately, she could brag about it only to her gynecologist. Her Hot Dreads went away, almost immediately with the Vivelle-Dot. Her next period had 50 percent less flow because of the ibuprofen.

She started biofeedback training with a psychologist and noticed a reduction of the intensity and frequency of her headaches. Her mood was still not up to par; therefore, she took a Carroll Rating (CR) Scale, a ten-minute test to evaluate the possibility of depression. She scored a minus 18 on the CR suggesting moderate depression. The test result, coupled with her complaints of crying, low energy, and loss of interest in her usual activities, made the case for trying a course of antidepressant medication. Brenda started taking Effexor XR 37.5 mg every morning, a low dose antidepressant (Chapter 12: Mood Matters).

Four weeks after starting the Womenopause Challenge, Brenda was almost where she wanted to be. She had no hot flashes/night sweats, and her headaches were almost gone. Her hemoglobin was up to 12.5 mg, and her energy had improved. However, she still had problems with crying around the time of her period, and her CR had improved to minus eight.

At this juncture, Brenda had choices. She had done very well on the lifestyle strategy and had done her part to change the things under her control. Because she was now officially a non-smoker, she could either go on cycle control hormone pills or vaginal NuvaRing, or go up on the dose of Effexor. Brenda decided to increase her Effexor dose to 75mg. A month later, Brenda declared peace with herself, her husband, and her job. Brenda had been smoke-free for two months; her hemoglobin was 13 g; her CR was minus 2; her last menstrual period was a breeze; and she had not cried every day. She took another wScore for comparison and was encouraged to find she had calmed down all the intrusive problems. Her score dropped from 50 W to 5 W.

LouAnn K.

When LouAnn K. says hello, everyone is immediately disarmed by her warmth and grace. At 50, LouAnn seems to have settled, peaceably, into the archetypical schoolteacher role; sincere, quiet, thoughtful, with a matronly figure, and some great dessert recipes. Her kids were grown and gone; she and her husband Jimmy had plans for an early retirement to Florida. Her health appears to be good. Unfortunately, none of it is exactly true.

Last year LouAnn's family doctor started treating her for hypertension, and this year she was told she had diabetes. LouAnn prided herself on being a premiere baker, and she steadfastly disdained exercise. With a BMI of 36, she had her work cut out for her to regain a healthful outlook. Her second daughter was going through a rough divorce, and she and her two children had "temporarily" moved back home five months ago. When she made her annual gynecology appointment, she was looking for a miracle.

LouAnn had undergone a hysterectomy (removal of the uterus), five years before for uterine fibroids (benign tumors in the uterus). Without a period to deal with, she had barely noticed her monthly cycles. LouAnn's mother at age 76 had recently been diagnosed with breast cancer, and LouAnn began her appointment with a statement about how glad she was she had not taken any of those hormones that would cause her to get breast cancer too. Initially, she insisted her life was grand, and she had not a care in the world. Slowly, the happy veneer began to peel off, and LouAnn confided about her problem with sex. She reported that she had been having vaginal discomfort for several years. It had gotten to the point that she had not been able to have intercourse for six months. She stopped intercourse because it was excruciatingly painful, and after sex, she would spot for days. She did not feel confident however that her husband had accepted the situation. Few had ever witnessed

LouAnn's crying and desperation.

LouAnn's physical exam demonstrated severe vaginal atrophy. The opening to her vagina had all but closed, and there was visible inflammation. The exam could not be completed even with a pediatric-sized speculum. Biopsies of the vagina were sent for pathology, as were vaginal cultures. Her primary care doctor had already performed routine blood tests, and a mammogram was ordered. LouAnn's FSH was 15 which implied she was still in perimenopause.

The wScore for LouAnn was as follows:

1. Hot Flashes: 4 W
2. Mood Matters: 5 W
3. Sexercise: 10 W
4. Vagina Sahara: 9 W
5. Skinny on Skin: 2 W
6. Insomnia Queen: 8 W
7. Plumbing and Pain: 2 W

Her total of 40 W is not extraordinarily high, but the concentration of problems on vaginal health and sex, was having a significant negative effect on her life. Although she had not volunteered any complaints about sleep, when she filled out the wScore, it was apparent that insomnia was a major problem.

LouAnn accepted the Womenopause Challenge. She was advised there were no miracles that could be given to her; there were only the little miracles she could create for herself. LouAnn was motivated to prove to herself she could control some aspects of her life that she had, up until now, pretended she couldn't. She was motivated to become the best spouse she could be. LouAnn began the Womenopause Challenge:

1. eating real food (Chapter 14)
2. taking supplements (Chapter 17)

3. exercising by joining an early morning aerobics class at the "Y" (Chapter 16)

4. starting marriage counseling with their pastor

LouAnn requested information about hormone therapy, and she was particularly interested in hearing about their effects on breast cancer. She learned that women who have had a hysterectomy can safely take estrogen alone (without progesterone), and the evidence reveals no increased risk of breast cancer.

LouAnn determined she was on wThursday, and by seeing the prompts on the Womenopause wTimeLine, she recognized she was having some other problems. She had been awakening at night with a wet nightgown. Lately, she had felt her head was in a cloud, and she just did not feel quite herself. All of these problems are common in perimenopause.

LouAnn elected to try transdermal estrogen (applied via the skin), Divigel. She had considered taking only a vaginal estrogen preparation instead because her primary problem was vaginal dryness. In the end she felt that the night sweats and Meno-Fog warranted systemic hormone therapy. Transdermal estrogen is known to improve diabetes and hypertension, two of her medical problems. Estrogen has the added benefit of reducing waist hip ratio, a fact she was glad to know. She chose to boost the treatment of her vagina with estrogen Premarin cream, once a day for a month.

Four weeks later LouAnn had made remarkable changes. The combination of her real food diet and aerobics class had already resulted in enough weight loss to decrease her BMI down two whole points to 34. Her vaginal exam demonstrated the return of a pink moist mucosa. She noticed improvements in areas where she did not realize there was even a problem, like her skin. On the estrogen gel, she already noticed her skin everywhere looked and felt smoother. With the help of their pastor, LouAnn and Jimmy were recovering emotionally and felt ready to consider bringing sexual intercourse back into their marriage. LouAnn was trained in Sexercise assignments (Chapter 18). Her wScore, after four weeks, had changed from 41 W to 9 W.

Each woman who enters perimenopause is unique, and when it comes to designing treatment, one size definitely does not fit all. The cornerstone to relieving menopausal problems resides in taking control of whatever can be controlled. In this world, there is very little that can be controlled. There are three lifestyle choices each of us can direct: what goes in the mouth, what activities are done (or not done), and what we choose to think. We should always try to maximize our influence over the variables that we can control. It would be shortsighted to rely entirely on prescription medications to straighten out perimenopausal problems. Hormone therapy has a place, and that place comes after controlling lifestyle choices.

Part V:
The Womenopause Challenge: Becoming Smoke Free

1. Write down on paper why you want to quit smoking and put it on your fridge.
2. Tell your spouse and your best friend you are quitting.
3. Pick a quit date: Friday the 13th, a birthday, or an anniversary.
4. Start Chantix two weeks before your quit date.
5. On your quit date, completely stop smoking: don't cut back, don't go to lites, just stop completely.
6. Avoid being in places where you know you like to smoke: at the table after dinner, out with friends playing pool, alone in the car; just stay away for a while.
7. Continue Chantix for three months after you quit.
8. Constantly review your list of reasons for wanting to

quit.

9. Remind your spouse and friends to continue to help you quit.

10. If you make a mistake and smoke, welcome to the human race; now try again.

11. Remember, the only people who successfully quit are the ones who actually try!

Chapter 6

Menopause: Kiss Your Periods Goodbye

Part I:
Grocery Shopping at Midnight

Menopause is not the "problem". Menopause is simply the term applied to describe the Final Menstrual Period (FMP), the pausing of menstruation. Women may experience irregular periods for between two and ten years leading up to the last period. At menopause, FSH no longer inspires the ovary to produce estrogen or to ovulate; low estrogen levels means low stimulation of the uterine lining. No ovulation also means no surge in progesterone; low estrogen and progesterone mean no uterine withdrawal bleeding. Very low estrogen with very low progesterone means no cycle and no period.

For most women the system runs down slowly, and like an unattended grocery cart scooting across the parking lot, at some point, it hits a flat spot and comes to a halt. Once the grocery cart stops it would take a pretty big wind to nudge it back into rolling, and the same principle applies to the ovaries. The ovary grocery cart starts out loaded with stuff and has enough momentum to overcome some hills and valleys. It slows down a little with each peak, and speeds up a little with the dips, but it runs out of steam eventually and comes to a complete stop.

That stop is termed menopause. Menopause, the permanent pausing of menstruation, occurs *w*Thursday at midnight.

The irregular menstrual periods of perimenopause occur *w*Wednesday and *w*Thursday. Menopause is the stroke of midnight *w*Thursday night (Figure 3-1: *w*TimeLine). One might be tempted to believe that determining midnight would be easy, just look at the clock. But in real life, it's not. Some women may have irregular periods for a decade or more, and during that time span, they may skip several periods. It is hard, during the time of unpredictable menstrual periods, to know precisely whether their *last* menstrual period was the *final* menstrual period. By convention, the FMP is considered to have occurred if there has been no menstrual period for one year — twelve consecutive skipped periods. If that grocery cart has stood in the parking lot and no storm in the past year got it to budge, it can be assumed that it's just not going to move again.

Part II:
Menopause by the Numbers

Because menopause is a single moment, women are said to have "reached" menopause. Technically, women do not "enter" menopause. For instance, on a road trip to the great white north, a person can reach the border with Canada, but you do not enter the border, do not begin the border, nor do you start the border. The border can be reached, but after the border is passed, you enter Canada. When menopause is reached, a woman enters her postmenopause time of life. The defining characteristic menopause bestows is cessation of fertility. Postmenopause is the rest of your long and happy life following cessation of menstrual periods. Perimenopause encompasses all the time of irregular menstrual bleeding leading up to menopause. The apparent overlap of these time designations can be a source of confusion. If you still have a question about this, review the *w*TimeLine (Figure 3-1).

There is a pretty wide age range for menopause: age 40 to age 58 is within the normal range. Six thousand American women reach menopause a day; that translates into two million women having their last period this year, and with the aging boomers, that number keeps getting larger. Less than 1 percent of women experience menopause earlier than the age of 40, and they are considered to have had a premature natural menopause.

Approximately 5 percent of American women have what is called an "induced menopause" when ovarian function ceases because of surgical removal, chemo, or radiation therapy. Menopause is typically reached earlier than average in women who have problems with smoking, hypertension, heart disease, thyroid disease, obesity with a BMI greater than 29, or diabetes. Other serious health problems such as cancer, HIV, and autoimmune diseases can also lead to an earlier menopause.

For some unknown reason, some unlikely factors such as living at a higher altitude or having been born during the springtime, result in slightly earlier menopause than average. Having one or more pregnancies also results in a slightly earlier menopause. Severe stress such as divorce, death of a loved one, or financial crisis, may move up the time of menopause.

The average age at which women reach menopause has stayed relatively constant over the past centuries, but the average life span has dramatically climbed. As a result, women now spend one third or more of their life postmenopause.

Part III:
The Menopause Banquet: A Look Inside the Kitchen

A successful dinner party is determined not so much by what the dining room looks like but by what goes on in the kitchen. The main course of menopause is the permanent cessation of ovulation. The foremost ingredient is declining estrogen. Estrogen levels fluctuate wildly early in perimenopause, wWednesday and taper down in later perimenopause, wThursday. During the last two years of perimenopause, there is a rapid decline of estrogen. At the time of menopause, estrogen levels plummet dramatically. The rapid descent of estrogen at menopause can cause the oven to overheat and dry-out the "meal". Hot flashes and vaginal dryness reach their peak when estrogen levels go down the drain. FSH is like the dinner guest who continues asking the kitchen for more food, but the cook is gone, and the kitchen lights are off.

Maria C.

Maria C. posed an interesting question when she asked about cancer of the uterus. Maria had reached menopause twenty months ago after finalizing a nasty divorce. Her three kids and her job as a county clerk kept her going. She had her menopause at age 46 without too much fuss and was taking no medications. After eighteen months of no bleeding, out of the blue, last month she had two days of bleeding along with some cramps. This month she had three days of cramping and bleeding with breast tenderness. Her mother saw this as warning bells and told her she might have cancer of the uterus and had better go get checked.

Maria looked great. Since her office visit last year when she started the Womenopause Challenge, she had made improvements in her eating and exercising to the tune of a 15-pound weight loss. She was happy and positively gushing about a new love in her life.

Maria's exam was normal. Her Pap test, pregnancy test, STIs, pipelle, thyroid, ultrasound and hemoglobin were all normal. By all accounts, it appeared that Maria had resumed normal menstrual cycles after "reaching menopause".

Her FSH level on day three of her cycle, a year ago, was 60 mIU/mL, clearly elevated and indicative of postmenopause. Another FSH level was ordered this year; and at 8 mIU/mL, it confirmed the probability that she had beaten the odds and had paused, but had resumed menstruation a year and a half later.

Maria's wScore total was 7 W. She was not having any significant physical or emotional problems that could be related to her endocrine rebirth.

Maria's youngest son was seventeen, and Maria decided he did not need a younger brother or sister. She chose to resume Yaz, a cycle control hormone pill, which would smooth out her cycles, as well as providing birth control in the light of her resurrected fertility.

Maria came to the opinion that her "first" menopause was due to her divorce stress. Once her ex was gone from her life and the stress subsided, she had resumed regular menstrual periods.

Elizabeth R.

Elizabeth R. had one question, was she in menopause? Elizabeth had undergone a hysterectomy for fibroids ten years ago that had successfully relieved her of what she termed "the monthly gushers". Her custom designer jewelry business had expanded to the point where she had recently leased new office space to accommodate her 12 employees. She was much too busy to be bothered by hot flashes that she swore occurred every 90 minutes. Her sleep was nonexistent. Her BMI had crept up one point every year for the past five years. Now at age 51, it pushed her into the full figured range. Elizabeth had been trying olive oil to relieve vaginal irritation and thought it helped somewhat, but her interest in sex had waned.

The exam for Elizabeth showed marked vaginal atrophy with areas of inflammation. All her tests were normal. Elizabeth examined the Womenopause wTimeLine (Figure 3-1) but was at a loss to know for sure whether she was on wThursday or wFriday. Without a uterus announcing the status of her hormones, it was impossible for Elizabeth to know if menopause, wThursday midnight, had passed or not. An FSH blood test could be ordered, but Elizabeth was advised the test would have virtually no bearing on the options she faced for treating her symptoms. Elizabeth was sure hormone therapy was out of the question for her. She reported that her mother had just finished treatment for ductal cell carcinoma of the breast, and her father had had a couple of heart attacks. Elizabeth had heard hormone therapy caused breast cancer and heart attacks.

Elizabeth completed the wScore:

1. Hot Flashes: 16 W
2. Mood Matters: 8 W
3. Sexercise: 6 W
4. Vagina Sahara: 8 W
5. Skinny in Skin: 2 W
6. Insomnia Queen: 7 W
7. Plumbing and Pain: 1 W.

Her total *w*Score was 48 W.

Treatment options for Elizabeth were considered. Lifestyle health habits were reviewed, and she recognized that she had probably devoted too much time to her career and not as much as she would have liked for her husband and friends. She was determined to change. Elizabeth considered treating her hot flashes with Pristiq, an anti-depressant, and her vaginal irritation with Estrace cream, the *w*BodyIdentical 17beta-estradiol, vaginal cream. Estrace cream is absorbed locally only and does not have a significant systemic effect. After a thorough discussion about the risks and benefits, Elizabeth began treatment with the one thing she thought she should never be able to use — estrogen. Elizabeth, like many women, was not aware that estrogen therapy, ET (estrogen therapy alone, not coupled with progesterone) has been found to reduce the incidence of breast cancer by 33 percent. Additionally, there is research to suggest that for women in Elizabeth's age group, initiating estrogen therapy near the time of menopause reduces the incidence of coronary heart disease by 40 percent. Estrogen therapy for *w*Wednesday through *w*Friday reduces women's total mortality by 40 percent.

Elizabeth began treatment with Evamist, a *w*BodyIdentical estrogen, 17beta-estradiol applied as a spray to the forearm. Because she does not have a uterus, the treatment for her would be the same if she were in perimenopause or postmenopause, estrogen alone. Therefore, she decided not to bother getting the FSH blood test. The Evamist, like the Vivelle-Dot and Divigel provides wBodyIdentical estrogen to the blood stream. These hormones are exactly like the estrogen Elizabeth's ovary used to make; they are wBodyIdentical (Chapter 21).

Four weeks later, Elizabeth returned, reporting a 90 percent improvement in hot flashes, better sleep, and a renewed enthusiasm for sex. She liked the way the Evamist was applied and wondered if she could go up on the dose to three sprays a day. She had hired a bookkeeper at work and found more time to devote to the things she really loved — her family and friends. Elizabeth's wScore declined from 48 W to 14 W in four weeks. Her BMI had already dropped one point. By reviewing the score, Elizabeth remarked how enthusiastic she was about keeping on track for the long haul.

Part IV:
The Pause That Refreshes

The Final Menstrual Period of menopause is a bit of an anticlimax. It's like getting the delayed report of an A+ on a term paper a year after graduation; it's like getting a coupon for something that is already expired; it's like finally getting an engraved invitation in the mail for a party in your honor that took place twelve months ago— and even worse, you were at that party but did not know it was all about you! Some think that menopause is a symbolic dividing line. It's not. The difference between wThursday and wFriday is just one little tick of the clock. The changes usually develop over a decade or more and continue onward for years. Your menopause makeover begins now.

Part V:
The Womenopause Challenge: The Punctuated Period

1. Like a small punctuation mark at the end of a beautifully crafted sentence, the final menstrual period may go by as

just a small dot, ending an otherwise glorious season of fertility. Spot your FMP on the wChart Figure 2-3.

2. Throw away all of your tampons, pads, and "period-days-panties".

3. Clean house to make room on the bathroom shelves for fun lotions, candles, and oils.

4. Now you are starting to stop pausing and start living!

Chapter 7

Postmenopause: The *w*UpSide of Menopause

Part I:
Defining the *w*UpSide of Menopause

The marketing genius who devised the term "postmenopause" should be let go.

Postmenopause *begins* a time when women report more fulfillment and happiness than they had ever experienced in their youth. Calling these years "postmenopause" makes the time sound like a leftover, an after thought. Nothing could be further from the truth. Womenopause prefers the *w*UpSide of menopause because that term describes what really happens, and it is mostly good. The *w*UpSide of menopause should be a time young women look forward to.

One could imagine the younger years as a long series of hills to climb. There are times of climbing up hill for days on end, followed by downhill slides into the valleys of relief. Great amounts of effort must be expended to get up the hills followed by minimal effort for coasting to the next one. Up and down, day-by-day and year-by-year, the female hormonal cycle leads women on a captivating ride. At menopause, a woman reaches new heights: a high healthy plateau. Up here, the terrain is smooth, and the views, magnificent. The difficult hill climbing days are in the past, but so are the days of downhill coasting. The high healthy plateau can be crossed if daily effort is applied, not the gut wrenching sweaty uphill grinds of youth, but a steady brisk hike will do nicely. Trying to coast may lead to a deadly standstill. Pick new challenges; the possibilities are endless; the choices are yours.

Part II:
Go Figure

The Womenopause *w*TimeLine (Figure 3-1) defines the *w*UpSide of menopause as beginning *w*Friday at 12:01 a.m. and continuing until last call *w*Saturday at midnight. Ninety percent of women enter the *w*UpSide by age 55. There are a few stragglers who continue to have regular periods even out to age 60. The *w*UpSide may well last a third or more of a woman's life (Figure 1-1). Therefore, it's a big deal. In the year 2000 there were 45 million women on the *w*UpSide. By the year 2030 that number will double to over ninety million women living in the US in their *w*UpSide. Two-thirds of *w*UpSide women will live beyond age 85. Wow! Unprecedented numbers of these women will seek answers to the questions about lifestyle choices and medical options for the alleviation of the consequences of living decades without estrogen and for the inevitable aging problems. Many women will ask, "Is this aging or is it menopause?"

During the menopausal *w*UpSide, the quantity and types of estrogen change. Regular reproductive cycles occurring on *w*Monday and *w*Tuesday consist of high amounts of estradiol (E2) ranging from 10 to 800 pg/mL and low amounts of estrone (E1) 30 to 180 pg/mL. Estradiol is predominately produced by the ovary, and estrone is predominately from the conversion of estradiol to estrone in adipose tissue. During perimenopause, the smooth cycling breaks down, and erratic high or low levels of estradiol can be seen at any time of the month (or day or hour!). Therefore, there is little value in checking estrogen levels in the blood (or saliva). It won't tell you where you are on the *w*TimeLine, and it won't help you know your average estrogen level. The extreme fluctuations (not the level) of E2 are believed to trigger the transition symptoms that most women experience such as Hot Dreads, Mood Matters, Meno-Fog, Insomnia Queen, and Vagina Sahara.

After menopause, during the *w*UpSide, estradiol (E2) precipitously declines to low levels in the 10 to 40 pg/mL range; while, estrone (E1) declines somewhat less, stabilizing in the range of 6 to 63 pg/mL. During the wUpSide, estrogen precursors are produced by the adrenal gland and converted into functioning estrogens by peripheral tissues (muscle and fat).

In wUpSide women, the ratio of estradiol to estrone flips from a greater estradiol level during perimenopause to a greater estrone level during postmenopausal, but there is far less of either hormone. Estrone (E1) is 80 percent less active than estradiol (E2). By the way, estriol (E3) produced by the placenta during pregnancy, is present in minuscule amounts in the non-pregnant woman. E3 is 95 percent less active than estradiol (E2).

Consistently low levels of estrogen generally result in diminishing hot flashes, mood swings, Meno-Fog, and insomnia. In contrast, vaginal dryness, osteoporosis, and other health issues all tend to accelerate during the wUpSide.

Women's testosterone is frequently overlooked as an important endocrine factor. Testosterone is not just a guy thing. Testosterone is produced in the ovary, but not by the follicle that is responsible for producing estrogen and progesterone. It is made from the supporting stromal cell tissue of the ovary, and some testosterone also originates from the adrenal glands.

Testosterone plays an important role in a variety of normal female functions. It is particularly important in a woman's feeling of well-being and in her sex drive. Some refer to sex drive as libido; a term usually associated with Dr. Sigmund Freud, the famous nineteenth century psychoanalyst. The term libido carries a lot a baggage and unnecessarily complicates a wonderful natural physical attraction.

During wUpSide, the free available testosterone declines in 40 percent of women, stays at the same level in 40 percent of women, or may even increase in 20 percent of women (Chapter 21). This increase is referred to as the "menopausal zest". A deficiency in testosterone may adversely affect sexual desire, arousal, and orgasms.

The hormonal stability seen during the *w*UpSide is responsible for the gradual improvement most women experience after the sometimes-chaotic years experienced during perimenopause. Hot flashes decline in severity and frequency but may not completely go away (Chapter 9: Hot Flash Fever). The transient memory malfunctions of Meno-Fog recede with time. Sleep patterns return to normal, resulting in improved energy and feelings of well-being.

Unfortunately, not everything reverts to what it was like before menopause. It is hard to clearly separate which physical problems are due to loss of estrogen from which physical problems are due to normal aging. Clearly, persistent hot flashes during the *w*UpSide are driven by inadequate amounts of circulating estrogen, as is vaginal atrophy and dryness (Chapter 10: Vagina Sahara). There is little dispute about the rapid loss of bone strength and bone mass, osteoporosis, which is directly attributed to lack of estrogen after menopause (Chapter 26: Boning Up).

It is clear, low estrogen during postmenopause contributes to the progression of thin wrinkling skin and to hair loss. It may also be a factor in memory decline, mood disturbance, and the general loss of vitality and strength some women experience. The long term effects of low estrogen as seen in menopausal *w*UpSide women has unknown and controversial consequences on the development of hypertension, heart disease, stroke, diabetes, hyperlipidemia, cancer, obesity, and longevity.

Part III:
More *w*UpSide

Many menopausal *w*UpSide women report improvement in all dimensions of their quality of life: physical, emotional, and spiritual. It may be that the wisdom gained through experience effectively counters any possible negative aspects aging might be expected to bring. For the most part, young women do not appreciate the things mature women value. Despite the fact that some wThursday women in the throes of hot flashes may cling to their youth, many would gladly age a little quicker to reach menopause early and obtain relief of their perimenopausal symptoms. Once hot flashes, Meno-Fog, and insomnia arise many women may begin to see 50 as a safe haven. Most wUpSide women report greater satisfaction with life than most women in their thirties do. The majority of women report the wUpSide of menopause as being the best time of their entire life.

For a woman to determine her best choices in managing problems encountered during the wUpSide, it is necessary to carefully consider many factors. Like trying on jeans, some sizes are too big and others, too small. Let's face it; some designer hip hugging tattered jeans with an embroidered human skull on the seat pocket are not the preferred style for some women, but they might be just the perfect pair for a discriminating few.

Veronica W.

Veronica W. presented with a single question; what happened to her sex drive? Veronica, a physician specializing in internal medicine, had experienced menopause five years ago at age 55. She and her husband, also a physician, had made a considered decision at the time, not to use menopause hormone therapy (MHT) because of newspaper reports of the WHI study that had been publicized in 2002. They believed the WHI study proved that health risks associated with MHT outweighed the benefits. In any event, her transition had been relatively smooth. She had required no specific interventions for any menopausal symptoms: no hot flashes, no insomnia, no moodiness, no sex problem, no "nothing". All was great until her hysterectomy six months ago.

Veronica explained that beginning about seven months ago she developed an ache just above her pubic bone. She had her urine tested, and it showed the presence of some bacteria. She took a course of antibiotics. She felt better for two weeks until the same discomfort recurred. She actually saw her doctor then, and her doctor discovered that Veronica was having some vague intestinal symptoms, cramps, and a little spot of blood after wiping for a bowel movement. Veronica was sent right over to the gastroenterologist (the specialty of stomach and intestines). After the colonoscopy, the doctor reassured her she did not have cancer of the colon or anything serious, just a small external hemorrhoid. Her symptoms persisted, and an ultrasound of her pelvis revealed a mass on her left ovary. An MRI confirmed the presence of a complex ovarian lesion but could not exclude the possibility that it was cancer. A blood test CA125, a marker for ovarian cancer, was borderline positive.

Veronica elected to have a total abdominal hysterectomy with bilateral salpingo oophorectomy (TAH & BSO, surgical removal of the uterus, tubes, and ovaries). Thank goodness, the ovarian mass turned out to be a six-centimeter benign tumor, called a serous cyst adenoma. Her hospital stay was brief, and she followed her surgeon's advice to stay off work and refrain from sex for six weeks. Six weeks passed, then six weeks more, and six weeks more with no sex.

It did not occur to her that she and her husband had stopped having sex until he finally had the courage to ask her about it. She was surprised to realize they had gone over four months without any sexual intercourse. Veronica asked her surgeon about it, but she did not feel like the question was taken seriously because it was not as if she had a fever or something important. At least that was how Veronica interpreted the conversation. Many women report improved sexual function after recovery from hysterectomy, and Veronica could not understand why it was different for her. After six months of going nowhere, Veronica made an appointment with a menopause specialist to get another opinion.

Veronica already understood how important lifestyle choices were for long-term health and well-being. She and her husband were great examples of people who took responsibility by eating right, exercising daily, and taking time to enjoy family and friends. She was fit and slim figured with a BMI of 20. Veronica had only one complaint; she had somehow completely lost interest in sex. Her exam was normal except for slight vaginal thinning. Her labs were all normal, and her mammogram was clear. Her bone density, however, had made a dramatic change. When Veronica had checked her bone density two years ago, the T score was + 0.4, but now it was − 1.9, putting her in the gray zone between normal and osteoporosis: osteopenia.

Sex drive is a complex interaction of body, mind, and spirit. Veronica was convinced, in her case, the only thing that had changed was her body. She loved her husband, and prior to the operation, she had fully expected the hysterectomy to have no effect on their excellent sex life. Veronica accepted information about menopausal hormone conditions. She was told her wUpSide ovaries must have still been producing enough testosterone to keep her sex drive active, and when they were removed at the time of her hysterectomy, her body could not compensate for the lack of testosterone. Her sex drive dwindled. Testosterone levels typically drop 50 percent after oophorectomy.

Options. Veronica wanted options! With the singular complaint of lack of sex drive, the simplest option would be to take a testosterone supplement. Testosterone treatment for women is a complicated social/political question, but it's not a particularly complicated medical question. Some women require low dose testosterone treatment for optimal functioning. There are currently testosterone products available for women in virtually every country in the world, but none are FDA approved in the United States. Veronica can receive a prescription for compounded testosterone in the U.S. or use, "off label", one to three drops (100 to 300ug) of an FDA approved testosterone gel approved for men (Testim). Men usually require 50 to 150 drops of the same gel.

There was another option that could address her lack of sex drive, thinning vagina, and osteopenia: estrogen therapy (ET). Initially, Veronica rejected the notion of taking ET because of her prior decision, when she believed the risks were prohibitive. Veronica sought additional information about hormone benefits and risks. She was advised, since she had already had a hysterectomy, she would be a suitable candidate for estrogen mono-therapy. Contrary to what Veronica and her husband had been led to believe, the WHI data brings to light evidence that estrogen therapy without progesterone actually reduces the incidence of breast cancer by 33 percent and reduces cardiac disease by 40 percent. Estrogen therapy for women in Veronica's age group according to the WHI study, reduces mortality from all causes by an astounding 40 percent. Estrogen therapy is a superior agent for preventing osteoporosis than any of the "osteoporosis" prescription medications. Estrogen therapy may or may not restore her sex drive, but it would reverse the dry thinning vaginal changes she had at present.

The wScore for Veronica demonstrated how impossible it is to compare total scores between different women. One might be tempted to recommend "stronger" treatments for women with high scores and try simpler remedies for women with low scores. That would be a mistake. Veronica's total wScore was a modest 14 W. Her before score was lower than some women's after score when they thought they were "cured". But Veronica's 7 W in the Sexercise box was, by itself, enough of a problem to warrant treatment.

Veronica elected to try vaginally applied testosterone cream three times a day for four weeks. She also resolved to take calcium citrate 500 mg three times a day and vitamin D 4000 IU a day. During her appointment four weeks later, she reported a definite renewal of sexual intimacy in both desire and orgasms.

After lengthy discussions and research, she and her husband decided to try estrogen therapy as well. Veronica began taking the Vivelle-Dot 0.05 mg, an estrogen transdermal patch that delivers wBodyIdentical 17β-estradiol (Chapter 21). During the next month she was planning to taper the testosterone to twice a day to see if she could eventually manage with the estrogen therapy alone.

Four weeks later, Veronica returned with some interesting observations. She felt she needed the testosterone cream only once a day. Since starting the estrogen patch, she noted improved sleep; and more importantly, she felt that the condition of her skin had improved. As an additional bonus, she noticed less arthritic knee pain and stiffness. Her wScore was lowered to 2 W. Veronica wanted to know how long she should stay on the estrogen patch? Good question. Perhaps the best answer is a return question: How long do you want the benefits? The current FDA approved recommendation is to stay on the lowest effective dose of menopausal hormone therapy for the shortest duration consistent with treatment goals and response. With current knowledge, it appears many women may safely choose to stay on hormone therapy indefinitely. It is advisable to reassess your personal health risks with your healthcare provider at least annually to determine whether or not menopausal hormone therapy is suitable for you to continue.

Part IV:
The Difference A Day Makes

The postmenopause wUpSide constitutes two days on the Womenopause wTimeLine (Figure 3-1). Menopause, the final menstrual period, occurs at midnight wThursday. Everything after midnight wThursday is the wUpSide. Early wUpSide women on wFriday may have different sets of problems than women living in the late wUpSide on wSaturday. Some refer to wSaturday afternoon as "geri-pause" combining the terms geriatrics with menopause.

Defining the differences may clarify which treatment options are preferred by some women and not by others. For instance, the WHI data demonstrated certain benefits of hormone therapy for women who started treatment before age 60 were not apparent if a woman waited to start therapy after age 70. For women over age 70, initiating hormone therapy 20 years after reaching menopause, actually posed increased risks for heart disease, temporarily, for one year.

All of these women are *w*UpSiders, but the best strategy each one might choose for treating an identical problem might be different. As an example, Hot Flash Fever, Vagina Sahara, and osteoporosis for an early *w*Friday morning woman would generally be treated differently than the same problems in a woman in her eighties living in *w*Saturday afternoon. As more data becomes available there might be reasons to divide *w*Saturday into specific subsets, like *w*Saturday morning, as distinct from *w*Saturday afternoon, and so on. For now, it is clear *w*UpSide women, including women up to age 60 or within ten years of menopause, are in some ways a special group and constitute *w*Friday women. Before and during *w*Friday, women have a "window of opportunity" in which MHT may be safer and more beneficial for long-term use than in any other women. *w*Upside women who carefully follow the principles of the Womenopause Challenge can be healthier and happier than ever. Become a role model by having the vitality, vigor, and relationships every woman in her thirties would envy. Postmenopause is overdue for a makeover too. Now is the time to stop pausing and start living.

Part V:
The Womenopause Challenge: *w*UpSide Essentials

1. Write a list of the top twenty blessings that have come your

way since age 30.

2. Buy a pedometer and write down how many steps you take each day. Shoot for 10,000-15,000 steps a day. The Sportline 4407 fits nicely into the pocket, purse, or even the bra.

3. Take a few minutes and put your favorite CD into the stereo and listen to three songs.

Chapter 8

Induced Menopause

Part I:
Patio Door

Menopause transition typically starts out with a few night sweats and hot flashes then gradually crescendos to full-blown mood-swinging-hot-dreads of perimenopause. This sequence usually allows women a chance to make adjustments and recognize the link between her biological and emotional patterns. Have you ever glided across the family room on your way out to the backyard deck, then smacked hard into the closed patio door? It's a shock to the system, isn't it? One moment you knew exactly what you were doing, then the next moment you had no idea. For many women, induced menopause is just like that.

Natural menopause occurs when the ovarian function declines naturally. Ovarian failure usually occurs in fits and stops over the course of three years to ten years. Leading up to menopause, estrogen may have erratic fluctuations, resulting in intervals of Hot Dreads, night sweats, Meno-Fog, Insomnia Queen and Mood Matters.

Induced menopause is the cessation of ovarian function by an external force. No, not Darth Vader. Most commonly, this means surgical removal of the ovaries (known as an oophorectomy) accompanied by surgical removal of the uterus (known as a hysterectomy).

Young women who require **chemotherapy** for cancer, such as breast cancer, may sustain an ovarian effect, which may induce an early menopause. If cancer of the pelvis is treated by external **radiation therapy**, it too may induce an early menopause. Induced menopause is an abrupt menopause, which is more pronounced when experienced at an earlier age.

In the US there are 45 million postmenopausal women. Two million of them had an induced menopause, which is about 5 percent. Which one is better? That is debatable. At Disney World you can choose between the Aerosmith Rockin' Roller Coaster that catapults you up and down for a mile and a half for two minutes, or the Twilight Zone Tower of Terror that simulates a ten story free-fall straight down in eight seconds. Which one is more fun? That is hard to decide since both can be pretty exciting and fun in different ways. Often, an induced menopause is more abrupt with more extreme menopausal changes than natural menopause, but there is not the long drawn out decade of irregular periods and perimenopausal symptoms. There is no obvious answer to which is "preferred" excepting induced menopause women are often times younger, and therefore, likely to have an even greater proportion of their lives with little or no estrogen.

Part II:
The Usual Suspects

Perimenopause (Chapter 5) brings forth a collection of symptoms that are related to the short-term withdrawal of estrogen. The same physical and emotional challenges can accompany induced menopause. Most of them are well-known to you now and are so important there is a whole chapter devoted to many of them:

- Hot Flash Fever
- Night sweats/ cold crashes
- Mood Matters
- Meno-Fog
- Insomnia Queen
- Headaches
- Palpitations

- Fatigue
- wWorry
- Vagina Sahara

The main difference between natural and induced menopause is that with induced menopause all the problems come, literally, overnight. As an example, a young woman may need a hysterectomy for fibroids (benign tumor of the uterus). In some cases, the surgeon says, "While I'm in there, I might as well take out the ovaries too." There are many legitimate reasons why the ovaries should be removed at the time of a hysterectomy. The ovaries may contribute to pain problems, PMS (premenstrual tension syndrome), Meno-Fog, crying spells, and ovarian cancer. If the ovaries remain after a hysterectomy, all of the hormonal cyclic effects will continue but without the bleeding. When normally functioning ovaries are removed, a woman may wake up from anesthesia with all the symptoms of menopause in full bloom: near incapacitating hot flashes, insomnia, meno-fog, and mood swings. Wham! Thank you very much.

Naturally occurring menopause will, at least, let you adapt to some of the changes. Often this is not true with induced menopause. The symptoms of induced menopause are often more intense and frequent than natural menopause.

The vagina may get hit the hardest with induced menopause causing Vagina Sahara. Vagina Sahara is often overlooked as an estrogen withdrawal problem and may catch many women off-guard. The high blood levels of estrogen during the reproductive years, sustains a healthy elastic and lubricated vagina. When that sustenance, estrogen, goes away, so may vaginal health (Chapter 10: Vagina Sahara). The resulting changes in sexual behavior, due to vaginal dryness, may have significant relationship implications, as well as loss of pleasure from sex (Chapter 18: Sexercise).

Part III:

Wait A Minute: Sometimes It's All Good

It might be tempting to think that hysterectomies (with oophorectomy) ruin women's lives. Not so. In fact, most women report an improved sense of well-being after a hysterectomy. More women experience orgasms (72 percent) after having had a hysterectomy than before (63 percent). Often, a hysterectomy is performed for seriously incapacitating problems like abnormal uterine bleeding, painful cramps, and general nuisance; thus, having the underlying problem gone comes as a relief. Occasionally a hysterectomy is done for cancer of the cervix, uterus, or ovary; and in such cases, there is really no other choice.

Part IV:
Induced Menopause: Crashing The Sex Drive

The ovaries produce the fundamental female hormones estrogen and progesterone. What is commonly missed is the role the ovaries have in producing testosterone. Women of reproductive age have all three hormones creating a uniquely feminine sexuality. At menopause, the ovaries stop production of estrogen and progesterone but *continue to make testosterone*. Hence, postmenopausal ovaries remain pivotal in certain aspects of sexual desire and arousal.

When the ovaries are knocked-out by surgery, radiation, or chemo, the amount of testosterone in the blood stream gets cut in half overnight — as in, immediately. Some women are very sensitive to this change and lose an important part of their sexual response. The long lasting effects on their desire for sex can be disruptive to a marriage and other relationships.

Loss of testosterone coupled with Vagina Sahara is a recipe for a disturbed sex life and possibly a diminished sense of well-being. Hot flashes usually go away, mood swings usually go away, meno-fog usually goes away, but loss of sex drive and vaginal dryness may not. They march on across the remaining years like soldiers of a losing campaign. Induced menopause, in this regard, is just like natural menopause.

Part V:
Top Ten Troubles

The short-term estrogen withdrawal symptoms are well-known and relatively easy to recognize. The long-term estrogen deficiency problems are more sinister (Chapter 22: Menopausal Hormone Therapy) and less well characterized. It is now known that induced menopause complicates these long-term problems. Current research adds clarity to this important health crisis. The following medical conditions are at risk with **long-term estrogen deficiency** as seen in young women who have an early, induced menopause:

- Osteoporosis
- Cardiovascular disease
- Sexual decline
- Premature death
- Psychological loss of well-being
- Dementia
- Parkinson's disease
- Dry eye
- Dry wrinkled skin
- Hair loss

It must also be noted that many women have a hysterectomy and removal of the ovaries for a serious medical condition. The course of the primary disease, as well as its treatment, will have its own complicating influences.

Part VI:
Modern Approach to the Treatment of Induced Menopause

If a healthy young woman has a hysterectomy with removal of ovaries for benign reasons, she would normally be an excellent candidate for Menopausal Hormone therapy (MHT). The long-term advantage of preventing estrogen deficiency has definite appeal especially when relief from short-term estrogen withdrawal is thrown into the deal. In times past, women having a hysterectomy were often advised not to take hormones because they were young, and they would have to be on them too long. In fact just the opposite is true. Women who experience induced menopause frequently require higher doses of estrogen because they are often younger than women who experience natural menopause. If hormones were offered, they were usually withheld for several weeks until healing from the hysterectomy was complete. The rationale was that the oral forms of estrogen are known to have a slight increase in the risk of blood clots. Since surgery also increases the risk of blood clots, it was regarded safer to wait until the surgery risk had past.

Transdermal estrogen (wBodyIdentical 17beta-estradiol) does not have an increased risk of blood clots. It may be started the morning of surgery in appropriate women.

Because the uterus is often removed with induced menopause, most women need to only take estrogen and can skip taking progesterone. Progesterone is paired with estrogen for MHT only to protect the uterus. If the uterus is gone, so is the need for progesterone with its side effects and risks (Chapter 22).

Vaginal atrophy and Vagina Sahara are well treated with systemic transdermal estrogen and local vaginal estrogen. If there is a reason why estrogen is not safe, as with women who have estrogen receptor positive breast cancer, local vaginal estrogen alone may be a safe option. If not, there are moisturizers and lubricants that help (Chapter 10: Vagina Sahara).

Impaired sexuality of induced menopause is a major concern. Absence of ovarian testosterone may adversely affect sexual desire, arousal, and orgasm. Testosterone therapy may be needed to restore normal function. Local vaginal testosterone 2 percent compounded cream may restore vaginal lubrication, and systemic transdermal testosterone gel may improve sense of well-being, sexual desire, sexual arousal, and orgasm. Local vaginal testosterone may also be considered a low risk option for breast cancer survivors with vaginal atrophy who are not candidates for estrogen therapy.

Unless the surgery is done for problems due to the ovaries, most surgeons examine the ovaries at the time of hysterectomy and try to conserve them if no abnormalities are found. Leaving in the ovaries has many positive health benefits for mood, cardiovascular disease, dementia, and osteoporosis.

Imogene M.

Imogene was a polite and soft-spoken career Salvation Army lieutenant. She was 39, never married, and had had no pregnancies. She had suffered from severe heavy periods for many years and eventually three years ago she had a hysterectomy. Her ovaries were removed at the time, and she experienced "fire and brimstone" hot flashes for more than a year. The flashes eventually calmed down to "just fire".

At the time of her surgery her OBGyn advised her to avoid hormones because she was so young, and the risks of taking them for a long time may not be not worth it. Three years later, she stated she would gladly exchange a few years of life for some relief.

Imogene's highly structured life left her little time to dwell on her own problems. She was in charge of several community programs with the mission, but the one that took up most of her time was the drug halfway house that she lived in and managed. The daily dramas of the characters that came and went over the years kept her very busy and on her toes.

Her overall health was good; although, she admitted she took advantage of it by not watching what she ate, and she never exercised. Imogene's BMI was an excellent 26, but her wScore revealed significant menopausal symptoms. Her total score was 42, and her Hot Flash Fever box accounted for 18 "W". She was not sexually active and chose not to fill in the Sexercise portion. She stated, "I can't stand it any longer. I don't care if I die next week. I have to have hormones even if they kill me."

Imogene believed her hysterectomy had ruined her life. The physical exam revealed severe vaginal atrophy making the pelvic exam difficult because of bleeding of the mucosa even with light touch. The rest of her exam and all of the routine annual tests were normal.

Imogene was offered information about benefits and risks of menopausal hormone therapy. She was surprised to learn that estrogen therapy would most likely eliminate her estrogen deficiency symptoms of hot flashes, night sweats, vaginal dryness, and Meno-Fog without causing her to immediately drop over dead. She had become convinced that she had to suffer hot flashes in order to become fully mature. Now she was not so sure. She obtained information about the various formulations of estrogen therapy, but her only concern was "which one will my insurance cover?" She was advised that although there were theoretical differences between wBodyIdentical transdermal estrogen and oral conjugated estrogens, the differences were subtle. Since she had no other underlying health problems she chose to take Premarin pills because she thought it was the only one on her health plan. She was glad to find out that the women in the WHI study who took only Premarin had a decreased incidence of breast cancer and a further decrease in breast cancer deaths (Chapter 20). She was offered a transdermal estradiol Climara patch that was also on her health plan and would decrease her risk of blood clots. Imogene elected to stay with

Premarin to avoid wearing a patch for the rest of her life. Her skin had always been extra sensitive.

Premarin 0.3 mg a day was the initial dose, but after four weeks there had not been much improvement in the frequency or severity of her hot flashes. The dose was increased to 0.625 mg daily for the next four weeks. At that appointment she reported about a 50 percent improvement; the dose was again adjusted upward to 1.25 mg daily. At that dose her hot flashes went away completely.

Imogene decided to go "all in" for the Womenopause challenge and recruited six of the women at the half way house to begin an exercise program with her. She made a decision to change all the food available at the halfway house to only real foods. Two years later Imogene looked and acted younger and healthier than she did the day she started the Womenopause challenge.

Induced menopause symptoms and medical troubles are preventable and treatable.

Part VII:
The Womenopause Challenge: Induced Menopause Worksheet

1. Are you having any menopausal symptoms like Hot Flash Fever, Insomnia Queen, Mood Matters, or Meno-Fog? Determine your *w*Score Figure 1-2 and add up the total W.
2. Determine your place on the *w*TimeLine by substituting your surgery date for the FMP.
3. You may be an excellent candidate for estrogen therapy if you have any of the following:

   • You have induced menopause for a benign condition
   • You have menopausal symptoms such as hot flashes, night sweats, or vaginal dryness

- You are under age 60.
- You don't have any contraindications (chapter 20).
- You are interested in a menopause makeover.

Chapter 9

Hot Flash Fever

Part I:
Nelly was Right

When a hot flash strikes, there's an impulse to "take off all your clothes"; but it's not always convenient to do so. When you're out with friends at a favorite restaurant, taking off all your clothes is technically illegal. Hot flashes can intrude at the most inconvenient times. It is a little like when your perfectly well-behaved child yells out an inappropriate word she has never used before, while you are waiting in a long check-out line. Thanks a lot, great timing. Hot flashes are the emissary of perimenopause – 85 percent of American women experience hot flashes, but other ethnic groups report significantly different rates.

There are some characteristics of hot flashes most women identify with, but there are great differences between women and between episodes in the same woman. A typical hot flash begins with tingling warmth on the chest or neck, then over a couple of minutes, it spreads to the head, arms, body, and the legs in succession.

Although most women categorize the sensation as an elevated temperature, there is often some degree of an emotional component. Sometimes the term hot flash does not do it justice. When the anxiety part of a hot flash takes over, it's more like a Hot Dread: a feeling like "I gotta get out of my skin". When a Hot Dread occurs, no amount of clothing adjustment can solve the problem. A hot flash may last from two minutes to thirty minutes and may occur up to dozens of times during the day or the night. Many women notice a higher frequency in the late afternoon or evenings.

Perhaps less known are the chills that frequently follow hot flashes. For some women, cold crashes are what bothers them the most, not the heat. Night sweats and drenched nightgowns are more likely to be blamed for disrupting sleep than a simple hot flash. They all stem from the same underlying physiology.

Just be aware that feeling hot is not always due to perimenopausal hormone changes. There could be other health implications. Thyroid disease is relatively common in midlife women, and a simple blood test could exclude that from the possible list of problems. Certainly, a fever from an infection can cause a hot feeling. Serious infections can progress to fever and chills that could mimic a hot flash/ cold crash cycle. Occasionally, out-of-control hypertension can cause a flushed fever-like feeling, and a blood pressure check is all that is needed to figure it out. Rarely, things like leukemia, epilepsy, TB, lymphoma, and other cancers may produce any number of weird symptoms. Some medications can trigger hot flashes. Drinking alcohol can frequently cause a flushed feeling. The breast cancer treatment drug, tamoxifen, commonly causes hot flashes. The osteoporosis drug Evista can cause hot flashes as well. Moderate and severe hot flashes warrant a medical evaluation.

Part II:
More Than Hot

Americans use the term hot flash, and the Canadians and British use the term hot flush to describe what is technically a vasomotor disturbance (Figure 9-1). Flash is useful in describing the rapid onset and relative short duration of a vasomotor event. Flush is closer in describing the unpleasant spreading wave of the vasomotor event. Many women report complicated sensations during a hot flash. Feelings like anxiety, frustration, embarrassment, nausea, irritability, depression, and forgetfulness are emotions commonly identified as related to hot flashes.

Interestingly, even though the vasomotor event is brief, lasting in the order of minutes, the emotional components may have persistent effects. During times of recurrent hot flashes, women report mood problems, sleep disturbance, and inability to concentrate. Simple hot flashes are not so simple. The unpleasantness witnessed by some women can be described as a Hot Dread because that term acknowledges the physical heat experienced and validates the important emotional component that fatigues and distresses women.

Estrogen deficiency of menopause that triggers hot flashes increases the risks of brain dysfunction. PET scans demonstrate changes in cerebral blood flow in many brain areas during hot flashes. Hot flashes may be representative of more than just an annoying symptom; they may be indicative of significant physiological changes in the brain as well as in other organs. Frequent and severe hot flashes may be a signal for cardiovascular disease, osteoporosis, cognitive impairment, and depression. It just might be serious.

Part III:
Go Buy a New Hat

Every once in a while, it's easy to think a woman's voice isn't heard, and nothing is ever going to change. Then something comes up, and you realize maybe there is some reason for hope. This is a true story that took place 30 years ago.

Katherine was a lovely sculptor married to a physician, and they had five children. At age 50, Katherine began to experience night sweats that progressed over the next year to incapacitating hot flashes occurring every 90 minutes. She explained it all to her local, well-respected OBGyn doctor. After hearing her complaints, he reached out, held her hand, and said, "Nothing to worry about, why don't you go out and buy yourself a new hat."

Today, hopefully, women realize there are many options for the management of menopausal hot flashes. If you like hats, by all means, get one. If you have bothersome hot flashes, you might want to start by taking off that hat.

Oh, and by the way, in case you were wondering, hot flashes are definitely not a psychological disorder, and retail therapy remains to this day, an unproven treatment for hot flashes. Thankfully, we now have very effective methods to successfully treat Hot Flash Fevers in just four weeks.

Part IV:
Anatomy of a Hot Flash

You might be surprised to know there are several laboratories around the world devoted to studying the physiology of hot flashes. Some experiments entail putting a subject into a space-suit-like device to tightly control the external temperature, then all sorts of physical parameters are measured while she experiences spontaneous hot flashes. Consistent patterns of physical changes occur in sequence (Figure 9-1).

Initially, the amount of blood flowing near the surface in the skin and underlying muscle increases. Soon after, a woman has her first conscious inkling that a hot flash might be starting. Within two or three minutes of the increased blood flow, the skin temperature rises up to ten degrees warmer than it was before the flash. As the skin temperature goes up, the body triggers a compensatory sweating. The perception of heat during a hot flash usually peaks about five minutes into the process. At the temperature peak, a woman experiences the most intense symptoms. At the same time, heart rate and metabolic rate (energy use rate) rise and max out at about the five-minute mark. The unpleasant hot feeling declines after the peak and typically disappears after ten to twenty minutes. The duration of a hot flash can be variable.

When the skin temperature starts to decline, there is a cooling of the surface due to evaporation of the sweat, and a woman may recognize this as a chill. After the cold crash sensation, the entire body cools off a degree. The increased blood flow, elevated skin temperature, increased heart rate, and elevated metabolic rate all wind down after about thirty minutes. Most hot flash episodes encompass approximately 30 minutes of measurable physical changes that coincide with a woman's ten-minute desire to take off all her clothes.

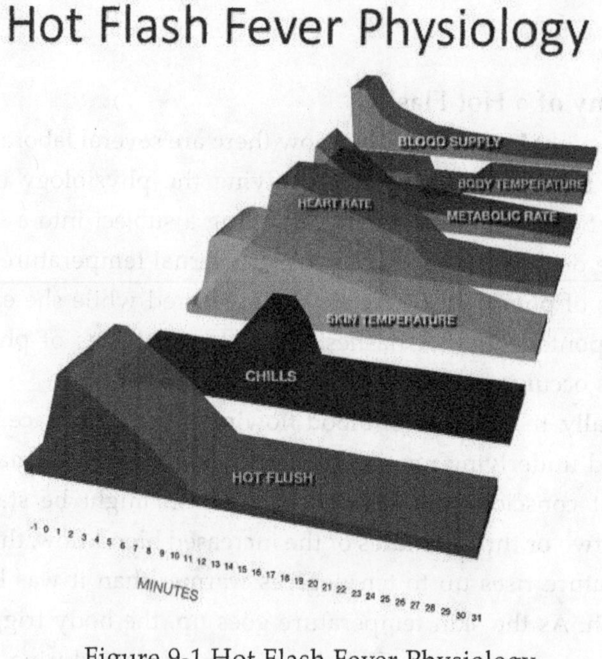

Hot Flash Fever Physiology

Figure 9-1 Hot Flash Fever Physiology

Part V:
Behind the Hot Flash Curtain

Hot flashes are the hallmark of perimenopause. Along with irregular periods, hot flashes define the start of wWednesday (Figure 3-1). Behind these physical changes are the endocrinological changes, notably alterations in ovarian function. During the reproductive years, wSunday, wMonday and wTuesday, the ovary produces predictable amounts of estrogen and progesterone cyclically. During this time, hot flashes almost never happen. After the ovary has exhausted a substantial number of eggs, there begins a time of unpredictable estrogen and progesterone release. Escalating levels of FSH and LH continue to stimulate the ovary to compensate for diminishing and/or erratic estrogen release. Measurement of circulating estrogen in the blood stream is not practical; as studies demonstrate perimenopausal women have wildly fluctuating blood levels of estrogen that might surge unexpectedly, many times a day. A *w*Thursday woman can have an estrogen level of 20, one minute, and an estrogen level of 600, the next.

It is during the years of erratic estrogen release from the ovary that the worst hot flashes occur. It is more accurate to think of hot flashes as being triggered by withdrawal of estrogen, not just by a lack of estrogen.

There is currently no test to identify who will suffer the worst symptoms of Hot Flash Fever. Hormone levels are not reliable markers, even though it is believed they govern the changes. The concentrations of hormones in other body tissues (such as saliva) do not correlate well with blood levels and have no known scientific usefulness. The theories explaining why hot flashes occur include: an alteration in the function of the temperature control system in the brain area called the hypothalamus, and a hormonally induced alteration in blood vessel response.

Part VI:
Be Cool

Women have successfully self-treated hot flashes since the beginning of time. After menopause, the permanent cessation of menstrual periods, hormone levels stabilize (at low levels), and hot flashes generally subside all on their own… or they may not; 30 percent of women are still bothered by hot flashes ten years after menopause; up to 20 percent continue to be bothered 15 years after menopause. For some women, hot flashes become a permanent part of their life.

The biggest no-brainers for taming Hot Flash Fever include strategies that have minimal risk and expense. It is useful to separate the no-brainer choices into two groups.

Group #1 includes the **bail-out** options: dress in layers, use a fan, take a cold drink, dunk your hands in cold water, go outside, and try to think about something pleasant.

Group #2 includes the **plan-ahead** options: stop smoking, exercise regularly, shape your waist (BMI less than 27). Practice a relaxation strategy you can use effectively even when the heat is on, such as yoga. Stay away from known triggers (like being caught in a small over-heated room with your in-laws), and avoid spicy foods.

For the next tier of hot flash control options, many people would list the nutritional herbs and supplements. It is felt they are low risk and not terribly expensive. Some women report improvement in hot flashes with the use of evening primrose oil, soy pills, and the herbal supplement: black cohosh. Scientific data is lacking concerning the effectiveness and safety of these supplements compared to placebo. A more expansive treatment of this subject is covered in Chapter 17. Vitamin E (200-400 IU per day) probably has some benefit in preventing Hot Flash Fever, but do not exceed doses greater than 800 IU per day.

Progesterone cream, herbal dong quai, ginseng, licorice, Chinese herb mixtures, acupuncture, and magnets are other alternative methods that have been reported to bring some relief. The amount of relief is about the same as placebo, which is 30 percent. However, the medical community cannot recommend those treatments for menopausal hot flashes at this time because proof of safety and/or effectiveness is lacking. The FDA has approved only menopausal hormone therapy (MHT) for the treatment of moderate or severe menopausal hot flashes.

Menopausal Hormone Therapy comes in three flavors (Figure 9-2): estrogen therapy (E) is, metaphorically speaking, the plain vanilla ice cream, progesterone therapy (P) is the plain chocolate ice cream, and estrogen plus progesterone (E+P) is like an ice cream swirl. MHT will relieve hot flashes for over 95-percent of women suffering from moderate or severe hot flashes, and MHT is effective in less than four weeks. MHT preparations are diverse and may be taken as a pill, cream, gel, spray, patch, or

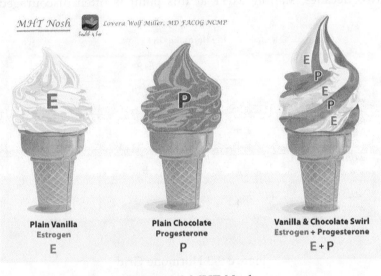

MHT Nosh   Lovera Wolf Miller, MD FACOG NCMP

Plain Vanilla	Plain Chocolate	Vanilla & Chocolate Swirl
Estrogen	Progesterone	Estrogen + Progesterone
E	P	E + P

Figure 9-2 MHT Nosh

ring. Deciding which one would work best, often takes careful investigation.

Perimenopausal women with a uterus, who suffer from hot flashes, frequently use a cycle control hormone pill (a birth control pill) such as Yaz; that is a swirl (E+P). Perimenopausal women without a uterus can generally be treated with the same treatments as postmenopausal women without a uterus, usually the plain vanilla option, transdermal (E), such as Vivelle-Dot, Evamist, or Divigel. Perimenopausal and postmenopausal women (wWednesday, wThursday, and wFriday women) with a uterus less than age 60, or less than ten years since menopause, may consider a different kind of swirl: transdermal E, such as Vivelle-Dot, in conjunction with oral P, such as Prometrium

(Figure 9-3: Hormone Grid).

Women, over the age of 60 with a uterus and more than ten years since menopause, have some risks associated with starting menopausal hormone therapy (but not *staying* on MHT). For women over age 70 who have not had hormones for more than two decades, *starting* MHT at this point is often discouraged

The Hormone Grid			
	E	*E+P*	*CCP* BIRTH CONTROL PILLS
Perimenopause with a uterus		**+**	**+**
Perimenopause without a uterus	**+**		*rarely*
wUpSide with a uterus		**+**	
wUpSide without a uterus	**+**		

Figure 9-3 Hormone Grid

unless significant modifiers are present (but *staying* on MHT is acceptable). Some do recommend having women take the lowest MHT dose for the shortest duration, but at this time, there are no studies to substantiate that recommendation. Both the dose and the duration are controversial topics that are discussed further in Chapter 22.

There are reasonable alternate medications for menopausal hot flashes if hormone therapy is not chosen or is not advisable. Several **anti-depressant medications** have been studied and found to reduce hot flashes independent of their effect on mood. Effexor, a mixed serotonin norepinephrine reuptake inhibitor (SNRI), has been found to reduce hot flashes in 60 percent of women. Pristiq has properties similar to Effexor. One might expect Cymbalta, from the same SNRI category, to have an equivalent effect as Effexor. Paxil, a different type of antidepressant, a selective serotonin reuptake inhibitor (SSRI), helps 50 percent of women with hot flashes but may cause weight gain. Gabapentin, an **anti-seizure medication,** also helps about 50 percent of the time. There is also evidence transdermal Clonidine, an **anti-hypertensive medication,** helps control hot flashes to some degree.

Just because these medications are not hormones, some mistakenly believe they are safer. They are not. Every treatment has it's own set of risks and side effects. Menopausal hormone therapy is roughly twice as effective in relieving hot flashes as any other second or third-line prescription therapy and without more risk. It is not easy to compare the overall health risks of medications from different classes of drugs like these.

Although hot flashes do not affect every woman during perimenopause and beyond, their presence may be a signal that significant physical and mental changes may be taking place. In other words, hot flashes are just the obvious outward sign of estrogen withdrawal that is being experienced by many organs of the body, notably the brain. As will be discussed in a later chapter (Mood Matters chapter 12 and Memory chapter 31), the degree of hot flashes may correlate with the extent of subsequent depression and memory malfunction. In a fairly predictable sequence, perimenopausal depression can be an important factor in marriage and relationship dynamics. Marital problems may eventually result in divorce. Divorce may be a factor in behavioral adjustment problems for the affected children, and so on. It is wrong to think of hot flashes as trivial.

Lana L.

At the age of 51 Lana L. is so elegant she could probably still get regular work as a runway model. Although she left that business over 25 years ago, her poise and posture suffuse sophistication. She worked as a freelance fashion writer, and her husband of 28 years sold real estate. Their two children were in a nearby college. She said her kids were more than happy to go off to college, so they could eat whatever they wanted. At home they had to follow their mother's rules. Lana was vegan. At six feet, weighing 118 pounds, Lana was off-the-chart slim figured (Figure 1-3: wBMI).

Lana had been experiencing what she called "burning hot oil showers", occurring about every hour for the past three months. Each episode lasted five minutes; then she was "locked in the freezer" for the next fifteen minutes.

She had never been really regular with her periods, but she had never gone four months without having a period before. She reported that the hot flashes and cold crashes had turned her world upside down. She wanted to know if she was "in menopause".

Menopause (Chapter 5) is the final menstrual period (FMP), the pausing of menstruation. A woman who has not had any menstrual flow for twelve months is considered to be postmenopausal. Lana studied the Womenopause wTimeLine, (Figure 2-1) and determined she may be either wThursday evening or wFriday morning. It is too early to tell for sure. In any event, she was definitely in perimenopause, which overlaps both wThursday and wFriday.

Seeing the other common symptoms on the wTimeLine chart, Lana realized she had been having other symptoms in addition to the hot flashes: memory problems, dry vagina, dry skin, mood swings, and insomnia. Lana had zero health problems and took no prescription medication. She took a soy capsule for hot flashes and lots of nutritional supplements. Her wScore was 61 W.

Lana's physical exam demonstrated moderate to severe vaginal inflammation but was otherwise normal. The following tests were ordered: pregnancy test, CBC, SMA, thyroid panel, FSH, LH, estradiol, mammogram, and colonoscopy and bone density. Lana was wary of entering into any form of medical treatment. Her previous experiences led her to believe medical doctors did not respect vegans, and they were likely to recommend dangerous and unnecessary drugs. Lana was assured her food beliefs would be respected, and she would never be encouraged to take any form of treatment she personally did not believe to be safe.

No treatment recommendations were made until Lana returned two weeks later with her test results. Lana was anemic with hemoglobin of 11.2 g. She had a low serum albumin level of 5.8 g. Her bone density was abnormal with a T score of -2.1. Her LH/FSH ratio was less than one, and her estradiol level was 20. Lana was informed her iron deficiency anemia and low albumin may be diet related. Her hormone levels suggested she was postmenopausal on the *w*UpSide of menopause *w*Friday. She was also significantly osteopenic, porous bones (much more on that later in Chapter 26: Boning Up 4 Osteoporosis).

A vegan diet can have health benefits but requires substantially more effort than an omnivorous diet. Lana confided she spent little time in meal planning, grocery shopping, and food preparation. Lana brought her bag of nutritional supplements she bought at a discount from her neighbor who was a regional distributor. She was taking many herbs but not any calcium, vitamin D, or iron.

Lana continued to express reluctance about agreeing to enter any type of formal program; she simply wanted the hot flashes to stop. She was counseled it might not be that simple. Lana presented with several unique factors that required consideration. The initial step was a recommendation for her to obtain professional guidance concerning healthful vegan nutrition. She readily agreed to a referral to a vegan specialist at a regional university center for diet recommendations. Next, Lana was given information regarding calcium and vitamin D supplementation and their effects in treating osteoporosis. Finally, Lana reviewed the *w*TimeLine (Figure 3-1) and was advised that her hot flashes were probably the result of a natural decline of estrogen production from the ovaries. She wanted to know how long they would continue and why the soy pills did not seem to work.

Hot flashes reach a peak in the first year to two years following the final menstrual period, but the duration is quite variable. Blood tests do not predict how bad or how long hot flashes will continue. Phytoestrogens from soy and yams have mild estrogenic effects and are ineffective for moderate or severe hot flashes. Although marketed as "natural", phytoestrogens are synthesized in a manufacturing lab with chemical reactions much like regular prescription hormones.

Lana expressed grave concerns about hormones because she believed they were products of horse urine. Premarin and Prempro were popular hormone therapy products, distilled from the urine of pregnant mares. Today there are several hormone therapy options derived from plant precursors (soy and yams) that have no animal products in their ingredients. In fact, most modern prescription MHT products made from plant precursors are the exact same molecular structure as the one synthesized by the human ovary, 17beta-estradiol (E2). That molecule is wBodyIdentical. wBodyIdentical prescription hormones are more natural to a woman's body than plant hormones marketed as "natural or bioidentical". Think about this, why would a human animal believe that a native plant hormone (phytoestrogen) would be more "natural" to a human than a human hormone (17beta-estradiol)?

At this, Lana said her head was spinning, and she needed more time to think things over. She decided to make a return appointment in two weeks and, in the meantime, begin the calcium citrate 1500 mg a day in divided doses, vitamin D 4000 IU a day, and iron supplements 300 mg three times a day. She would see the nutritionist and research the hormone topic. It was recommended she consider using olive oil for her vaginal dryness.

Two weeks later Lana returned. Her hot flashes continued unabated. She had joined a vegan cooking club at the recommendation of the nutritionist and found the meetings very informative. She had researched the menopause topic and, initially, could not find an authoritative source. It seemed every website she found was selling herbs like those she had already tried, until she found menopause.org, the official site for the North American Menopause Society. That site was a gateway to an enormous cache of medical research about menopause and hormones. Lana decided plant hormones were not really more natural to her human animal body. It was a revelation that required Lana to re-evaluate some fundamental self-perceptions. Lana needed relief from her hot flashes in order to resume her normal life. She decided to try wBodyIdentical hormones because she believed they were the most natural hormones for her and still consistent with her vegan principles.

Lana began treatment with Vivelle Dot 0.05, a transdermal estrogen, which provides 17beta-estradiol that is wBodyIdentical. To protect her uterus, she elected to use oral wBodyIdentical progesterone, Prometrium. Starting on new MHT, she was advised she might experience some light irregular vaginal bleeding for the next three to six months.

Four weeks later, Lana was happy to report zero hot flashes, no vaginal dryness, improved skin, razor sharp memory, and much better sleep. Her wScore improved from 61 W to 8 W. She felt okay about gaining four pounds because her nutritionist recommended a slightly higher BMI for optimal health. Her sex life was better than ever, and she had experienced only brief vaginal bleeding during the first week of therapy. Her hemoglobin had improved to 13.5.

Lana stated that if she ever decided to enter into a medically supervised menopause program, Womenopause would be the one.

Bev B.

Bev B. was not sure she should have made the appointment to see a new gynecologist, let alone actually come to the office. She was an unmarried executive secretary at age 67, who had reached menopause 12 years ago. She had initially been treated with Prempro, an oral combination E+P, for four years until her doctor advised stopping it in 2002 right after the breast cancer scare from the WHI news (Chapter 19). For the next six years her doctor kept reassuring her, the night sweats would eventually stop. They had not stopped; and if anything, they bothered her more now than ever. Two or three times a night she would wake-up soaking wet and cold. She would get out of bed and change her nightgown. Sometimes the sheets were so clammy, she had to change them in the middle of the night too. On top of that, she just could not get back to sleep. She felt progressively exhausted because of lack of sleep. Bev wanted to know if she could get a prescription for a sleeping pill.

Bev was a very private person, and it was clearly distressing for her to discuss health issues with a new doctor. After examining the wTimeLine (Figure 3-1), she determined she was a wSaturday early morning woman, and somehow, that recognition alone allowed her to drop her guard. Bev did not want to come across as being superficial; but after some hesitation, she confessed her most important physical problem was her thinning hair. She felt completely unattractive because she was going bald. Her hair had been noticeably thin for more than a decade. Her one and only medical discussion about balding five years ago had been a disaster. She had seen a local dermatologist who, after about a three second exam, told her "get a wig". He had also encouraged her "be bold, go blond". That did not go over well with Bev's proud African-American heritage.

She gave up on the idea of even trying to have this sensitive discussion. Bev had gradually withdrawn from all her usual social activities; she even stopped going to church. She lived alone, and her two adult daughters had taken jobs out of state.

Other health issues had crept onto the scene over the past three years. Bev's internist had started medication to help her control hypertension (lopressor) and diabetes (insulin). She was not doing herself any favors by her lack of exercise and poor food choices. At 5'4" weighing 202 pounds, Bev was full figured with a BMI of 33. The wScore total equaled 38 W with high scores in Insomnia Queen, Skinny on Skin, and Hot Flash Fever. A Carroll Rating Scale, a brief objective measurement for depression, had a score of 24, indicating significant depressive symptoms. Bev's physical exam confirmed alopecia, scalp hair loss, on the top and front of her head with preservation of her forehead hairline. Bev reported absence of sexual activity for seven years. Her pelvic exam demonstrated moderate vaginal dryness. She pointed out skin changes on her face which she found distressing, "crows feet, and eye bags". Routine tests included: Pap test, STI cultures, CBC, thyroid test, mammogram, a recommendation for a colonoscopy, and a bone density. All of her tests returned within normal limits except her thyroid function was low.

The wUpSide of menopause coincides with natural aging; and therefore, assigning a hormonal cause for all health problems is unwarranted. That being said, Bev's night sweats may be attributable to low estrogen, and her hair loss may be attributable to high hormonal androgens (masculine hormones). Bev was now motivated to make changes to start feeling and looking better. She reviewed the information about real food (Chapter 14), supplements (Chapter 17) and the Vitamin-X exercise (Chapter 16). She agreed to institute the Insomnia Queen sleep recommendations (Chapter 11).

Bev readily admitted her social life restrictions were self-imposed, but she lacked confidence and was unsure how to change anything. She asked if she should go back on Prempro to relieve her night sweats but questioned if it was too dangerous.

She also wanted to know if there was anything she could do about her thin hair.

Information about MHT for wFriday was reviewed. Initiation of menopausal hormone therapy on wSaturday has risks that are not present for wFriday women, such as increased risk for cardiovascular disease during the first year of therapy. Those risks do not appear to be present for women under age 59 or less than ten years since menopause. Because Bev is over age 60, more than ten years since menopause, has hypertension, and diabetes, she probably would have developed some sub-clinical cardiovascular disease by now. That may make her slightly more vulnerable to a cardiac event during the first year of MHT.

After careful consideration Bev chose not to try MHT for her night sweats. As an alternative, Bev received information about Pristiq (desvenlafaxine) and its effectiveness for reducing hot flashes and night sweats for approximately 60 percent of women. Pristiq would also be indicated as a treatment for her depression and social anxiety, "a two-fer", as Bev later described it.

The causes of hair loss for women were reviewed. Bev learned that thinning hair is as common in women as in men. Fifty percent of women notice significant hair loss by age 50, but men may have more extreme frontal loss. The most common mechanism is probably the same for men and women: genetic predisposition, hormonal changes, and age. It is easier to prevent hair loss than to get it back.

Bev accepted the Womenopause Challenge. She started Pristiq 50 mg once a day in the morning. She made herself a promise to follow the exercise, eating, and supplement guidelines of the Womenopause Challenge. For her social project, she made a plan: during week #1, she was going to contact her pastor and arrange a home visit; during week #2, she was going to visit both of her daughters; during week #3, she was going to take her best friend, Lucille, out to dinner; and during week #4, she was going to organize a carry-in luncheon with everyone at work.

Bev agreed to keep a careful diary of her sleep patterns for the month. She decided to trial Rogaine 2 percent (minoxadil), a topical hair loss over-the-counter product; 100mg of vitamin B6 daily; and drink green tea. Bev also agreed to meet with her internist to discuss her hypothyroid lab result and inquire about the advisability of changing her hypertension medication.

Four weeks later Bev had good news to report; her wScore had dropped from 38 W to 12 W; her Carroll Rating Scale had improved from 24 to 8; and her BMI had gone down one whole point to 32. She had been awakened only three times this week with night sweats instead of three times a night. She was particularly happy about her visit with her daughters. They gave her high marks for her new hairpiece.

Bev had grocery shopped five times this month, more than she had in the past year. She felt that eating at home helped her to eat real food instead of the fast processed food to which she had been accustomed. She had started her exercise program by walking the neighborhood twice a day for 30 minutes for the first two weeks, and then, added an exercise video three times a week at home. Bev's internist had repeated the thyroid test and agreed she should consider thyroid replacement therapy, which she did. Bev was also given the option to switch her hypertension medication to a different class of drug; she stopped the lopressor and began lisinopril. Bev was using the topical hair loss preparation Rogaine recognizing it may take months to have an effect.

Part VII:
No Joke

For some unknown reason, people like to make jokes about menopausal hot flashes. Stand-up comedians and cartoonists love to poke fun at the subject. It might be funny for someone who has never had one, but for the roughly 30 million perimenopausal women in the US, it's no joke. Hot flashes, hot flushes, and Hot Dreads can take a toll on an otherwise, well-grounded mature woman. It is totally treatable, and no one needs to suffer unnecessarily. Many women have been misinformed about the safety and effectiveness of menopausal hormone therapy. For most women, it is safe to take estrogen to relieve the symptoms of moderate to severe hot flashes; and if not, there are other options. All of the benefits and risks of menopausal hormone therapy are covered in Chapters 21 & 22. Non-hormonal medical alternatives are covered in Chapter 24.

Part VIII:
The Womenopause Challenge: Hot Stuff

- Practice the following breathing relaxation exercise three times a day for four weeks.
- Sit in a comfortable chair in a quiet place.
- Take off your shoes.
- Listen to Vivaldi or Chopin (or anything you find calm and relaxing).
- Light a vanilla scented candle (or similar).
- Place your hands across your abdomen.
- Breathe in allowing your belly to move outward with each breath.
- Count silently to five on each inhale and slowly exhale counting to seven.
- Let you shoulders relax down and breathe ten times.
- Now take your left index finger and press the side of your left nostril closed.
- Breathe five times through only your right nostril.
- Now switch and close your right nostril and breathe five times only through your left nostril.
- Breathe ten times through both sides of your nose filling your lungs and moving out your belly.
- Wiggle your toes on the floor and feel the ground.

• Release your shoulders down and breathe.

See how much calmer and clearer you become with only ten minutes of practice. No matter where you are, if you begin to experience a Hot Dread, imagine you are home in your practice chair, and do the breathing. Relaxation can be learned, just like learning to shoot a free-throw. The more you practice, the more likely you will make it during the pressure of a big game. The more you do the more you can do.

Chapter 10

Vagina Sahara

Part I:
Soooo, How's Your Vagina Doing Today?

Everybody knows: hot flashes mean menopause. Hot flashes get all the headlines, TV specials, and book covers. Nobody seems to know a dry vagina means menopause too. Apparently, it's a well-kept secret. Probably as many women experience menopausal vaginal dryness as menopausal hot flashes (75 percent); and get this, if left untreated, hot flashes usually go away with time, but vaginal dryness frequently gets worse.

It could be said that vaginal dryness flies under the radar, simply, because it's "down there". Women generally do not discuss their vagina with their spouse, family, friends, or even their doctor. Estimates suggest less than a quarter of women with clinically significant vaginal dryness ever seek help for their condition. Why is that? Why is there so little awareness about vaginal dryness? There are, perhaps, two reasons: sex organs are taboo subjects even in our enlightened modern culture (men do not talk about penis health in public either; at least, polite men do not talk about it), and vaginal health just has not caught the public's attention, yet. It will.

Although erectile dysfunction commercials are ubiquitous, no one has ever seen one for Vagina Sahara treatment. Vaginal health is an under-appreciated component for midlife women. Because the vagina is essential for sexual pleasure, a malfunction may initiate a domino effect leading to alterations in relation-ships in a complicated way that hot flashes may not.

Most doctors do not ask, "How's your vagina today?" Most women do not volunteer, "By the way, my vagina hurts." Who knows why, but it has to change. For many women; vaginal dryness, itching, and pain come on unexpectedly. Unlike hot flashes, which every woman knows to expect, vaginal symptoms sneak up slowly; and most women do not link the vaginal problem to their menopause. There are many possible causes for a dry, itchy, or painful vagina; all of them are treatable; and when we say all of them, we mean 100 percent. Every woman should have a regular vaginal health exam because vaginal problems have verifiable physical signs the doctor can identify and treat. Vaginal dryness and itching are sometimes a short hand way of describing a problem with the entire female vulvovaginal region, also referred to as the introitus. The vulvovagina encompasses the vagina, internal labia, external labia, clitoris, clitoral hood, and the exiting urethra. All of the structures participate in various changes referred to as vaginal dryness. More on that later.

Part II:
Atrophic Vaginitis: Is It Just Dry or Is It Something Else?

In perimenopause, menopause, and beyond (wWednesday through wSaturday), the leading cause for vaginal discomfort is vaginal atrophy due to changes of circulating estrogen. There are certainly other causes that will be discussed shortly; but for now, the concentration will be on the role of estrogen in vaginal health.

A woman's vagina is somewhat like a small soft purse. When it is empty, it collapses down, and the interior space is minimal. When the purse is packed with a billfold, cell phone, lipstick, compact, keys, brush, lotion, and other essential items; the little purse expands generously to accommodate all the stuff.

The thicker, softer, more flexible fabric with folds and pleats can expand greater than thin, stiff inelastic, material. The vagina is like that in a way. The vagina owes its soft expandability to the healthy tissue layers that comprise the lining. There is connective tissue scaffolding, supportive muscles, and a moist mucosa. Health of these tissues depends upon an adequate blood supply delivering nutrients, water, immune fighting equipment, and hormones. All of these structures and tissues are loaded with estrogen receptors. Beginning in perimenopause, estrogen changes can begin to adversely effect physical changes in the composition of the vagina.

Changes in estrogen, as seen in perimenopause and beyond, result in dramatic changes in the tissues in and around the vagina. Early changes involve, first, delayed lubrication during sexual arousal; and then later, diminished, sometimes zero, sexual lubrication because the small glands within the vaginal wall require estrogen stimulation to produce the slippery stuff. Subsequently, there is a measurable decrease in vaginal blood flow impacting the health of all of the tissues. Gradually, the surface of the vagina becomes thin; the color turns from pink to pale; the stretchy elasticity stiffens-up; the rugae or small folds go away; and the size of the vagina and vulva begin to shrink like a favorite wool sweater accidentally sent through the washer and dryer.

The interior of the vagina is not the only thing affected. Over time, low estrogen results in atrophy of the external structures such as the labia, clitoris, and the opening of the urethra. Coupled with vaginal drying, shortening, and narrowing; the small stiffened introitus becomes itchy, irritated, inflamed, and in no mood for fun. In fact, the labia and vulva, which surround the vagina with erogenous structures, may atrophy to the point of disappearing completely. When the opening of the urethra becomes atrophied, like the vagina due to changes in estrogen, symptoms such as increased frequency of urination, urgency of urination, and burning with urination can occur. All of those symptoms are similar to a common urinary tract infection; but treating non-infected, hormonally induced urinary tract atrophy with antibiotics will not work. Infections of the urinary tract are common during the *w*UpSide because there is hormonally induced atrophy of the lower urinary tract mucosa similar to what happens in the vagina when there is colonization by bacteria from the colon. That type of infection will be temporarily better with antibiotics.

As the mucosa of the vagina decreases its secretions, the micro-environment changes. The "good" bacteria, which normally inhabit the area, do not behave well because of the change of moisture and a rising pH (the normal vagina has an acidic pH of around 3.5 - 4.5). The good bacteria clump-up, creating "clue cells" (smelly cells), and cannot defend the vagina from bacteria who migrate in from the colon (yuck) and bladder. As might be expected, there is a marked difference between which animals live happily in the tropical Amazon Forest compared to those which live in the Sahara Desert. Certain bugs can take over in a dry high pH vaginal environment, leading to infections and more irritation. Ironically, women often try, on their own, to combat this problem by adding an additional problem such as applying baby oil, Vaseline, or douching. It seems sensible, but it does not work. Those three solutions tend to irritate the vagina and make the problem even worse.

When the vagina is dry, inflamed, thin, and infected; bruising (petechiae), tears of the mucosa, and bleeding may occur, even without trauma. Sex may become difficult, unpleasant, painful, or just completely out of the question. Dyspareunia means painful sex. Research indicates 75 percent of *w*UpSide women have vaginal atrophy, 40 percent have dyspareunia, and 15 percent have continuous vaginal pain. Dyspareunia may lead to no *"pareunia"*.

Part III:
Something Else

The symptoms that may emanate from the vagina are clues to the underlying cause. Sensations such as dryness, itching, irritation, burning, and pain are common. Discharges such as blood, slippery clear fluid, white thick mucus, white cheesy stuff, frothy grey bubbles, or even, purulent yellow pus, frequently can be noticed on light day pads or lingerie. Since the urinary bladder empties out through the urethra at the front edge of the vagina, sometimes the discomfort is predominately felt as a bladder problem rather than a vaginal problem. Dyspareunia, painful sex, often accompanies vaginal maladies.

For midlife women, the most common cause of vaginal problems is lack of estrogen. It is not the only cause, by any means. The following list covers many of the non-hormonal perpetrators of vulvovaginal discomfort. These conditions may be chronic and progressive and may lead to significant disabilities. They require expert evaluation and treatment:

- **Infection:** Some pelvic infections are sexually transmitted, and some are not. The common sexually transmitted ones are 1) herpes, which often causes a sharp burning pain with small blisters, 2) mycoplasma, which may be silent or cause cramping discomfort, spotting, or infertility, 3) chlamydia, which is often similar to mycoplasma, with more severe cramping, pain, and scarring; leading to greater infertility, 4) gonorrhea, which is similar to chlamydia, 5) trichomonas, which has a distinctive frothy smelly discharge causing vaginal irritation, and 6) HPV, which may cause warts, externally, or cervical dysplasia and cervical cancer, internally. The common non-sexually transmitted infections are thought to be opportunistic overgrowth of bugs that normally reside in the vagina or GI tract. These infections include: 1) candida, commonly called yeast, which results in an itchy white cheesy discharge and 2) bacterial vaginosis, which has a distinctive foul smelling discharge and irritation. Any of these infections may cause itching, burning, pain, dyspareunia, and bleeding or spotting.

- **Allergy**: Our environment is packed with pollens, spores, no-see-ums, and whatnots. Then, we bring into that mix, a boatload of chemicals and detergents. It's a wonder everyone doesn't suffer from some kind of allergy. Fortunately, the human body defends itself well from most external allergens. Vaginal allergies are like other allergies; they cause a puffy inflammation and itching. It may be next to impossible to track it down and identify the exact cause.

- **Irritants**: Unlike allergens, irritants are compounds we supply to ourselves and, unwittingly, cause an irritation. The vaginal symptoms are the same, burning and itching. It is relatively easy to start eliminating things applied to the vagina that are known common causes of irritation such as Vaseline, baby oil, dryer softener sheets, shower gels, and douching products. It's a good idea to modify or eliminate anything that might contact the vagina through sex, shower, bath, hot tub, toilet, or clothing.

- **Diseases**: Rarely, systemic diseases may manifest as vaginal dryness: Crohn's disease, diabetes, and auto-immune diseases such as Lupus or rheumatoid arthritis.

- **Vulvodynia:** Vulvodynia literally means pain in the vulva, which is the external part of the female genital tract. It commonly causes pain at specific locations on the labia without itching or pathological findings.

- **Lichen Sclerosis**: White areas of the vulva produce an itchy wrinkled patch that are so thin, they are vulnerable to tears and bleeding. The labia minora may adhere, atrophy, and then disappear. This disorder may reoccur after successful treatment.

- **Lichen Planus**: Rarely, the entire vulva may be afflicted with this condition, causing a stiff white thickening of the mucosa that progresses to vaginal adhesions and stenosis (narrowing or closing). The surface becomes fragile, tearing and bleeding easily.

- **Squamous Cell Hyperplasia**: Overgrowth of the top layer of skin cells produce an irritating white thickening that may be pre-cancerous.

- **Radiation and Chemotherapy**: Radiation of the pelvis for any type of cancer may damage the vulvovaginal area, causing scarring, pain, and bleeding. Some chemotherapy drugs are known to accelerate vaginal atrophy such as tamoxifen and raloxifene.

- **Pelvic Floor Muscle Dysfunction**: Several distinct bands of muscle support the floor of the pelvis and may become involved in spasm and pain.

Vivian C.

Vivian C. had made her first appointment to discuss menopause at the age of 84. Her main concern was her golf game. She had taken up the game twenty years ago when her husband retired. She was accustomed to playing a round of golf with him five days a week. Since his death two years ago, she had maintained her golf activity by organizing a senior-singles group at her country club. Her concern was she often felt like going home at the turn on nine, instead of finishing the usual eighteen holes. She felt like stopping half way, but she never actually did. She walked eighteen holes of golf five days a week; she babysat her toddler great grandson three afternoons a week; she remained active in her sorority and did about a hundred other things. She also mentioned having a sore back.

Vivian listed her height as being five feet four inches, and she was surprised to know she now measured to be only five feet one inch. On examination, Vivian had a severely atrophic vagina with areas of inflammation and several white patches on the mucosa. Although she had not volunteered any complaints about it, after questioning, she admitted her vagina has made it almost impossible to sleep because of the burning. She continued, that since her husband's death, she had had a progressive problem with sleep. She now leaves all the lights on and runs the TV continuously. She has had recurrent urinary track infections for years, but she thought it was normal. Her pelvic and rectal exams were otherwise normal. Vivian did not require a Pap test because she was over 70 and had never had an abnormal result. She was not sexually active. All of her blood tests were normal from her primary care doctor, two months ago. Vaginal cultures were done to check for yeast and bacterial vaginosis. A biopsy of the white lesion was sent to pathology. Colonoscopy, mammogram, and DEXA (bone density test) were recommended. A plain x-ray of her spine was ordered.

The *w*Score indicated the following:

1. Hot Flash Fever: ☺
2. Mood Matters: ☺
3. Sexercise: blank
4. Vagina Sahara: 9 W
5. Skinny on Skin: 8 W
6. Insomnia Queen: 7 W
7. Plumbing and Pain: 5 W

Some single, divorced, or widowed (or not), women find it impossible to discuss sex even with their gynecologist. Vivian chose to leave the items pertaining to sex blank. Her big-ticket items were vaginal burning, insomnia, wrinkles, back pain, and bladder infections.

Results of Vivian's tests confirmed the presence of significant osteoporosis with a DEXA T score of -3.0 and healed vertebral compression fractures at T 10, T 11, and T 12. The vaginal biopsy showed a benign condition, lichen sclerosis. All of the cultures were negative.

By all external accounts, Vivian was living a grand wUpSide life, and no one but her gynecologist knew of any problems. Vivian was determined to keep it that way. She had every intention of living past 100 and being the first centurion at her golf club to shoot a hole-in-one. Vivian sought information about how to improve her energy. After reassuring her that her activities already exceeded 98 percent of her peers, her specific problems were addressed.

Daytime energy is often best improved by improvement of night time sleep. Vivian had two fundamental aspects she could attack. First, she was given information about sleep hygiene: how to control the sleep environment to make it more conducive for sleep (Chapter 11: Insomnia Queen).

Next, a detailed treatment option list was assembled to compare the available treatments for Vivian's painful vagina. Vivian decided to begin treatment with Estring, a small flexible ring-shaped device placed in the vagina that releases topical wBodyIdentical estradiol, E2. The Estring treats only the vaginal mucosa and does not have enough absorption to affect the rest of her body. It is replaced every three months. Along with the topical vaginal estrogen, Vivian was going to try applying olive oil to her vagina twice a day. It was her idea to use only "extra virgin" olive oil.

The incidence of osteoporosis in the US is of epidemic proportions. Osteoporosis (the loss of bone strength) is preventable. Osteoporotic complications are a leading cause of mortality in women, resulting in 50,000 deaths per year. Vivian had already experienced an osteoporotic spine fracture, and she was lucky it did not lead to any serious incapacity. For some women, a fall leading to a fracture is the first big step toward loss of independence. Vivian was encouraged to make every effort to reverse her bone loss. She began taking 1,500 mg of calcium citrate a day along with 4000 IU of vitamin D a day. Vivian's T score of -3.0 indicated she should consider prescription therapy, and she decided to begin Boniva because she loved Sally Fields and thought she could remember to take a pill once a month. Her three-hour golfing walk also improves her chance of growing stronger bones.

Four weeks later Vivian reported improvement in her energy that she attributed to better sleep. She had turned off the TV and lights and doused her vagina with olive oil each night. She rated her vagina as 90 percent better since starting the Estring, and for the most part, she forgets it is even in her vagina. She had not missed taking her calcium or vitamin D except once when she had six grandchildren as overnight house guests. She took her second Boniva pill the morning of her follow-up appointment.

Vivian was evaluated monthly for six months until her vaginal mucosa recovered. She elected to stay on the estrogen ring for three months; then converted to intermittent Estrace cream 1 gm. once or twice a week. A year later her bone density improved to -2.6 (better but not yet great, Chapter 26). Her calcium, vitamin D, walking, and Boniva were doing their job. The most unexpected result, in her mind, was the remarkable reduction of bladder infections. As her vagina recovered, her infections went away.

Vivian stills plays golf and continues to chase that ace.

Part IV
The Fix

It is no secret. Estrogen is the predominant hormone for

sexual characteristics in women and is integral to the development and continued health of female specific organs: uterus, breasts, vulva, and vagina. Estrogen works inside certain tissue cells only if those cells have receptors for estrogen. All the female specific structures are loaded with estrogen receptors. It is surprising that vaginal atrophy goes largely unnoticed as an important consequence of estrogen loss during menopause. The vagina possesses estrogen receptors that stimulate normal growth and maintenance. When estrogen levels begin to change in perimenopause, the vagina loses one of its main supporters and starts to atrophy. In some women, it may be the first change she notices during wWednesday or wThursday but not realize that it is a sign of hormone change that accompanies perimenopause.

During the reproductive years, the vagina has a thick moist lining with abundant elasticity. The blood supply delivers ample nutrients and fluids, and when stimulated with the friction of sexual intercourse, the vessels dilate during arousal allowing the vagina to secrete additional lubrication. As estrogen declines in perimenopause and later during the wUpSide, many women experience changes in the structure of their vagina. The surface layer of the vagina becomes thin with reduction of blood flow. The supporting connective tissue cells produce less elastic fiber. The entire organ and surrounding tissues begin to shrink. In fact, seventy-five percent of women note new vaginal problems during perimenopause and the wUpSide.

Have you ever noticed that sometimes the most direct way to get somewhere fast actually requires you to turn around and go back to where you started? Treating vaginal irritation is like that. Step one: stop using everything you are using right now that makes contact with your vulvovaginal area. Specifically, stop using douches, baby oil, Vaseline, clothes dryer softener sheets, scented toilet paper, scented tampons, scented shower gels, powders, perfumes, and scented anything else. It may not be causing the problem, but it is better to be absolutely sure. Step two: wash yourself only with pure clean water or Cetaphil cleanser to help restore proper pH, pat dry, not rub, and double rinse your clothes in the washer.

Moisturizers for the vulvovaginal areas should be used daily for maintenance purposes, just like you would apply moisturizers to your face after bathing. All of the following work well, so choose the one you like best: RePhresh (word play indicating that the product can refresh the vagina and restore it to a proper pH), Replens, K-Y Moisturizer, olive oil, or generic mineral oil.

Lubricants are different from moisturizers. Lubricants are more useful to aid sexual intercourse. These should be applied before sex and do not need to be used everyday (unless, of course, you have sex everyday!). There is one exception, plain mineral oil works very well both as a lubricant and as a moisturizer. Try a combination of some of the following: Olive oil (okay, use the extra virgin), vitamin E oil, K-Y Lubricant, Lubrin, Silk E, Astroglide, Moist Again, and Intimate Options. For variety, you might try making your own by adding a drop of vanilla to your bottle of mineral oil.

Regular sexual activity stimulates renewed blood supply to the vulvovaginal area and indirectly leads to improved natural lubrication.

Sometimes the vulvovaginal area has other disorders. If an infection is present, antibiotic creams or pills are necessary. If white lesions are detected, they need to be biopsied and are usually treated successfully with Temovate cream, a prescription anti-inflammatory vaginal cream.

The treatments for chronic vaginal infections, vulvodynia, Lichen Planus, Lichen Sclerosis, squamous cell carcinoma, and pelvic muscle dysfunction are serious, complicated, and beyond the scope of this book. Seek expert professional advice for these conditions.

Part V:
The Cure

The logic behind treating estrogen depleted vulvovaginal atrophy by restoring estrogen is self-explanatory. Not some, but all of the menopausal vaginal symptoms caused by inadequate circulating estrogen can be reversed by taking estrogen, either systemically, locally, or both. This is how estrogen heals the vagina:

- Estrogen **restores the blood flow** to the vagina and vulvo-vaginal structures including the labia, clitoris, opening of the urethra, and the vulva. ·
- Estrogen **increases the secretion** of vaginal lubricants, both the maintenance type and the sexual arousal type.
- Estrogen **lowers the vaginal pH** back to normal, allowing the good bacteria to take back over and evict the bad ones.
- Estrogen stimulates **growth of vaginal mucosal cells**, making the vagina wall thicker.
- Estrogen increases the **production of elastic fibers** within the vaginal wall, making it flexible.
- Estrogen improves the **immune system** within the vaginal environment, reducing infections.
- Estrogen restores the health of the vagina and **stops tearing and bleeding**.
- Estrogen **re-grows** atrophied clitoris, labia, and vulva back to normal.
- Estrogen **relieves** the vaginal symptoms of burning, itching, and pain.
- Estrogen **restores the erogenous sensory nerves** in the vulvovaginal area allowing pleasurable sex and enhanced arousal.
- Estrogen works in less than **four weeks**.

Estrogen may be taken in any number of forms to get the

healing effect. wBodyIdentical estradiol may be used systemically through the skin by patch, gel, spray, ring, or cream, manufactured by pharmaceutical companies with brand names: Vivelle Dot, Divigel, Evamist, Femring, Estring, and Estrace Cream. wBodyIdentical vaginally applied is believed to have predominately only local effects with very little or no systemic effects (with the exception of Femring). Such products as Estring, Estrace Cream, and Vagifem tablet are put directly into the vagina. These products may be considered low risk for women with estrogen positive breast cancer who continue to suffer estrogen deficiency vaginal atrophy. Oral systemic and local vaginal MHT such as Premarin (conjugated estrogen) are also effective. Systemic estrogen and local vaginal estrogen used together can be even more effective. Chapters 21 & 22 detail the benefits and risks of the preferred hormone options.

Recent studies demonstrate that the effects of topical testosterone applied directly to the vulva and vagina are similar to the positive restoring effects of estrogen. More on testosterone later.

Part VI:
When the Rivers All Run Dry

Vagina Sahara can be a debilitating condition; it may cause both medical problems (bleeding and infection) and emotional distress (pain and disruption of normal sexual relations). Vagina Sahara is in need of a Menopause Makeover.

Of all the problems that come with menopause, vaginal dryness is the most persistent. It is 100 percent treatable. Frequently, women ask, "How long should I continue the treatments for Vagina Sahara?" To that, the response would be, "Treat it as long as the distressful symptoms last... and continue for as long as you want to feel fit, feminine, and fabulous."

Part VII:
The Womenopause Challenge: Scratch Resistant

1. This is going to be educational...get a mirror and look at your vagina.
2. The folds of skin going up and down along the outside of the vagina are the external labia.
3. The smaller folds of skin inside the external labia are the internal labia.
4. Near the top of the vulva is a very sensitive hump; the clitoris.
5. With your fingers, spread open your labia and look at the lining of the vagina.
6. The lining of the vagina should be moist and pink with a lot of small folds.
7. The urethra is a tiny hole exiting above your vagina and below the clitoris.
8. The rectum is a larger hole exiting behind your vagina. Okay, we're done with the mirror.
9. Even "normal" vaginas appreciate moisturizers, apply mineral oil twice a day like this:
   - Transfer six ounces of mineral oil into a wide-mouth travel container.
   - Add two drops of vanilla extract (or any essential oil that you like and does not cause any irritation).
   - Dip two fingers up to the second knuckle into the mineral oil mixture.
   - Gently rub the oiled fingers along your labia on both sides, up onto the clitoris, and then up inside the vagina.
   - It takes just about 15 seconds to become scratch resistant.

Chapter 11

Insomnia Queen

Part I:
Sleeping in the Kitchen

Like so many other things of our youth, sleep was automatic and effortless. We could play all day, eat whatever we wanted, and sleep like a log every night. The only interruption was being roused from a perfectly wonderful dream by our mother, claiming we had better get going, or we would be late for school. Remember those days and those glorious nights?

Well, those nights are not likely remembered because two minutes after our heads hit the pillow, the brain's sleep system turned on; and nine hours later, it turned off. Many perimenopausal and postmenopausal women experience a significant decline in their ability to obtain a decent night's sleep. Hormones play a big part in the sleep process. If a box of hot flashes is mixed with a cup of family stress, a teaspoon of spousal snoring, and a pinch of high BMI (overweight), it is a recipe for insomnia. Fortunately, as is true of most good cooking, with careful attention to the ingredients, sleep can be changed from a frozen dinner to a seven-course feast at a five-star restaurant. Like everything else in this world, nothing worthwhile is easy. Sleep patterns definitely can be rehabilitated, but it takes some planning and effort.

Insomnia describes a group of related problems that results in sleep that does not refresh. Difficulty going to sleep, difficulty staying asleep, waking during the night, and awaking early in the morning are typical complaints of insomniacs.

For menopausal women the universal question remains, "Is it menopause, or is it aging?"

Discussions about sleep generally fall into one of two camps:

1. sleep is a mystical and magical interlude between periods of hopeless awakening or
2. sleep is a progressive series of brain wave patterns that integrate memory and restorative functions.

The two views of sleep translate into two approaches people commonly take to solve sleep problems. First, one might take the poetic /philosophical route and plumb the depths of the enigma of sleep and conclude that it is fundamentally unknowable and beyond human control. Or second, one might consider insomnia strictly as a medical disease for which the only reasonable cure is a prescription. There is, however, a third route, which strikes a balance. The third or "middle way" emphasizes practical steps every insomniac can take to improve her sleep, even though sleep remains forever somewhat mysterious. A few sleep disorders require expert medical attention. Most sleep problems can be improved and even fixed by implementing the suggestions found in this chapter.

Part II:
A Brief Look into the Black Box We Call Sleep

A fun road-trip vacation is the result of a car, like sleep is a product of the brain. Even if we knew everything about how the car works, we still could not easily explain what "fun" means. So it is for sleep. Understanding everything about the neuronal structures which drive sleep (which we don't by a long shot) still leaves us grasping for how and why sleep is so important. For now, we have to accept that sleep is important on the order of magnitude as air and water.

The science of sleep has exploded in the past 25 years. Sleep study laboratories measure EEG (electrical brain waves), EKG (electrical heart waves), EOG (eye movements), EMG (muscle movements), respirations, blood oxygen concentration, body positions, and snoring.

Normal sleep has been divided into stages, depending upon the variations of these recordings:

- Awake: Although we take being awake as self-explanatory, it is better to describe it as a state in which a person is consciously aware of stimuli in the environment and responds to those stimuli. Brainwaves are fast and random (like our thought?) during wakefulness.

- Stage 1 (light sleep): Brainwaves slow down; the eyes rove around under the eyelids; tension in the muscles lightens up; and sounds fade out during the transition from awake to asleep.

- Stage 2 (continued light sleep): Brainwaves begin to show bursts of activity called spindles, and the body becomes less sensitive to the environment.

- Stage 3 (deep sleep): Brainwaves change to slow deep oscillations, and there is a deepening disconnection from environmental stimuli. The heart and lungs slow down.

- Stage 4 (deeper sleep): Brainwaves are slower and deeper; muscles become slightly more relaxed; blood pressure drops; heart rate declines; body temperature declines; and the body is maximally insensitive to the environment.

- REM Sleep: An hour and a half or so after going to sleep; the brain works its way down through the first four stages into REM stage sleep. The brainwaves have random fast "saw-toothed" shaped spikes, and during this time, the body is close to awakening. The muscles of the body in REM sleep are almost completely paralyzed while the muscle around the eyes contract wildly.

In normal sleep, a person progresses through the four stages and REM sleep, three or four times a night, before awakening after eight hours (don't you wish) of sleeping. Mundane dreaming occurs in deep sleep stages 3 and 4, and dreaming vivid dreams occurs in REM sleep. Scientific theories about the purpose of sleep, describe sleep's "restorative" function with the physical *body recovering* during stages 1 – 4 (referred to as Non-REM sleep), and the *brain becoming restored* during REM sleep.

What is most surprising is the incredible complex of activity in distinctive brain areas that must coordinate with each other to allow normal sleep to transition from one stage to the next. It is surprising that anyone gets the job done right.

The average adult requires eight hours of sleep a night for optimal performance – preferably as a continuous rather than broken stretch. The evidence is overwhelming; the evidence is clear: eight hours, not six hours, not four hours plus a nap, but eight continuous hours.

When we wake up (hopefully refreshed after our eight hours of sleep), we accumulate one hour of sleep debt for every two hours we are awake. After being awake for 16 hours we have to "pay back" half of that, eight hours, to the ZZZZZs accountant. Interestingly, we do not get sleepier and sleepier as the day progresses. This is because there is an alerting system superimposed on the sleep debt system that counteracts the accumulating sleep debt. The alerting system gets stronger as the day progresses with a little sag in the afternoon (about that time a siesta would be nice), a big surge in the evening, then a quick drop-off just in time for bed.

The alerting system is strongly influenced by exposure to light. Light entering the brain through the eyes directly influences the alerting and sleeping systems. It sets and maintains the day/night biorhythm which is called the circadian rhythm.

Part III:
Women, Insomnia, and the Five "P"s

There are five discrete times when women are vulnerable to

sleep disturbances related to changing hormones. The five "P" times of insomnia are:

- PMS
- Pregnancy
- Post-Partum
- Perimenopause
- Postmenopause

That just about sums up a woman's entire life! The simple strategies that are effective in straightening out insomnia during PMS are equally effective for the insomnia during perimenopause and all the other "P" times.

Estrogen receptors are located in virtually every region of the brain. It is no wonder that a complex function such as sleep that requires so many different brain systems to work together, can get thrown off when estrogen levels change so drastically from one day to the next during the reproductive years, and from one minute to the next in perimenopause. Sometimes it is difficult to separate run-of-the-mill sleeping problems from hormonal sleeping problems.

The clues most women find useful are the ones found in their calendar. If menstrual cycles are plotted on a calendar (Figure 2-3: wChart) along with troubled sleep nights, it is pretty easy to spot a common hormone induced sleep disorder. At the end of the menstrual cycle, just before the period, for wMonday and wTuesday women, progesterone becomes dominant and then withdraws along with estrogen (luteal phase). At this time, some women notice difficulty with sleep accompanied by pimples and a grouchy mood. Sleep is often fine the whole month except during PMS. Similarly, many women sleep well until they hit their forties in wWednesday and wThursday; then, out of the blue, sleep may become progressively difficult. Hot flashes and night sweats may throw-off sleep. During perimenopause, estrogen levels fluctuate wildly and may trigger sleep problems. It is worthwhile to interject briefly here; just as was seen with estrogen induced vaginal dryness in the previous chapter, the most effective treatment for hormone induced insomnia is Menopausal Hormone Therapy (MHT). Insomnia and mood swings of perimenopause can be effectively managed with cycle control pills (birth control pills) or with MHT, for instance, Evamist in conjunction with Prometrium (E+P) (Chapter 21). There are other factors that may impact the ability to get a good night's sleep.

Part IV:
Scared Sleepless

Everyone's sleep problem is unique, but there are some common insomnia scenarios that crop-up frequently and might prove helpful to know about.

Top Ten Other Sleep Troubles Seen in Perimenopause and Postmenopause:

1. **Neglect**: By far the most common reason people are tired all day is they neglect to consider how important sleep is to their health and well-being. It is extremely important.

2. **Situational Insomnia**: Brief periods of poor sleep (a few days to a few weeks) as the consequence of a specific problem, like a death in the family or stress at work, are common and, to a degree, normal.

3. **Protracted Situational Insomnia**: This is what sleep experts call psychophysiological insomnia. Usually, after a few weeks of poor sleep, these insomniacs start worrying about sleep itself, rather than the problem that caused them to have lousy sleep in the first place. There is a snowball effect: the worse they sleep, the more they worry about not sleeping, and the worse sleep becomes,

and so on.

4. **Out-Of-Sync Insomnia**: Keeping odd hours can throw-off the circadian (the daily natural brain and hormone) rhythm and seriously disturb sleep.

5. **Moody Insomnia**: Significant mood disorders, like depression, have a direct line to the sleep department, and they usually call each other at night. Marital discord is a special category of mood matters, which may effect sleep.

6. **Serious Health Disease Insomnia**: Many serious health problems: heart disease, COPD, diabetes, peripheral vascular disease, dementia, chronic pain, and obesity, alter aspects of sleep.

7. **Substance Use Insomnia**: Cigarette smoking (another reason), excessive alcohol consumption (more than three drinks), all of the bad illegal drugs, and some prescription medications interfere with normal sleep.

8. **Movement Insomnia**: Restless leg syndrome (RLS) and periodic limb movements disrupt sleep. They are more common than physicians used to think but much less common than the public thinks, due to the advertising for RLS treatments.

9. **Sleep Apnea Insomnia**: Obstructive sleep apnea is a dangerous condition. Restless sleep and daytime drowsiness coupled with snoring should be evaluated.

10. **A Million Other Insomnias**: OK, that is an exaggeration; there are only a hundred thousand other less common sleep disorders.

Some sleep problems require an evaluation by a sleep expert and a formal sleep study may be required to sort out everything. There is no risk in implementing the following strategies to improve sleep for perimenopausal and postmenopausal women.

Part VI:
Insomnia Queen De-throned

Normal sleep is dependent upon the proper quality and quantity of sleep. A night's sleep is considered "a good night's sleep" if it results in adequate alertness during desired waking hours. Poor sleep has known physical and mental consequences such as: hypertension, cardiac disease, depression, impaired thinking, pain, and increased injuries from accidents.

Seventeen Secrets for Successful Sleep:

1. Reserve eight hours for sleep.
2. Go to bed at the same time each night.
3. Wake up at the same time each morning.
4. Expose yourself to bright lights first thing in the morning.
5. Expose yourself to dim lights in the evenings.
6. Use bed for sleep and sex only.
7. Control room temperature and room darkness.
8. Take the TV and computers out of the bedroom.
9. Avoid daytime naps.
10. Avoid eating a heavy meal or alcohol just before bed.
11. Avoid nicotine all day and all night.
12. Avoid caffeinated drinks after 12 o'clock noon.
13. Exercise every day so that you are physically tired.
14. Practice a relaxation technique daily, like yoga.
15. Drink a glass of milk or chamomile tea at bedtime.
16. Take ibuprofen if not contraindicated.
17. Go to another room for a relaxing activity if unable to fall asleep within 30 minutes.

Part VIII:
Hormones, Hot Flashes, and Slumberfest

In Chapter 8, the sleep disturbance associated with hot flashes was detailed. It is not just hot flashes that wake women up from a sound sleep. Sleep studies have identified several interesting facts about menopause and insomnia. Poor sleep is more common in women than men, and 40 percent of perimenopausal and postmenopausal women have a documented sleep disturbance. Women are more likely to wake up during the chilling time of their night sweat rather than during the hot time. They may sleep through both, or be awakened before, during, or after their hot flashes, or during other parts of their sleep cycle.

It is now believed the architecture of normal sleep is disorganized when there are changes in estrogen whether or not it is causing hot flashes. Some aspects of the poor quality of sleep reported by menopausal women are not completely explained by current sleep study technology.

Many see relief of insomnia by estrogen as a happy side effect, but more research is pointing to the use of estrogen as a stand-alone treatment for perimenopausal and postmenopausal insomnia. wBodyIdentical 17beta-estradiol, when taken in the morning, restores sleep patterns independently from relieving hot flashes. Micronized progesterone taken by mouth at night has a relaxing effect and improves sleep quality. Non-micronized oral progestin (Provera, medroxyprogesterone acetate) and all topical progesterone creams do not improve sleep.

Many clinicians prescribe antidepressants for perimenopausal insomnia such as Prozac, Effexor, or Pristiq, and those drugs have some usefulness in that regard. However, when compared to estrogen therapy, antidepressants are less effective in treating perimenopausal and postmenopausal insomnia. As a little preview to the next chapter, it can also be argued that estrogen treats perimenopausal mood matters better and more safely than antidepressants do too. Antidepressants are a good choice for insomnia and mood matters for women diagnosed with estrogen-positive breast cancer for whom estrogen MHT is contraindicated.

Some may need to use sleeping pills after exhausting all of the simpler and safer remedies. Ambien, Lunesta, and Sonata have a place in the treatment of otherwise resistant insomnias. But 90 percent of the time, upgrading lifestyle choices such as careful application of sleep hygiene (17 Secrets), hormone therapy, and reversal of underlying health problems will work.

More research is needed; but at this point, if a healthy perimenopausal woman is treated proactively with cycle control pills or MHT, she will most likely avoid developing insomnia because she will never experience hot flashes, night sweats, sleep disturbance, mood swings, and all the rest. Prevention is better than treatment every time.

Allison K.

Allison was at the end of her rope, and the first thing she said was, "I could live with all this stuff if I could just get a little sleep." At age 45, she was overweight with a BMI of 33 and had never met a hamburger she didn't like. She and her husband, Mike, owned an ice cream shop and spent the winter months in their condo in Florida. They had returned from Florida early this year because Allison hoped her bed at home could help her sleep better. It didn't. She also complained of night sweats and occasional hot flashes. The *w*Score for Allison demonstrated a total score of 44 "W". Hot Flash Fever and Mood Matters were all significant problems, but the one she was desperate about was Insomnia Queen; that was a perfect 9 "W".

Allison reported she had always been the one to fall immediately to sleep "within 2 milli-seconds" of her head hitting the pillow. In fact, a pillow was not even necessary. She used to sleep anywhere she liked: couch, chair, or car. Now, she believes she has not had more than two hours of decent sleep for the past three months.

Healthy lifestyle choices were not Allison's forte, and considerable time was spent covering some of the important variables that may contribute to insomnia. Important information about

Real Food (Chapter 14), Vitamin-X Exercise (Chapter 16), and Mood Matters (Chapter 12) were explained to Allison, but she did not welcome the advice. Allison admitted she had "zero interest" in going on a diet or exercising, she just wanted sleeping pills.

It is common in our culture to look for a seemingly simple medical "cure" for what ails us. Sometimes healthcare providers lose interest in emphasizing lifestyle changes because almost no one values it. It takes a lot of time that could be spent taking care of more patients. Insurance companies do not value health maintenance either, and healthcare workers usually cannot get paid for teaching nutrition or exercise. In Allison's case, she had a multitude of personal health factors that were no doubt contributing to her insomnia.

Insomnia is common in perimenopause, and Allison determined that she was in wThursday (Figure 3-1). Her full figure and lack of exercise had at least as much to do with her poor sleep as her hormones. She was counseled to consider modifying as many variables as she could in order to resume better sleep.

Allison accepted the Womenopause Challenge. In addition to swearing off hamburgers for a month, she was determined to drop one BMI point in four weeks by eating Real Food and joining an exercise class.

She reviewed the Seventeen Secrets For Successful Sleep and identified several points where she could improve. Over the past ten years, she and her husband had used the bedroom for watching TV, and they usually fell asleep with it left on. Lately, since she could not fall asleep or stay asleep, Allison had been staying up all night watching classic movies with the bedroom lights on "for security". She made at least four snack runs to the kitchen each night to do "quality control work" on the ice cream that they made.

Allison had a lot of room for lifestyle improvements, and she took aim at the obvious ones.

After Allison agreed to work on controlling her sleep environment, there was a discussion about cycle control pills and MHT. Estrogen withdrawal during perimenopause may disturb sleep, and it is a confounding factor with women who have poor sleep habits in the first place. After a thorough discussion about the benefits and risks, Allison elected to start cycle control pills. Her main reason for this form of therapy was to reduce risk of pregnancy. She reasoned that once she started sleeping better, eating better, and exercising, her husband would not be able to control himself. "I'm likely to wake up trim, rested, and pregnant all at the same time!"

It all worked out, and she did not get pregnant. Four weeks later Allison was getting adequate sleep; she had lost two points on her BMI and gained some new friends at the aerobics class. She and her husband had actually used the bedroom for sleep AND SEX instead of TV viewing. Her hot flashes were gone, and she had stopped bringing home samples from the ice cream shop for "quality control testing".

Part IX:
The Womenopause Challenge: Sleep More/Worry Less

1. Write down a list of your top three most annoying problems. Now put those problems away because there is nothing more you can do about them tonight. Choose not to think about them until tomorrow when you are going to do something about fixing them.

2. Turn down the lights, take a warm bath or shower, and listen to some of your favorite music.

3. Lie flat on the floor with your arms at your side. Take three slow deep cleansing breaths. Now, contract EVERY muscle of your body and squeeze it all for five seconds then release. Go completely limp. Now take three more deep slow cleansing breaths and contract everything as

hard as you can for five seconds then let go. Let every-thing go. Lie calmly for a minute listening to your own breaths.

4. Try a drop of sandalwood or lavender essential oil on you pillow or sheets for a sleep-friendly aroma.

5. When you turn off the lights, choose to construct a pleasant dream and let your imagination take you to your favorite mountain top, beach or...

Chapter 12

Mood Matters

Part I:
Normal Is Over-Rated

Happy and sad are *not* two sides of the mood coin. Happy and sad are more like stripes of color on a beach ball with alternating red, yellow, green, white, and blue stripes. As the ball rolls around, there are times when it looks a little redder rather than blue. If "normal" has to be defined, then bouncing between periods of happy or sad is about as normal as it gets. In perimenopause and postmenopause, *w*Wednesday through *w*Friday, the ball just bounces to more extreme levels than usual: higher and lower. Many women express a vague sense of not feeling quite themselves. This change in mood is not exactly depression, although some women clearly are depressed. It is more of a pervasive unsettling than a deep blue. There is not really an accepted medical term to describe the most common mood disorder of perimenopause and beyond. We call it Womenopause *w*Worry. *w*Worry has an onset in perimenopause, a peak near menopause, and it mostly goes away during the *w*UpSide. Does that sequence sound familiar? The pattern of Hot Flash Fever, night sweats, Cold Crashes, Insomnia Queen, Meno-Fog, and *w*Worry all track together. Hummm... perhaps they are all related in some way. *w*Worry is almost universal in perimenopause, and frank depression may have an incidence as high as 20%.

When is a mood normal or abnormal? In fact, there is a family saying, "The only people who are 'normal' are the people you don't actually know well enough!" A persistent change in mood is a problem only when it interferes with a person's relationships and personal expectations. There is no standard; there is no absolute normal. If you have noticed your usual sunny disposition with your husband, kids, or co-workers has changed to a fretful-stressful-tension, then this chapter will bring some sense to the mystery.

Part II:
Defining Depression

How would you define a fine sunny day? Is it more like 72 degrees with a clear sky walking through the woods, 85 degrees with a soft breeze on the beach, 90 degrees with low humidity sipping a margarita, or 96 degrees with 80 percent humidity and no air movement stuck in traffic with no air conditioner? When is too much sun, too much heat, or too much humidity a problem? Of course, there is no exact cut-off. The same applies to depression. It's when the heat is of such intensity, you cannot get anything done, and your thoughts get messed-up because you just can't stand it any more. At some point along that continuum, it would be reasonable to go cool off somewhere. We can tolerate the heat for a while; just like, we can tolerate a mood problem for a while. If it lasts, then we need to do something about it.

Major depression can be correlated to major surgery. Major surgery is anything that happens to you or to someone you love, and minor surgery is what happens to everyone else. Major depression is a serious problem most people do not take seriously enough.

Womenopause *w*Worry is not major depression, although they share some of the same features. At any one time, about 3 to 6 percent of American women suffer from major depression (approximately twice the incidence seen in men).

The symptoms of major depression include both body and mind disturbances:

1. depressed mood

2. loss of interest or pleasure
3. weight loss or gain
4. psychomotor agitation or retardation
5. insomnia
6. low energy and fatigue
7. feelings of worthlessness or excessive guilt
8. diminished ability to think or concentrate or complete tasks
9. thoughts of death, suicide, or a suicide attempt

The causes and risk factors for depression are complex:

1. hormonal
2. genetic
3. sleep disturbance
4. personality make-up including passive, dependent, or learned helplessness
5. social stressors such as poverty, domestic violence, abuse, caretaking burdens, gender discrimination, and divorce
6. previous history of mental illness
7. certain medications

Major Depressive Disorder, sometimes referred to as clinical depression, appears to be driven by changes in certain neurotransmitters in the brain; serotonin, norepinephrine, and dopamine. A psychiatrist should evaluate a life-threatening major depression.

During the time period of perimenopause the incidence of depression may be 14 times higher than it is during premenopause. The reasons for that include:

- Hormone flux
- Hot flashes
- Insomnia

- Stressful life events
- Changes in lifestyles
- Body image (yours and his)
- Onset of chronic diseases (diabetes, hypertension, COPD, arthritis)

Estrogen may be an effective antidepressant in perimenopausal depression 60% to 80% of the time. Of particular interest is the recent data indicating hormone therapy during perimenopause may prevent the onset of depressive symptoms. This is important because depression by itself conveys an increased risk for several illnesses relevant to women at midlife including: osteoporosis, metabolic syndrome, and cardiovascular disease (the #1 killer of women).

Estrogen initiation later in postmenopause has not been found to be as effective as it is in early perimenopause for the treatment of depression. Evidence that treating depression earlier rather than later has significant benefits because depressed postmenopausal women have a 50% higher risk of death from cardiovascular disease than non-depressed women.

Part III:
Womenopause *w*Worry

Upwards of 75 percent of *w*Thursday and *w*Friday women have menopausal mood matters affecting their daily life. Their previous normal swings between happy and sad may morph into *w*Worry: "not quite feeling myself", anxiousness, sadness, tearfulness; and for almost no reason they feel tired, tired, and more tired. Many women notice changes in their mood before they have menstrual irregularities, insomnia, and hot flashes. Mood matters may be the first sign of a hormone shift. There is a cluster of associated findings that arise around and contribute to the genesis of *w*Worry:

- A family history of depression

- Personal history of post-partum blues
- Rising BMI (body mass index)
- PMS (pre-menstrual syndrome)
- Change in marital/relationship status
- Poor health (diabetes, hypertension, heart disease)
- Smoking (yet another reason to quit)
- History of physical or sexual abuse
- No children
- Previous need for anti-depressants
- Poor social and spiritual support

Womenopause wWorry has an onset with fluctuating hormone levels, beginning on wWednesday in early perimenopause. It is not so much a matter of too high or too low levels of a certain hormone; it is more a matter of erratic ups and downs of hormones that used to cycle more smoothly. For that reason, measuring hormone levels does not help identify who has what degree of wWorry. The hormone turbulence peaks at menopause, the final menstrual period, at about the same time wWorry is maximal. Just as we have seen with hot flashes, night sweats, and insomnia, wWorry gets better with time after menopause, but that is not the end of the story.

Part IV:
No Worries

Womenopause wWorry can be restrained with simple self-directed strategies that pose little to no risk or expense. Yeah. The first step is to recognize that our body and mind are united. How our body feels affects our mood, and our mood effects how our body works. Proper nutrition (Chapter 14: Real Food) and exercise (Chapter 16: Vitamin-X Exercise) are an integral part of feeling well. Daily vigorous exercise produces natural substances in our brains that takes away some of the wWorries. Another step is to recognize that we have control of our own thoughts.

In fact, there is precious little in this world a person does control. We do not control the weather, our cranky neighbor, or the stock market. We control what we physically do, what goes into our mouth, and the thoughts we choose to think. We can choose to think better thoughts (or not). Thoughts are not beamed into our skulls from a transmitter in outer space, and thoughts are not implanted into our brain by our spouse. Our thoughts are absolutely our own.

Consider the following **cognitive example**:

Imagine two people in a car stopped at a railroad crossing. There is a giant train coming down the track.

One person in the car says, "Shoot, we are going to be delayed by that lousy train."

The other person says, "Whoa, that's a really cool train."

Both of them are experiencing the exact same moment in time and space. One of them is viewing the train as a negative event, and the other is viewing it as a positive or neutral event. It is their *choice*. The train is just doing what a train does, going down the track. It is not *for* them or *against* them. If a person assigns a negative feeling to that train, it does not affect the train one bit. A negative feeling, however, does affect the person who thinks it, by turning on the flight or fight response in their autonomic nervous system, revving up the pulse, elevating the blood pressure, and cranking up the anxiety and pain, and to what purpose? The train is going down the track, and even if you stepped in front of it, nothing would change. For the most part, we do not control things or persons outside of our self; just as, they do not control our thoughts. When we think it through, everything outside of us is neutral until we assign a value to it. We can *choose* to see things as neutral, negative or positive. That is our choice. Choosing a positive thought turns on the relaxation response in our nervous system, which in turn, coaxes our body into peace.

Consider this **behavioral example:**

Stand bare-footed in a quiet room. Gaze at a spot on the floor 10 feet in front of you. Feel your toes touching the floor. Slowly bend your right knee, and stand just on your left leg. Raise your right foot, until it is resting on the inside of your left knee. Stand on one leg still gazing at the floor at one spot. Now raise both arms and fold your hands across your belly. Breathe. Move your belly in and out with each slow breath; feel your breath in your nose. Stand strong on your one leg. Wiggle your toes and feel the floor. Move the air into your lungs through your nose. Breathe. Feel the air sliding smoothly through your nose, down your throat, into your lungs, and pushing your belly out. Drop your shoulders a little with each breath. Extend through your legs and through your spine. Keep your focus on the floor and breathe. Take twenty slow breaths and change legs.

The preceding is an example of a relaxation technique. There are an unlimited variety of possibilities to try. For most women, it is impossible to hold that pose, and breathe those breaths without first abandoning all the mental clutter. The balancing and deep breathing occupies so much consciousness; it frees us from wWorry. Try it.

wWorry frequently becomes apparent when women feel out of control or overwhelmed with tasks that used to be routine. Serious consideration of priorities can pare down an overwhelming number of perceived obligations to a manageable few. Superwoman is a comic-book character; she is not real. For many women, learning to relax is harder than learning to play the violin. Daily exercise has many positive mood effects, and exercising through yoga combines both the physical part and the relaxation part. There may not be a better way to invest in your health and well-being than an hour of yoga each day. Reading reputable self-help books can be useful. There is a reason why writers like Dr. Phil and Dr. Laura are respected; they give good advice.

Midlife may be an uphill challenge. If we coast in our relationships, then we are most certainly going to slide downhill, not climb up to a better view. There is nothing more important to a person than an intimate relationship with another person. Relationships with your spouse, children, and friends are worth the effort. Nothing improves our own mood faster than helping someone else's. Sending a card, stopping by to say hi, burying a hatchet, and arranging social gatherings are all positive acts of kindness. Thoughts of kindness are not as effective as acts of kindness!

Part V:
Hormones and wWorry

By now, it probably comes as no surprise to hear wWorry is largely an estrogen driven problem. Bear in mind, wWorry is distinctly different from major depressive disorder. Womenopause wWorry has the same health implications as hot flashes, cold crashes, night sweats, vaginal dryness, and insomnia; they won't kill you; you have reasonable time to sort through your options. The previous section of this chapter sketched out the no-brainer, self-help tricks many women find useful for managing wWorry. If the mood matter persists and interferes with your otherwise perfect life, then consider the following information.

In perimenopause, wWednesday and wThursday, estrogen release from the ovaries becomes progressively unpredictable. This results in irregularities of the menstrual cycle with short or long periods and cycles. As many women notice edginess in their mood with PMS, that same kind of disturbance can progress and persist. What starts out as a tolerable and predictable hormonal mood fluctuation, may become an unpredictable intolerable persistent problem. For women who are still having periods, cycle control pills (often referred to as birth control pills) or a birth control hormone vaginal ring can smooth out the estrogen fluctuations and return the mood back to normal.

In perimenopause and the *w*UpSide, menopause hormone therapy (MHT) can hasten the improvement of *w*Worry. Transdermal estrogen may work better than oral estrogen by producing a more consistent blood level of estrogen (Chapter 22 and 23). For women who have had a hysterectomy, estrogen alone is sufficient. Oral non-micronized progestin tends to worsen the mood, but micronized progesterone does not. If the uterus has been removed there would be no reason to take progesterone.

Although there is no accepted standard measurement for menopausal mood matters, some researchers have used screening tests for depression to evaluate the mental health of postmenopausal women. What they found was no surprise. Women aged 50 to 59 who were on MHT scored consistently better on depression tests than matched women who were not receiving MHT. Another important study looked at *w*UpSide women over age 60, *w*Saturday. Women tended to have a gradually higher incidence of depression with age except for those women who continued on MHT. Menopause hormone therapy reverses *w*Worry and helps prevent the development of depression in women who stay on it.

Melinda M.

Melinda M. could be featured in an Oil of Olay commercial. At age 53 she appeared to be a "transposed dyslexic" age 35. She was trim (BMI of 22), fit (yoga four times a week), and successful (hospital manager). Melinda reached menopause 18 months ago and because her hot flashes were manageable with wardrobe modifications, she elected not to take menopausal hormone therapy. She was completely healthy, physically. At her annual appointment she found it difficult to bring up the problem that bothered her most. With some reluctance, she said, "I think I am losing my mind."

Looking back on it, she felt the problem had been percolating for a couple of years, but lately it had transformed into a roaring geyser of grief. She said she was "drowning in worry". She could make no sense of it, whatsoever. She had never been depressed, and she did not think the current problem was depression either. She noticed she was constantly worried about everything, and most distressingly, she was on the verge of tears all the time. She thought she had become forgetful and impatient, particularly with the employees working under her direction. In a meeting at work yesterday, she could not remember the name of her new boss, and she became so distressed she had to leave the room right in the middle of an important discussion because she was on the verge of tears. She thought she was making her family "walk on egg shells" around her, and at work she had to put up a " big disguise to hide her secret". All of it was wearing her out.

Melinda's physical exam and routine annual tests were normal. Her wScore was impressive with 21 "W" in the Mood Matters box (Figure 1-2) and a total score of only 27. She reported 3 "W" for vaginal dryness. She took a Carroll Rating Scale to measure depression, and the score was 9 suggesting possible mild depressive symptoms but certainly not a major concern. Melinda was tested with a simple memory test and passed with 100 percent accuracy. She was sleeping well; she had not changed weight; and she maintained all her usual duties and recreational activities. She just did not feel herself and had "worries for little or no reason".

The mood matters of menopause are under-appreciated. It is not dementia, it is not depression, and it is not made-up. wWorry defines a condition very frequently seen in perimenopause and postmenopause. It is more disconcerting than dangerous. It is presumably driven by estrogen withdrawal, and is therefore, more common in perimenopausal *w*Thursday. It is not uncommon after menopause, as is Melinda's case.

Although not much of an issue in Melinda's situation, most women can greatly improve their mental health by taking optimal care of their physical health. Thirty minutes of exercise daily is superior to Prozac, and maintaining a BMI under 29 helps mood disorders better than counseling.

Melinda was reassured her worries were not uncommon, and there were treatment options for her to consider. She could get a psychiatric consultation to rule out serious problems. To that she recoiled, "No way, I'm not crazy, and I know it's not really a serious mental illness, and I wish now I hadn't mentioned it." She was advised referral for psychiatric evaluation was not intended to imply that she was crazy. It was meant to mean her problem was taken seriously, and every means of investigation and treatment should be considered. Standard antidepressants may also help the problem, and one such as Pristiq (desvenlafaxine) an SNRI, would be a possibility. If she wanted to consider a treatment that would help both her mood and her vaginal dryness, menopausal hormone therapy (MHT) should be considered. Melinda was not interested in antidepressants because she had never been depressed, and she felt the problem was due completely to menopause and her hormonal change.

Melinda expressed an interest in MHT and was given extensive information about benefits, risks, and side effects (Chapters 21 and 22). Because Melinda was healthy and less than five years from menopause, MHT posed few risks and many benefits. She began therapy with transdermal *w*BodyIdentical 17beta-estradiol (Divigel 0.5 g applied to the skin of her thighs each morning) paired with oral progesterone (Prometrium 100 mg) nightly. She was coached on deep breathing relaxation exercises and encouraged to practice them four times a day plus every time she felt things were getting out of hand.

Four weeks later she was improved but not quite where she wanted to be. She expressed confidence that she was "returning to her usual self". Her wScore improved from 27 to 15, and she had complete elimination of vaginal dryness. She had had a few ups and downs with her worries, and they were tamed somewhat. She found it difficult to do the breathing exercises when she was most distressed. Melinda accepted the option to go up on the dose of Divigel estrogen to 1.0 g daily (rather than add a low dose antidepressant), keeping Prometrium the same.

By the time of the next appointment Melinda had been on MHT for two months. She reported significant improvement in all the menopausal mood matters and was surprised to note that her spider veins on her thighs had disappeared. Her wScore was now 5; her Carroll Rating Scale was 2; and she remarked that her family had, in jest, given her a welcome home party.

Part VI:
Uplifting News About Antidepressants

When hormone therapy is not advisable or a woman simply does not want to take hormones, standard antidepressants are frequently used to treat wWorry. Antidepressants are indicated for major depressive disorders and have a long clinical experience of effectiveness for menopausal mood matters as well. Both estrogen and antidepressants can be used effectively for menopausal mood matters. Both can potentiate the other and may reduce the dosage needed for each. MHT is not indicated as a primary treatment for major depression.

Because wWorry resembles some aspects of depression, antidepressants are effective treatments. Modern antidepressants work by:

1. Raising the neurotransmitter serotonin (SSRI's like Prozac, Paxil, Lexapro, and Zoloft)
2. Raising both serotonin and norepinephrine (SNRI's like

Effexor, Cymbalta, and Pristiq)
3. Raising dopamine and norepinephrine (DNRI like Wellbutrin)

These neurotransmitters are distributed in many regions of the brain and are involved in the processing of diverse functions, not just mood. Modern antidepressants are highly effective in treating depression and have a good safety profile. When antidepressants are combined with professional counseling, upwards of 80 percent improvement in major depression is seen in four months. Antidepressants are an effective alternate therapy for wWorry and hot flashes in women for whom hormone therapy is contraindicated. Most women who take wBodyIdentical Hormone Therapy for wWorry have mood matters well in hand in less than four weeks.

Part VII:
The Womenopause Challenge: Mood Mending

1. Go for a walk, go for a bike ride, go for a swim, go do something fun and physical, for 30 minutes. Sweat that wWorry right out of your pores.
2. Find a peaceful place and practice the one-legged breathing exercise for 15 minutes.
3. There is someone out there (you know who it is) who needs your forgiveness. Send her a card, give her a call, or go stop by to say hello.
4. Since you were created by a loving creator, don't hold back; there's beauty in the making; find all the love that's meant for you.

Chapter 13

Testing, Testing, One—Two—Three, Testing

Part I:
Doctors Love Tests

Doctors love getting tests on their patients. The absoluteness of an objective test result can be so comforting to them. Sometimes the doctor's interest in tests diverts her attention away from the thing that matters most, the person with a problem for whom the test is being done. For the healthcare provider, there is really no downside to ordering a zillion tests. And besides, the doctor does not have to pay for them. That being said, let's get on with the tests!

The testing discussed in this chapter are the medical tests that directly pertain to the usual care directed toward perimenopause, menopause, and wUpSide women. It is beyond the scope of this chapter to discuss every conceivable medical test for all health problems. There will be no discussion about who should get an EKG or chest x-ray, but that does not mean they are not important. They are just not important to the management of menopause.

Part II:
The Cavalcade of Tests

Part III and IV of this chapter will deal directly with hormone testing specific for menopause. The following list covers the more general tests women should undertake for the evaluation of their menopause health.

- **Self-Breast Exam**: All women are encouraged to perform a systematic self-breast exam every month, just after their

145

period ends. Women may detect a suspicious lump by knowing what their breasts usually feel like.

- **Clinical Breast Exam**: All women should have a breast exam by a competent medical practitioner every year as part of their annual exam.
- **Mammogram**: All women should have yearly mammograms after age 35, or younger if certain risk factors are present (Chapter 27: Breast Cancer Prevention).
- **Pap Test**: All sexually active women should have a Pap test every year. Some experts disagree, but there are numerous reports of women whose Pap test changes from normal to cancer in one year. It makes sense to leave nothing to chance.
- **Vaginal and cervical cultures for STIs** (sexually transmitted infections): All sexually active women should obtain annual cultures if multiple sexual partners are, or could be, involved.
- **Pelvic exam**: All women should have a complete examination of the vagina, cervix, uterus, and pelvis done annually.
- **DEXA**: All women should undergo a test for osteoporosis at menopause and every one, two, or three years after that depending upon the results and risk factors (Chapter 26: Boning Up).
- **Stool occult blood test**: All perimenopause and wUpSide women should have a rectal exam and, starting at age 50, a test for invisible blood in their stool every year as part of their pelvic exam. It is a simple screen for cancer of the colon, the second most common cancer found in women (the first is lung cancer, another reason to quit smoking).
- **Colonoscopy**: All women should undergo a screening colonoscopy by a Board Certified Gastroenterologist at age 50 and at intervals thereafter, determined by the GI doctor.
- **Cholesterol panel**: All adult women should have their

lipids checked at intervals depending upon their lifestyle and family history.

- **Blood pressure**: All women should have their blood pressure checked with every healthcare appointment or at least once a year.
- **Visual acuity**: All women should have an eye exam at a minimum of every three years.
- **Dental exam**: All women should have a dental exam every six months.
- **Blood sugar**: All women should have a test for diabetes, a fasting blood sugar level, every three years.
- **Thyroid blood test**: All women should have their thyroid function checked every three years.
- **Weight**: All women should be weighed every year. It is hard to think of this as a medical test, but weight has enormous health implication.
- **Vitamin D blood test**: All women should get their 25(OH)D blood level checked annually.

Part III:
Salivary Hormone Tests

Simply put, hormone levels in saliva have no clinical value. To say it another way, salivary hormone testing is useless. The amount of hormones in saliva is not representative of the blood level or any known medical condition. In spite of what Suzanne Somers says, and yes, in spite of what even Oprah seems to say, salivary hormone testing is simply a waste of money.

There are certainly a vocal few who are proponents of hormone testing of saliva, but The Mayo Clinic, The University of Chicago, NYU, Stanford University, The Cleveland Clinic, The University of Alabama, and any other certified hospital clinical laboratory are *not* among them. Not the hospital clinical lab in your hometown, not the one from across the river, none of them test saliva for hormones. How could all of them have missed something so important? They didn't.

Saliva is tested for hormones by certain pharmacies that compound replacement hormones that only they can make. Do you see the problem? There is a built-in conflict of interest. Some compounding pharmacies want to sell you the test in order for them to sell you the treatment. Women would do well to consult a NAMS Certified Menopause Practitioner before agreeing to undergo salivary hormone testing. The tests are useless, expensive, and may possibly lead to unwarranted and unproven treatment.

Part IV:
Blood Hormone Tests

In contrast to saliva, there are legitimate reasons why blood levels of reproductive hormones may need to be checked. However, unlike the thyroid gland that releases a slow steady amount of thyroid hormone, the ovaries release pulsating, variable amounts of estrogen. The amount of estrogen in the blood stream is highly variable from woman to woman and varies within a single woman depending on the time of day, her time of the month (Figure 2-1), her place on the wTimeLine (Figure 3-1), her emotional state, her food and wine, her smoking habits, her BMI, and probably a dozen other variables we have not yet identified. The estradiol level may vary from as low as 10 to as high as 800 pg/ml in the same woman depending on the time of day and the day of the month.

A perimenopausal wThursday woman with Hot Dreads, Cold Crashes, Insomnia Queen, Vagina Sahara, and Mood Matters, may sensibly inquire about "getting her hormones checked". It is reasonable to expect her hormones are behind the changes she is experiencing. However, performing a blood test to check her estrogen level may not add anything to her medical care, only to her medical bill. Her symptoms clearly demonstrate her estrogen blood levels are all over the place. For a woman experiencing those symptoms, the estrogen level in the blood may vary as much as 300 percent up or down during a single day, even moment-by-moment (Figure 2-1). If her blood sample were to be taken when the estrogen was at a peak, the conclusion might be that her estrogen level was too high. If her blood sample were to be taken when the estrogen was at the low point, then the conclusion might be the opposite; her estrogen is too low. In fact, her problem is *erratic fluctuations* of estrogen, and there is no way a blood sample can capture that. Clearly it is not related to what ends up in a drop of saliva either. Usually, a woman's *symptoms* are the best measure of her hormones and blood tests are mostly unnecessary.

There are several exceptions to the preceding comments. If a woman stops having menstrual periods altogether, amenorrhea, before the time of natural menopause (age 40 -55) or never starts having regular periods, then a full reproductive endocrine workup would be indicated.

If there are some confusing circumstances surrounding menopause such as a woman who was believed to be in the *w*UpSide resumes bleeding, then an FSH level might help clarify the situation. Recall that FSH released from the pituitary gland stimulates the ovaries to release estrogen and progesterone. As the ovaries age, erratic amounts of estrogen gets released, and FSH tries harder and harder to stimulate it. Through perimenopause the FSH levels in the blood begin to go up slowly. A trend of rising FSH is present in perimenopause, and a permanent sky-high elevation of FSH is seen in postmenopause when estrogen production from the ovaries all but ceases. If the FSH level is greater than 30mIU/mL on two or three separate blood samples, then most probably she's had her final menstrual period. Women must keep in mind that a high FSH level does not guarantee that menopause has permanently occurred; and therefore, fertility may still be possible. FSH peaks midcycle in *w*Sunday through *w*Thursday women during the normal menstrual cycle each month (Figure2-1). The blood level obtained during that peak could be misleading in diagnosing menopause.

Testosterone blood levels in women may need to be determined if there are symptoms of androgen excess such as unwanted hair growth, acne, or deepening of the voice. Some women require testosterone therapy and use a prescription testosterone (off-label only in the US) and may need to have their levels checked when starting therapy, more on that subject in Chapter 17: Sexercise.

Another time that hormone blood levels may need to be checked is when standard Menopausal Hormone Therapies (MHT) fail to resolve the menopausal problem even after several dosage and product adjustments.

The majority of women reaching menopause, suffering from the usual suspects: hot flashes, night sweats, insomnia, dry vagina, and mood swings, needs no expensive hormone blood tests to confirm what the problem is. If a car is driven for days and days then sputters to a stop, there is little to be gained by taking apart the gas tank in order to look inside to see how much gas is there. It is simply not enough to make the car go.

There is zero medical literature supporting the notion women should get their hormones tested while they are young to determine what "kind of woman" they are hormonally or to determine what hormones they will eventually need. She would be a different "kind of woman" each time of the day or month she was checked. According to unsupported theories, this early test factors into what hormones they should take after menopause; it doesn't. There remains no known medical reason for testing progesterone blood levels.

Theressa W.

Theressa was an attractive interior designer at age 48, who owned and managed a large office design company. She had recently moved her residence away from downtown Chicago where she had lived near her work for the past 20 years. At her inaugural gynecology office visit "in the outback", she rather impatiently inquired about needing to make arrangements to have her salivary hormones tested to find out, "what kind of woman I am". Theressa was a well-informed medical consumer and immediately began to have doubts about her new doctor because there was not a single copy of any of Suzanne Somers' books in the waiting room.

Twice divorced, Theressa described herself as "more than a little OC" (obsessive compulsive), and she apologized for being impatient (even before she had actually been impatient). For the past two years she had been taking increasing doses of compounded hormones prescribed by her former doctor based upon frequent salivary hormone tests. She believed the tests had been inaccurate because she "felt terrible all the time, and my temper is constantly on the verge of eruption". Her periods were gone, but the hot flashes and drenched nightgowns were worse. Frequent "vaginal infections" made sexual intercourse "prohibitive".

With some difficulty, the ingredients of her custom compounded hormones were obtained by phone with her pharmacy. Although they would not release the exact recipe because of "proprietary" concerns, she was taking a topically applied cream containing 80 percent estriol, E3 (the low activity estrogen of pregnancy which has never been tested in women for safety or effectiveness), 10 percent estrone, E1 (the low activity estrogen of postmenopause), and 10 percent estradiol, E2 (the normal potent estrogen of reproductive years) along with progesterone and testosterone. (Figure 9-3)

Theressa insisted new salivary tests be done so that an adjustment in the hormone dose would, "stop all this madness". She was rather desperate and intentionally dramatic.

Because of several popular books and TV personality endorsements, many women have come to believe menopausal hormones should be tested in their saliva, thinking personalized hormone therapy can be devised to "correct" their imbalance. In fact, there is not a single recognized medical society promoting saliva testing for hormones, certainly not the most influential scientific societies: The North American Menopause Society (NAMS), American College of Obstetrics and Gynecology (ACOG), and The Endocrine Society (ES). No licensed clinical laboratory performs routine saliva hormone tests. Interestingly, only pharmacies that compound hormones test saliva for hormones. Hummm.

Theressa underwent a full medical history and physical exam. She had quit smoking ten years ago and had a tubal ligation 15 years ago. She had no children but was very close with her five nieces and nephews, who were the five main reasons she had moved. Her BMI was 23; her blood pressure was high at 140/88; and her hemoglobin was 13 g. Her wScore was 34 W. She reported decent food habits and regular exercise at an upscale health club downtown. She had neither a mammogram nor a Pap test for over 3 years.

Those tests were performed along with a measurement of FSH (the brain hormone that tells the ovary to make estrogen and progesterone), TSH (an indicator of thyroid function) and cholesterol. Her vagina was atrophic, pale, and dry. Routine cultures were taken. Theressa was not interested in taking on any more projects and politely declined participation in the Womenopause Challenge. She was advised to stop her present compounded hormones for two weeks before getting her blood tests just before her next scheduled appointment.

Two weeks later Theressa returned for her first follow up medical visit. Her blood pressure remained elevated at 146/86 and her total cholesterol was on the high side, but in the normal range, 188. She was referred to an internist for evaluation.

Since stopping her hormones she did not notice anything different about her symptoms except she was "possibly a little more relaxed and oh by the way, I had a menstrual period last week for the first time in two years". Her blood test showed an FSH of 10 indicating that Theressa was perimenopausal, wThursday. Her hot flashes, night sweats, and mood swings may all be related to ovarian changes and erratic estrogen levels. She was advised that her compounded hormones were not usual medical care. The topical progesterone was particularly troublesome because topical progesterone is not well absorbed through the skin and may not adequately protect the uterus from the estrogen she was receiving. She was further advised that treating her symptoms solely with medication was going to have limited long term benefits if she did not combine it with lifestyle improvements.

She said she "would think it over". All of her vaginal cultures were negative, and she was advised that Vagina Sahara was probably the culprit of her "infections". A pipelle was performed for her irregular bleeding which proved to show no abnormal cells.

Theressa was given the option of treating her perimenopausal symptoms with either cycle control pills or MHT. Both would be expected to have similar effectiveness in relieving her most troublesome symptoms. She elected to begin daily therapy with Yaz, a cycle control pill. Four weeks later, Theressa reported mixed results. Her hot flashes and night sweats were much improved, but she felt her mood and insomnia and sexual desire were the same or worse. A decision was made to go to "plan #26", MHT. She was switched from Yaz to a combination of trans-dermal 17beta-estradiol wBodyIdentical estrogen (Vivelle Dot 0.1mg) with oral wBodyIdentical progesterone (Prometrium 100 mg) (Chapter 22). Four weeks later everything had improved, except she had more frequent hot flashes than she had while taking the Yaz but still much better than they had been on the compounded hormones. Her Vivelle Dot was increased to 0.125 mg (one patch at .1 mg plus one patch at .025 mg).

Finally, "after three years of trying with compounded hormones, it only took two months of *regular* hormones to straighten me out". Theressa's *w*Score improved from 34 "W" to 8 "W". Everyone at work believed there must be a new significant other in the picture because she acted so much happier. She reported zero hot flashes, excellent sleep, and just felt better all around. Her vaginal health was improved, and she considered dating again for the first time in two years. Theressa came to the conclusion that even in the "out back", there is a possibility of improving her health and well-being. She decided to look into the Womenopause Challenge to see if she agreed with anything else.

Part V:
The Womenopause Challenge: Test Check

1. If you have not had your mammogram this year, please make arrangements.
2. If you are menopausal, please make arrangements for a bone density test.
3. If you have not had a Pap test this year, make an appointment.
4. If you are over age 50, please make arrangements to have a colonoscopy.
5. If you are having Hot Dreads, get your saliva tested (JUST KIDDING).
6. Please make an appointment with your eye doctor and dentist.

Chapter 14

Real Food: Fake Food

Part I:
Putting Food Back Into The Diet

It is tempting to present a breakthrough nutrition plan that would guarantee 20 pounds of weight loss in just four weeks. By following a few previously unknown quasi-scientific principles, every reader of this book could get a six-pack, improve their stamina, and get promoted. Wouldn't that be great! Actually, at last count, there already are 1,584 books (okay, that's an exaggeration) promising exactly that. Funny, it does not seem to be working. In fact, the opposite effect has been noted; the more books and magazine articles that are written about nutrition, the worse everyone's waistline gets. What is going on? *Womenopause* will not be recommending a new "diet plan" because dieting does not work. *Womenopause* is recommending a new *"eating plan"*.

Let's take a field trip to Meijer's store in Michigan City, Indiana. Along the front wall, across from the checkout lanes, notice a series of enlarged photographs taken in downtown Michigan City about 80 years ago. Each picture is interesting, but there is one that is emblematic of an important point about diet. In this particular picture, ten male road workers apparently stopped their labors for a moment to pose for the photograph. They range in age from teens to forties. Strikingly, every one of them was thin. Now, where could we find ten guys or gals working together today who are all thin? Where could we find three working together who are thin? Nowhere. A good 70 percent of adults in the U.S. are overweight and according to strict interpretation of the BMI charts, almost 40 percent are now obese (full figured, Figure 1-3). Yikes! Why are all of these guys in the photograph so thin? Were they on a special diet? Were they calculating the glycemic index of all their carbs and counting the milligrams of their cholesterol? Did they know something about food we don't? Of course not. Those guys were not on a diet; they were not counting calories; they were not "watching what they eat"; and yet, they were all skinny. How can that be? Eighty years ago adult obesity in the U.S. was rare, probably less than 5 percent.

Many experts believe "back in the day", everyone was thin because the only food they had available to eat was "real food". Real food is the food God put on the planet for real people to eat. Real food comes in real serving sizes not super sizes. Why does it matter? People are meant to come in all shapes and sizes, and the diversity inherent in the human form is an important part of its beauty. Obesity matters only for two reasons. First, obesity is correlated with poor health; and second, obesity is correlated with poor personal body image. The following information may be useful if you feel you want to improve your health and well-being. Everyone has, at one time or another, tried to diet. Temporary success typically leads to backsliding, which leads to falling completely off the wagon, leading to weight gains beyond the original problem, leading to guilt and doubt, which further leads to renewed commitment for a new and improved diet plan, in an endless perfect circle. Almost everyone has failed at dieting. *Womenopause* does not recommend dieting.

Part II:
What Not To Eat

In some ways it is easier to understand what TO eat by knowing first what NOT to eat. It seems backwards to look at it that way; but hopefully, it will become clearer when it gets to the part about what we should eat.

Fake food-like substances are the opposite of real food. Fake food-like substances are everywhere. They are on TV, radio, magazines, newspapers, pop-ups, billboards everywhere. Everywhere food can be marketed to consumers, there is marketing for fake food-like substances. There is virtually no marketing for real food. No wonder there is so much confusion about food. A reasonable person struggles to ignore the non-stop bombardment of advertising for fake food-like substances. Fake food-like substances are killing our children and us. Here are a few rules to consider when choosing what *not* to put into your mouth.

1. If it has a label on it describing its contents, don't eat it.
2. If the package has a marketing slogan on it like "eat me and get healthy", don't eat it.
3. If it wasn't eaten 100 years ago, don't eat it.
4. If the food can be gotten without leaving the car, don't eat it.
5. If the food is "convenient", it's probably deadly, so don't eat it.
6. If the food is white, don't eat it (except low fat cottage cheese or white meat).
7. If the food is a favorite craving, don't eat it.
8. If the food is eaten as a substitute for happiness, it's not really helpful, so don't eat it.
9. If the food is easy to eat while watching TV, don't eat it (and turn off the TV).
10. If knowing how the food is prepared seems gross, don't eat it.
11. If children go crazy for it, don't eat it.
12. If the food is sold at a gas station or convenience store, don't eat it.
13. If a celebrity recommends eating it, don't eat it.
14. If you have ever seen an advertisement for it, don't eat it.

After removal of all those wonder-foods, what's left?

Real Food.

Part III:
Real Food: It's Not Rocket Salad

Now it is easy to describe what is meant by the term "real food". Real food is whole food that does not get modified by a food company into a fake food-like substance. Take carrots, for example. Carrots do not have a label on them describing the contents or ingredients because carrots are just carrots. Carrots have a nice color and are not sold at drive-thrus or gas stations; they are not advertised on TV by a movie star; and kids generally don't ask for them. Take salmon, as another example. Salmon has no label either because it is just salmon; it's pink, it's sold at the back edge of a grocery store, and it has no extra ingredients. You get the idea.

In some circles, real foods are considered un-American. Real Food is not cheap; it takes time to prepare; it is inconvenient; it is not new; it is not improved; and it has no catchy marketing slogan. Real food is the food everyone knows they should eat, but somehow they just don't. It's not complicated. It is not rocket salad. Real food is the stuff humans were made to consume, and they did so, just fine, for thousands and thousands of years. Probably, we may eat as much real food as we want: broccoli, beans, eggs, spinach, rice, bananas, steak, cucumbers, squash, asparagus, chicken, edamame, cauliflower, cheese, melons, tomatoes, apples, pears, fish, and nuts. Imagine the possibilities of real foods combined with other real foods: limitless!

Drink is not food, but it deserves as much consideration. Many people consume vast quantities of carbonated pop, coffee, tea, sport drinks, and alcohol each day. Sugar in sodas and pop adds up quickly to the calorie count and comes with no nutritional value. Artificial sweeteners have uncertain health risks. High intake of caffeine has adverse effects on anxiety, sleep, and blood pressure. Excessive alcohol undermines performance. A glass of fruit or vegetable juice a day has beneficial effects for the prevention of Alzheimer's. Green tea is good for you. Skim milk in moderation has nutritional value. The human body was designed to run on water: drink it up.

Gloria E.

Gloria E. managed a home that was populated by a husband, three sons, two daughters, two dogs, a cat, and a hamster. She managed her husband's dairy farm populated by 150 Brown Swiss cows and four cats, possibly five. She also took care of her in-laws and her brother, "the artist". In her spare time, she was a managing owner/broker of a successful real estate firm and a regular soloist in the local opera company. At age 53, overweight with a BMI of 33, Gloria had stopped having periods and started having hot flashes. Although she never smoked around the children, she somehow found the time to consume a pack and a half of cigarettes a day. Gloria was a beautifully full figured clash of overachieving contradictions.

Gloria insisted the family eat only "organic" foods grown by someone whom she knew personally. What that meant in practical application was, she served meat and potatoes 90 percent of the time, and she categorized the other ten percent of her meals as "bad-for-you food". She was too busy taking care of everybody else to have any time for exercise. By the time she got around to make her "annual" gynecology appointment, three years had lapsed.

The physical exam for Gloria was unremarkable. Pregnancy test, Pap test, mammogram, STI check, thyroid, colonoscopy (colon cancer screening test due at age 50), DEXA (bone density test), and CBC were all fine. She reported 12 hot flashes a day and two to three drenched nightgowns every night. She wanted them stopped, and she wanted to do it "naturally". She also wanted to stop walking into a room and forgetting why she went there in the first place.

The *w*Score at the initial visit were as follows:

1. Hot Flash Fever: 20 W
2. Mood Matters: 11 W
3. Sexercise: 1 W
4. Vagina Sahara: 4 W
5. Skinny on Skin: 10 W
6. Insomnia Queen: 6 W
7. Plumbing and Pain: 3 W

Gloria's *w*Score total was 55 W. Gloria initially resisted participating in the Womenopause Challenge. She was sure there must be a non-hormonal supplement she could swallow that would cure hot flashes. She was certain smoking kept her from weighing even more than she already did. Gloria sought information about the efficacy and risks of complementary and alternative treatments for *w*UpSide hot flashes. She compared the overall health benefits of alternative treatments to lifestyle and complementary changes including eating real food, exercising, relaxation, and taking vitamin E and fish oil.

With some hesitation Gloria opted to make some changes in how she lived instead of trying to rely exclusively on a health food store miracle. Gloria was given further advice on how to "be cool" (Chapter 9: Hot Flash Fever).

Chantix, a prescription medication to assist people who want to quit smoking, was chosen by Gloria as her first step. After enlisting the help of her family, she made a list of the reasons why she wanted to quit smoking and attached it to the fridge, so she would have it to remind her why she was quitting. Gloria did not quit smoking because her doctor wanted her to quit. She quit because she wanted to do it for her kids. She took Chantix for one week and threw her smokes away for good. She continued taking the Chantix for three months.

She believed there was no way she could find the time to go exercise, but her teenage daughter convinced her to buy a yoga exercise DVD they could do together every day after school. It worked, and the two of them really enjoyed it.

Gloria also decided to consciously add a "food with color" to every meal, make the protein part of the meals more like the size of a side dish, and mix things up a little by serving fish and poultry instead of non-stop beef. She was surprised how much the whole family enjoyed the changes.

Four weeks later Gloria was happy to report she was down to six hot flashes a day and one drenched nightgown per night. She thought they were less severe and still improving. Even if they did not get much better, she could at least live with these. She had learned the art of dressing in layers, and the fan on her desk at work was a brilliant addition. She was elated to be smoke free and weigh five pounds less. Her family had noticed less coughing, and Gloria was certain that her voice was in better shape too. Her wScore improved to 38 W, and she was pleased with the progress.

Part IV:
Think Green

Before everyone moans about another politically correct "green" scam, please give a moment to consider two green ideas. First: green as a food color really works. Green is not white, and green foods are never sold at convenience stores. Whenever green foods are seen, think real, think healthy, think nutritious, think eat. "Green is good" has a nice sound to it. Spread the word. Second: green is the dominant color of our planet, and we should try to keep it that way. Fake food-like substances take an enormous amount of energy to produce. A fast food burger costs a lot more than you might think. The feedlot cow that produced the meat consumed a lot of grain. The grain was farmed a thousand miles away by a farmer who had to spread tons of fertilizers and gallons of insecticides by driving a giant tractor, just to compete with all the other farmers who are growing a zillion acres of wheat the same way. Feedlot cows produce mountains of waste. Meat is transported hundreds of miles and frozen stiff "for freshness". It all takes a lot of energy. It is a big mess. Ironically, processed foods cost the planet dearly; while, the fast-food eater gets a bargain price. Green foods can be locally grown, fresh, and reasonably priced. Environmentally green foods can even be a cow if it is local and pasture-raised.

Part V:
Food Pyramid: Extreme Makeover

All school children know about the food pyramid. The bottom of the pyramid consists of six to eleven servings of bread, cereal rice, & pasta; the second level recommends two to four servings of fruit and three to five servings of vegetables; the third level recommends two to three servings of meat and two to three servings of dairy; and the top level recommends using as little fats, oils, and sweets as possible. Whew. It's fuzzy math that adds up to 26 servings a day. (Are you still gasping at the recommended six to eleven servings of bread a day?)

Most children agree the first problem with the pyramid is that it is too much trouble to keep track of all those servings; and besides, there is no place for macaroni and cheese. The purpose of the structure, no doubt, was to foster an appreciation for non-meat foods as the foundation for healthful nutrition and encourage a diverse diet. Another problem all kids noticed with the food pyramid, is that it always just looked like a plain flat triangle.

Womenopause proposes converting the classic food pyramid into the Real Food Wheel. The Real Food Wheel looks like the Wheel of Fortune on the TV show. The Real Food Wheel has an almost endless number of slices, each one containing a real food. Simply spin the wheel and eat whatever comes up. Any combination is fine. The more varied the mixtures of foods selected, the better. Obviously, random selection of real food is superior to self-selected burger-fries-pop. The chance of coming up with eleven servings of bread on the Real Food Wheel would be next to zero.

Part VI:
Food First

Eating food is one of life's great pleasures. Celebrations and feasts throughout history invariably had a meal as a focal point. There is something deeply relaxing about sharing food with family and friends: Thanksgiving, Christmas dinner, Fourth of July picnics. Religious ceremonies such as Ramadan, Passover, and Communion are intimately connected with a meal. People are meant to enjoy food in the company of other people. Perhaps one of the things our society has lost is the value of a meal by focusing, instead, on "value meals".

Many families, at the end of a day, come home seemingly exhausted from work, school, and other activities. Each one passes through the kitchen just long enough to microwave a quick so-called-meal on the way to their bedrooms to "relax" and watch their favorite TV shows. Since none of them like the same shows, they all disperse into different rooms of the house for the evening. Parents end-up interacting with their children only to ask them to remove their ear buds, turn off the TV, and go to bed, (and stop texting).

Eating should be fun. With a little planning, meals can regain their proper family and community importance. Consuming real foods in a relaxing environment with a real conversation is good for the body, mind, and soul.

Part VII:
Real Food Shopping List

Free-range eggs
Cold water fish and lean fish (salmon, trout, orange roughy,
    halibut)
Soy
Almonds & walnuts
Lentils
Wild game (buffalo & ostrich)
Fat-free milk (Okay, Okay, some white foods are good for you)
Organic chicken
Organic turkey
Soy/whey protein powder
Low-fat yogurt (white)
Low-fat cottage cheese (yes, more white)
Flank steak
Artichokes
Kiwis
Blueberries
Kale / greens
Beets
Cauliflower (off-white!)
Garlic
Sweet potatoes
Spinach
Cabbage
Broccoli
Edamame
Brussels sprouts
Apples (green and red)
Peppers (green, red, and yellow)
Cranberry juice
Beans
Tomatoes

Red skin potatoes
Whole wheat bread
Whole wheat pitas
Quinoa
Carrots
Oranges & tangerines
Grapes
Bananas
Green beans
Asparagus
Flax seeds
Avocados
Natural peanut butter (look for the no-stir kind)
Almond butter
Extra virgin olive oil

Part VIII:
Size Matters

When it comes to food at least, size *does* matter (for the other size-matter, check out Chapter 18: Sexercise). Whether we eat 20 percent protein or 40 percent protein, it hardly makes any difference. Eat ten percent fat or 30 percent fat; it matters very little. What matters most: how *much* of it we eat. "Generous" serving sizes are doing no one any favors. If the average American adult woman wants to lose weight, she has to eat about half of what she is currently eating. "But I already eat only half of what I used to eat." Yes. Yes. Now you have to eat half of that. Eating food is great. Enjoy it to the max—for as long as possible. Eat Real Food.

One odd finale, Womenopause recommends staying away from eating grapefruit and grapefruit juice. It's sad, but there is something in grapefruit that interacts with the liver and alters how several drugs get metabolized including common medications like estrogen and Lipitor. To be safe, just stick to oranges, lemons and tangerines.

Part IX:
The Womenopause Challenge: Eat It

1. Get a Hefty garbage bag (or two) and completely purge your home of fake food-like substances.
2. Make a shopping list and go to the local grocery store or farmers market and stock your home with real food.
3. Notify your family about the "new deal for meals" – everyone eats the same great food together at the table.
4. Everyone gets to help with the preparation for meals because everyone eats (everyone cleans up together too).
5. Enjoy your family's company. Repeat everyday.

Chapter 15

Shape Your Waist: Exposing The Metabolic Syndrome

Part I:
A Waist Is A Terrible Thing to Mind

Women near menopause endure some of the most intolerable problems: Hot Dreads, Vagina Sahara, Insomnia Queen, Meno-Fog, and Mood Matters, and they endure some of the most intolerable health changes: osteoporosis, hypertension, and diabetes. But what menopausal women find unbearable is weight gain. Invariably, many women voice more concern over their weight than they do over any other single thing. Right or wrong, almost every adult woman wishes her waist would shape up.

A preoccupation with the waistline does not, by itself, improve the waistline. Adult women in North America and the UK almost universally gain weight after age 20, and during perimenopause, women gain about a pound a year. Usually that weight is added to the waistline more than to the hips and thighs. Getting a handle on the waist situation is more complicated than cutting back on donuts, and it is more important than just improving your good looks. Weight gain during perimenopause and beyond has serious health consequences. For instance, the 20/20 rule: gaining more than 20 pounds after menopause increases the risk of breast cancer by 20 percent. Conversely, losing 20 pounds reduces the risk 20 percent.

Part II:
Thermodynamics Makes Us Honest

Trying to figure out all of the things that go into weight gain during menopause is complicated. One thing is not complicated

– the energy equation of thermodynamics. The energy equation says that if a person eats the same number of calories they burn, then they stay the same weight. No exceptions. If a person consumes more calories than they burn, then there is weight gain. If a person consumes fewer calories than they burn, then there is weight loss. Many may want to say, "Well, I did not eat anything for two weeks, but I still gained four pounds." Of course, that is a violation of the energy equation, and therefore, impossible.

Part III:
Metabolic Syndrome: MBS

In times past, 20 or 30 extra pounds were considered merely a cosmetic problem. Today we know differently. If those pounds are concentrated at the waist, it may mean a serious health problem: The Metabolic Syndrome (MBS). MBS affects 25 percent of Americans: 10 percent of women in their 20's and 40 percent of those over age 60. The characteristics of Metabolic Syndrome diagnosis for women must include any three of the following five:

- **Waistline** greater than 35 inches (measured right at the top edge of the belly button)
- **Triglycerides** greater than 150 mg/dL (one of the bad blood lipids)
- **HDL-C** less than 50 mg/dL (the good cholesterol)
- **Blood pressure** greater than 130/85 (hypertension)
- **Fasting blood sugar** greater than 100 mg/dL (diabetes)

MBS is a silent partner working behind the scenes. It slowly undermines the health of the cardiovascular system and turns, what looks like merely a figure problem, into a life and death struggle. The following are known health problems that cluster around persons with Metabolic Syndrome:
- 400 percent increase in heart disease (heart disease is by far

the #1 killer of women)
- Increased risk of dementia
- Increased risk of depression
- Increased risk of sleep apnea
- Increased risk of cirrhosis of the liver
- Increased risk of stroke
- Increased risk of vascular disease
- Increased risk of type II diabetes
- Increased overall mortality
- Increased risk of *not* owning a swimsuit

In fact, there is not a single positive thing that comes from an enlarging waistline.

Part IV:
Life Is Waisted On The Young

If a woman eats the same amount of food when she is 50 as she did when she was 20, she will most definitely gain weight to the tune of more than a pound a year. Sad but true. Many theories abound as to why that is so. The fundamental difference between a woman in her 20's and a woman in her 50's centers on the muscle tissue. Young women, before *w*Wednesday, tend to make more muscle and engage in more physical activities than those near menopause. It is not that menopausal women cannot make muscle; it just tends to require greater conscious effort. Muscle is a calorie burning tissue. Muscle burns calories even when we sleep, but fat, adipose tissue, burns very few calories by comparison. The proportion of muscle to fat declines in the average woman as she ages. This decline in lean muscle is the result of a combination of age related hormonal changes and reduced physical activities. Reduced muscle mass with increased adipose tissue results in a decreased basal metabolic rate (the amount of calories burned at rest). It becomes a vicious circle — the fewer the activities are done, the fewer the calories it takes to put inches on to your waist.

Absolute weight, however, does not always predict metabolic rate or the presence of Metabolic Syndrome. Chapter 1 examined a short cut for the determination the Body Mass Index (BMI) using only height and weight (Figure 1-3). A more accurate determination needs to include waist measurement. Consider the difference between the next two examples who have the same BMI. Two 5 feet 3 inch women may weigh the same 135 pounds but may have considerably different shapes and metabolic rates. If woman #1, Ellen, is an exercise queen who eats real food, her body fat may be as low as 15 percent, and her lean muscle mass may be high as 40 percent. If woman #2, Eileen, instead, watches 12 hours of TV a day and eats mainly burgers, fries, and a Coke, her body fat may be as high as 40 percent, and her lean muscle mass may be as low as 15 percent. Ellen has a waist measurement of 29 inches and a calculated basal metabolic rate of 2500 calories a day. On the other hand, Eileen has a 36-inch waist and a basal metabolic rate of 2200 calories a day. Here is the apparent irony: even though both women weigh the same, the "thin" small waisted one, Ellen, can eat more food in a day than the thicker waisted Eileen and still not gain any weight. In fact, Ellen should eat more. The reason Eileen needs to eat less each day is because she has considerably less calorie burning muscle.

Chalking up weight gain to menopause is everyone's favorite rationalization. It has a truth, in so far as menopausal women frequently gain weight, but it is not true that reaching menopause *causes* an expanding waistline. Like many things, when we were young, being thin was effortless; but also, when we were young, we were across-the-board clueless. Fretting about not being young may sabotage the joys of maturity and is pointless. Remaining trim or regaining a trim figure is absolutely achievable by every woman, but it does not happen by wishful thinking. Waistlines are created like a sculptor creates a fine statue: she keeps chipping away day by day, hard little chip after hard little chip.

Part V:
The Causes Of Metabolic Syndrome: MBS

Metabolic Syndrome (MBS) is the result of a confluence of, shall we say, less than optimal lifestyle choices. At the top of the cause-list is weight gain. Women with a Body Mass Index (BMI) greater than 25 (Full Figured) are at risk for Metabolic Syndrome (see Figure 1-3 to calculate your BMI). Women who are over age 50, postmenopausal *w*UpSide and have low estrogen levels, are at risk for developing Metabolic Syndrome. Smoking increases the risk of having Metabolic Syndrome by 600 percent, yet another reason to become smoke free. A diet high in carbohydrates, especially at the expense of quality protein, leads to Metabolic Syndrome. Women with Metabolic Syndrome are less physically active than their normal counterparts. Interestingly, being alcohol free, a teetotaler, has a slightly higher chance of developing Metabolic Syndrome. No surprises really. Anything that might lead to an expanding waistline fits the bill, which is why measuring the waistline is a convenient method for following the progress of women fighting the battle of the bulge.

Menopause is the most identifiable physical event that contributes to Metabolic Syndrome. Whether or not it is aging or menopause hardly matters. All women who live long enough and reach menopause have the privilege of aging. Metabolic Syndrome affects almost half of all *w*Friday women. The intersection of decreased physical activity, uncompensated calorie intake, and hormone changes usually spells gradual increases in BMI. An elevated BMI, associated with an increasing waistline, reliably predicts changes in lipid and glucose metabolism that define Metabolic Syndrome. Although you cannot change your chronological age, every other factor that plays into the development of Metabolic Syndrome is completely under your control. It is time to take control of the few things in this world that we actually do control. Having Metabolic Syndrome is optional. Womenopause recommends opting out.

Part VI:
Fast 4 Fit

There are no magic wands for Metabolic Syndrome. There are, however, direct and practical ways to reverse the process. Some women prefer to jump start their recovery program because immediate gratification encourages long term discipline. For those who desire an urgent exit from MBS consider the following **Fast 4 Fit** for four weeks.

1. **Walk 15,000 steps a day** (that is fifteen *thousand* steps a day). That's a lot of stepping. The only way to achieve 15,000 steps is to count them precisely with a pedometer. Pedometers are cheap, under $20, and serve as a constant reminder to take the extra step every moment of every day. For the average step length, 15,000 steps add up to be around seven miles. Very few people get that many steps in their usual daily activities. It requires getting up and consciously walking for time and distance every day.

2. **No sugar drinks.** Do not consume any beverage that contains any sugar of any kind; no pop, no sweet tea, no so-called energy drinks. Corn syrup is as addictive as cigarette nicotine and just about as deadly. It is amazing how many unnecessary calories can be eliminated, by making this one simple switch. Drink all the water you want.

3. **No potatoes.** Americans love all forms of potatoes, particularly the deep fat fried ones and the ones smothered in butter and sour cream. Potatoes can easily be eliminated from the diet because they are easy to spot; they look just like potatoes every time.

4. **No bread.** Bread means white bread, brown bread, black

bread, green bread (if there is such a thing), whole wheat bread, rolls, pastries, anything made mostly of flour. All bread has to go.

Fast 4 Fit is so simple it is ridiculous – it is so effective it is delightful. Three diet *don'ts* and one activity *do* can make significant changes in four weeks. Particularly notice that taking a diet pill is not a recommended simple or direct method for reversing Metabolic Syndrome. By the way, if there was such a thing as a safe and effective diet pill, wouldn't everyone know about it and already be thin? As will be detailed in the next chapter, performing a lot of abdominal exercises does not guarantee a trim waistline either.

Part VII:
Designer Bellies

This is the naked truth about metabolic syndrome; it is not a disease that we get by chance, accident, or bad luck. Metabolic Syndrome is not contagious, and it's not our spouse's fault that we came down with it. We get Metabolic Syndrome only when it is earned. Decisions about what we do and what we eat determine whether or not we develop the cluster of problems that define the Metabolic Syndrome. Look on the bright side. All of these problems can be improved, reversed, and even eliminated by carefully committing to apply the following principles for the long haul.

- **Weight loss.** Lowering your current BMI one point has a direct positive effect. The long-term goal should be a BMI under 25.
- **Regular vigorous exercise.** Find something you like, or better still, a combination of activities you like doing and do them faithfully, building up to six days a week. Consider yoga. It is a great way to tone and shape the

physique.

- **Smoke free.** Enough said.
- **Real food.** Eat real food not fake food-like substances.
- **Menopause Hormone Therapy.** In addition to all the usual benefits it endows, MHT actually decreases waist measurements in women who do not exercise or diet. Imagine what it might do for a motivated woman who does all three.
- **Fish oil.** Omega 3 fatty acids are deficient in the diets of most women in North America. This is simply remedied by taking 2 grams of fish oil supplement each day. Look for a quality "de-odorized" brand. It seems like a contradiction — eat fat and lose weight, but it's not. Omega 3 fatty acids are essential to making healthy cells and consuming them helps you lose weight. Flaxseed oil is excellent too. Better yet, go to the source and eat deep water ocean fish like salmon and tuna twice a week.
- **Folic acid.** Ditto. Supplement with 800 mcg a day.
- **Hypertension medication.** When the blood pressure consistently measures greater than 130/85 it is time to start medication. Even mild elevations in blood pressure can double the risk of stroke.
- **Metformin.** Metformin is a standard medication for diabetes and is prescribed for elevated blood sugar. Sometimes it is a valuable treatment for MBS even when the blood sugar levels are borderline.
- **Lipid-lowering medication like Lipitor.** Lipid lowering drugs are used to lower the LDL (bad cholesterol) and raise the HDL (good cholesterol). A 25 percent reduction in total cholesterol can reduce heart disease risk by an amazing 50 percent.
- **Benecol.** Benecol Light Spread (a butter substitute) helps block the uptake of cholesterol, therefore, reducing the level of cholesterol.
- **Triglyceride-lowering therapy.** If the triglycerides are

elevated over 150 mg/dL, then medication should be considered.

Consultation with an internist or family doctor would be prudent to assure proper coordinated care for lipid, hypertension, and diabetic disorders. Estrogen therapy for menopause, MHT, is not generally used or recommended for the treatment or prevention of lipid disorders, hypertension, and diabetes leading to cardiovascular disease. However, it is well-documented for women who do use MHT, there are positive changes noted in their lipid profiles, hypertension, and diabetes. MHT raises HDL (good cholesterol), decreases LDL (bad cholesterol), and decreases total cholesterol. Furthermore, transdermal wBodyIdentical 17beta-estradiol favorably affects blood sugar levels and decreases blood pressure and triglycerides (bad lipids). Many women who initiate menopausal hormone therapy during wFriday along with the Womenopause Challenge improve all of the Metabolic Syndrome risk factors to such a degree they do not require antihypertensive medication, Lipitor or other lipid lowering medication, and Metformin.

Part VIII:
It Is Never Too Late

We cannot change what happened yesterday, and we know nothing about what tomorrow might be. Today is all we ever have. There will never be a better day than today to start living like we mean it. Each day is the moment of our liberation from neglect and bad habits. In that moment, time stands still, and we glimpse the person we were meant to be.

If you are starting with a BMI of 28 or 48 it does not matter; the principles are the same. Know what you are this morning and make an improvement before you go to bed tonight. Each day is an opportunity to exercise right and to eat right. If you make a mistake, welcome to the human race; then get back on track. Women of North America, Australia, and Great Britain have an expanding life expectancy, and many will live into their nineties. Just how healthy we may be is, to a large extent, dependent upon how well we take care of ourselves, not so much, how well medical science takes care of us. Now is the time to stop pausing and start living.

Sky K.

Sky, at age 52, was a married mother of four who worked part time as a nurse in the psychiatric ward. After 30 years of psychiatric nursing she had seen a lot of odd stuff happen. She thanked God every day her husband of 34 years remained the salt of the earth guy she had met in high school. Their life together was a remarkable rags to riches success story. Everyone loved Sky and her husband Frederick. They were kind, loyal, generous, and always ready for fun.

Menopause had been reached at age 49, and Sky was determined to go through the transition without medical intervention. She had seen first hand what the best of medical intentions do to some patients, and she wanted to avoid becoming a "chronically complaining patient". She "never saw doctors professionally, only socially".

At her first official gynecology appointment Sky was not her usual relaxed self. Sky related four years of hot flashes, night sweats, insomnia, and progressive dyspareunia. "None of that really matters, what matters is my weight," she said through tears. At 5 feet 9 inches, weighing 209 pounds, Sky's BMI was a full figured 31 (Figure 1-3). Her waist measurement was 44 inches, and her hips were 43 inches. Her total wScore was 37 W (Figure 1-2). She had weighed about 160 pounds for two decades prior to menopause "then, whamo, 40 pounds, overnight". She never exercised because a doctor had told her in junior high school she had "exercise induced asthma". He took her permanently out of school gym classes and advised her to avoid all physical activities or else she would die. At least, that is what she remembers him saying. No one would have guessed she had asthma, and she had never taken any medication for it. She lived in fear of triggering an attack like she had once at age 13. She had never had another attack during her entire adult life and attributed this luck to staying away from physical exertion.

The physical exam demonstrated normal heart and lungs, a pale, dry vaginal mucosa, and a small normal uterus. Her blood pressure was 132/88. Pap test, cultures, mammogram, bone density, and colonoscopy were ordered. A battery of blood tests was requested, and she accepted a referral to a pulmonologist specialist in asthma.

Sky received information about real food and vitamin supplementation. She returned in two weeks for the results. There was good news to report. Her Pap test and cultures were negative. The pulmonologist had found no evidence for asthma after a careful history, review of the medical records, examination, x-ray, and pulmonary function tests. He gave her a clean bill of lung health and advised her that what she had experienced as a single episode in her youth was more likely an allergy response and not asthma. After that good news, all the rest was a little bad.

Sky's blood tests showed 1) an elevated fasting blood sugar of 117, 2) high total cholesterol of 269, 3) high triglycerides of 264, 4) marginally low hemoglobin at 11.7, and 5) low bone density with a T score of minus 1.9.

Sky had a lot of serious things going on behind the scenes. By all external accounts she was simply a fantastic woman who managed her home, worked, and socialized. She was just a little over weight, but who isn't? In truth, Sky was a set up for developing diabetes, hypertension, heart disease, stroke, and osteoporosis. Sky had some big decisions to make.

Fortunately, Sky chose to act in a positive way toward all the negative news she had received. Often, there is an unconscious urge to reject health advice when there is no dire emergency at the moment. Sky wanted to out-live her husband "so he's not left home alone to mess up the house."

Sky actively participated in a discussion about the metabolic syndrome. She met all the criteria for the diagnosis, and she would need a health care team to help her turn things around. She made an appointment to see a family practice doctor in a neighboring town, one she had never personally met. She asked if she could take hormones to control her hot flashes.

Sky started the Fast 4 Fit plan to jump-start her recovery. Now that she could safely exercise, she bought a pedometer, eliminated carbonated drinks, eliminated potatoes, and eliminated bread from her diet. After a thorough discussion about the benefits and risks, she elected to begin menopausal hormone therapy (MHT) with Evamist (wBodyIdentical estrogen) three sprays in the morning, and Prometrium (wBodyIdentical progesterone pill) at bedtime. Because she had never exercised, Sky was advised to count her steps for two average days then advance the number of steps by 10 percent every couple of days until her next appointment.

Four weeks later Sky was anxious to get on the scales and to have her waist measured (not exactly the way she had been on the original visit). Her weight had dropped 11 pounds, and her BMI dropped two points. Her waist had shrunk an inch, from 44 inches to 43 inches. Her initial waist/hip ratio was greater than one (meaning her waist was bigger than her hips); and now, it was equal to one. Having a waist smaller than the hips is a positive predictor for improved health (and looks). Sky had started walking 3,000 steps a day and was now up to 6,000 steps. She was certain she could advance to 10,000 steps a day within the next month. Her new family doctor had consulted with her gynecologist, and Sky began treatment with Lisinopril 10 mg a day for blood pressure.

All of Sky's menopausal symptoms were completely gone, hot flashes, night sweats, and vaginal dryness. Her wScore improved to 4 W.

Frederick had taken her out to their favorite restaurant last week and had made advanced arrangements to have the waiter NOT serve any of their favorite bread to help her keep to her four week plan. Sky looked at the first four weeks as a trial to see if anything could be done to shape her waist. It had been such a success she did not want to stop there. This Sky had no limit.

Part IX:
The Womenopause Challenge: Shake-up to Shape-up

1. Go to: www.bmi-calculator.net/body-fat-calculator (or similar).
2. Determine your percent body fat.
3. Determine your basal metabolic rate (BMR) and see how many calories you need to survive (and how many calories you can do without).
4. Shoot for a body fat under 25 percent.
5. Shoot for a body mass index (BMI) under 25.
6. Shoot for a waistline that is smaller than the one you have today.
7. Shoot for the sky!

Chapter 16

Vitamin-X: Exercise

Part I:
It's Not Fair – Brad and Angelina Have Personal Trainers

Granted, if we all had a personal trainer to gently rouse us from sleep at 9 AM by handing us a hot cappuccino and coaxing us out of bed into a pair of designer sneakers for a brief targeted personal morning workout, we would probably do it. That's not going to happen, so we have to get over it. Very few adults love to exercise, and scarcely any like exercise enough to do it regularly. Almost everyone thinks they should exercise more than they do. If you identify with the latter group, this chapter is for you.

The human body was built for movement. Ironically, the human mind has spent most of its efforts trying to figure out ways to minimize movement. In this regard, the mind has temporarily triumphed over the body to the detriment of the body's health. People living in North America, Australia, and the UK may function adequately with their family and jobs and never be required to do any real physical work. Trains, planes, and automobiles have eliminated long distance walking. Phones and mail have eliminated short trip walking. Wi-Fi access has virtually eliminated the need to even stand up. This was not true 50 years ago. As a result, many have gravitated down the path of least resistance and acquiesced to becoming a "chair pear", the working woman's equivalent of a couch potato.

Most people think they know how to exercise, but very few have ever read anything about it or have spent any time with a real expert. If you have studied exercise, taught yoga classes, and have pumped iron for years then, okay, great, skip this part, give our regards to Arnold, and go on to the next chapter. If you are a little unsure about why you need to exercise let alone have no clue as to how to start or maybe just want a little guidance about how to tweak your current exercise routine, then follow the Vitamin-X suggestions.

Part II:
Why Exercise?

There are legitimate competing theories about the relationship between the body and the mind. Without getting too far afield, many experts believe the mind and body are united in a complex way. It follows, that how the mind "feels" effects how the body "works" and vice versa: how the body "works" effects how the mind "feels". They are thus unified into one being. In this simple regard, most women accept the first premise; how we feel impacts our physical health and well-being by affecting how our body functions. For example, a high-strung, type I executive probably drives herself into having a heart attack. Unfortunately, few women recognize the opposite argument: a chronically de-conditioned woman becomes vulnerable to depression, but it is just as likely. Fullness of life always encompasses mental-emotional-spiritual health coupled with physical health. Either one alone, or significantly out of balance with the other, predisposes to a lack of ease with life, or what might be termed, disease.

Regular exercise can have positive observable effects within four weeks for women in the perimenopause and *w*UpSide. Certainly, many of the symptoms identified with menopause are understood as problems arising from changes in hormones, and it is not known exactly what exercise does to hormone levels. What is known, however, is that exercise reduces the intensity of many of the commonly encountered transition troubles. It is good to know that Vitamin-X, exercise, *decreases* the following:

- Hot Flash Fever
- Night Sweats
- Cold Crashes
- Osteoporosis
- Insomnia Queen
- Meno-Fog
- Body Mass Index (BMI)
- Depression
- Mood Matters
- wWorry
- Breast Cancer
- Heart Attacks
- Strokes
- Dyspareunia
- Loss of sexual desire
- Diabetes
- Fatigue
- Dementia
- Wrinkles
- Waistline

On the other hand, Vitamin-X, exercise, *increases* the risk of:

- Feeling Fit
- Feeling Feminine
- Feeling Fabulous
- Wearing a swimsuit in four weeks

Part III:
Common Exercise Myths

Some medical myths are so entrenched it takes a stick of dispute dynamite to dislodge it from our brain. Take, for example, the commonly held belief that being wet in a drafty cool temperature causes a person to catch a cold. Not so. A cold is an upper respiratory track infection caught by being exposed to someone who has a virus you have not seen before. It is called the germ theory, and everyone, except moms, has accepted it as true for over 100 years. There are some equally held false beliefs about exercise that deserve explanation.

Consider these **myths:**

1. **You can exercise yourself thin.** An average woman who has a family, home, job, and a real life does not have enough hours in a day to exercise herself thin. An average sized woman may have a basal metabolic rate burning 1,500 calories a day at complete rest. Walking briskly for 30 minutes burns only an additional 100 calories. Since one pound of body fat stores 3,600 calories a woman would have to walk continuously (without eating) for 18 hours to burn-off one pound of fat. It is not likely to happen.

2. **You can target exercise and reduce belly fat by doing a lot of abs** (abdominal exercises such as sit-ups). Careful exercise can build muscle tone, strength, endurance, and size. Exercise decreases the risk of getting diseases like heart disease and diabetes. Fat is not directly affected by exercise at all. If the only exercises you did were abs, there would be no change in your waistline except, perhaps, enlarging your abdominal muscles. Consuming fewer calories than you burn decreases fat. Sorry, no exceptions. The only proven exercise that reduces belly fat is pushing back away from the table.

3. **You get enough exercise just doing your job and housework.** Of course if that were true, you would not be reading this chapter, and your BMI would already be less than 25. Office-type jobs and housework burn less than 130 calories an hour, not enough to make any meaningful change in your overall net energy expenditure, and therefore, weight.

4. **You should not exercise because you do not want to look muscle bound.** We have seen what some extraordinary male athletes look like, and we do not want a body like that; therefore, we delete exercising from our schedule. Women have a unique female genetic make-up and do not make muscle like men do. Exercise shapes a woman's figure into an in-shape womanly figure not into a man's shape.

5. **Sweating is unattractive.** But a 38-inch waistline is?

6. **Exercise takes too much time.** Everyone gets a full and perfect amount of time each day to complete all of the things they *want* to do. At last check, everyone still gets 24 hours.

7. **Exercise equipment is expensive.** Exercise equipment is fun but completely unnecessary for a good workout.

Part IV:
The First Step Is, Well, First

If you are not currently exercising or have never really exercised, today is an exciting day. The first step to take is literally the first step. Walking, according to the clock, or better yet, according to a pedometer, is the best first step you can take. Keeping track of every step you take in a journal is an important part of the first step. Adding steps or minutes to your walks, over time, will give you concrete evidence that your physical capacity is on the mend. Easy? Not exactly, but it's definitely do able. Thirty minutes of brisk walking is about 3,200 steps or about a mile and a half. Once you have built up the endurance to walk continuously for half an hour, it is time to graduate and take exercise to the next level.

When starting out, it is critical to keep track of the amount of exercise you do every day. Resist the temptation to over-do on good days and under-do on bad days. Just do the same as you did yesterday plus a little bit more. Pace yourself. Of course, if you have serious health problems, check with your doctor before beginning anything strenuous.

Part V:
The Part After The First Step Is Harder

If you want easy, you will need to move to a different universe. Nothing worthwhile in this one is easy. Many women mistakenly believe walking 30 minutes a day is exercise enough, and nothing else needs to be done. Who knows where that idea came from? It is a little like saying that wading on the shore is all that can be done to enjoy the lake; what about swimming, sailing, water skiing, jet skiing, snorkeling, and what about parasailing? Why stop with wading when there is all of the other fun stuff to do? Vitamin-X, exercise, means much more than walking. Walking is the equivalent to a baby crawling. With time she needs to get up on her little feet to begin walking, eventually, skipping and dancing.

There are five types of exercise that should be included in a complete exercise program. At first it may seem a little overwhelming, but after the parts are analyzed individually, it will be seen they combine seamlessly in many exercise routines. The following exercise groups are called the **phys-ed-5**.

1. **Aerobics**: The extension of walking into a complete fitness program could constitute the aerobics section. Activities such as biking, swimming, and running are commonly used aerobic activities. The purpose of aerobics is to push the level of fitness higher than can be achieved by ordinary daily activity. The word aerobics comes from the word air. In a roundabout way, aerobic exercises are supposed to get you exercising enough to breath heavily. Becoming relatively short-of-breath is a good thing. Breathing heavy is linked to increases in heart rate (heavy breathing is a

different thing altogether, see chapter 18: Sexercise). Exercise of an intensity that causes a stimulation of the pulmonary and cardiovascular system will make you sweat. Exercise that makes you sweat will make you tired: hot and tired. The usual immediate effect following sweating-hot-tired is an incredible feeling of energy and joy, the exercise high, caused by the release of endorphins. There are hundreds of activities women may choose to get a good aerobics workout. Casual walking while chatting away with friends probably is not intense enough to get the job done unless at some point along the way you are too tired and winded to keep up the conversation. Gyms typically have elliptical trainers, treadmills, recumbent bikes, upright bikes, stair steppers, rowing machines, and cross country skiing equipment. You can improvise with hiking, biking, swimming, tennis, golf, volleyball, dancing, cross-country skiing, racket-ball, and basketball; you name it. Notice, no gym membership is required for many of these activities. Remember: hot and sweaty. Taking aerobics to the third level requires slightly more thought and planning. Although slow or moderate continuous aerobic exercise for 30 to 60 minutes is good, high intensity interval training for 20 to 30 minutes is great. Interval training is anything like sprinting for a minute, jogging for a minute to catch your breath, then sprinting for a minute etc. High intensity interval training maximally stimulates aerobic conditioning and gets you the highest reward for the amount of time devoted to exercise.

2. **Resistance Training.** Surprising benefits come to those who push and pull their body parts through resistance training. Whereas, aerobics can improve body *size*, strength training by lifting weights can improve body *shape*. There are many runners who get into good running condition, but who maintain their original chair-pear shaped body,

just a smaller version of the original. Resistance training, on the other hand, transforms the body into a sculpture-form, even the Greeks would admire. It is the most direct type of exercise to build lean muscle. Remember, muscle is a calorie-burning machine that increases metabolism and burns fat. Women can define their legs, arms, and abs better with resistance training than with only aerobics. Although there are several classic weight training schemes, many experts recommend starting out with free-weights like dumbbells. Standard gym weight machines are a good alternative. Beginners should concentrate on developing as perfect a technique as possible for maximizing the results with a few basic movements. There is no substitute for getting some hands-on advice from a trainer to learn proper and safe strength training. Some women have obtained satisfactory information about strength training from books, magazines, DVDs; and there are a couple of on-line sites with instructional videos. Again, like the aerobics portion of your exercise plan, writing down everything you do in a journal has tremendous advantage. For beginners, combination moves with lightweights and perfect technique will pay great dividends. Chatting on the phone through a blue tooth while lifting weights will not produce optimal results. Intensity matters. Make every minute of your workout count. After six months or a year of basic resistance training, it would be appropriate to advance your workout to the third level, consisting of more isolated muscle routines. No normal person needs to spend hours a day in the gym. Targeted intense workouts take a maximum of 40 minutes. Exercising the whole body with each workout probably has advantages over concentrating on just legs one day and arms another.

3. **Stretching.** Hands down, the most overlooked part of an

exercise routine for most women is stretching. Exercise depends upon contracting muscles to get them to work harder than they did before; but afterwards, the muscles need to be stretched-out to maintain their length and tone. Exercise without stretching may lead to imbalances of muscle groups and can affect basic posture and stance. Consciously stretching every muscle after a workout helps restore proper muscle coordination and feels great. Working on muscle stretching is the best thing to do to reduce uneven wear and tear on the major joints like the knees, hip, and shoulders.

4. **Core Muscle Development**. Core Training has become a trendy phrase lately and has been used to market certain programs and products. It's great this critical component of exercise has finally seen the light of day and gotten the recognition it deserves. Some exercise routines leave out strengthening the deep trunk muscles that support the spine. The core muscles can be targeted with specific "bridging" exercises, yoga poses, and free weights. Everyone should become familiar with them. There are several standard exercises for core training, and like all strength training, it is best to change-up the exercises you do from time to time to keep your mind and muscles challenged.

5. **Balance and Coordination**. Dancers are made, not born, and you are an amazing learning machine. Everyone can improve their balance and coordination, just like they learned the multiplication tables: practice, practice, and more practice. There are sensors buried within our muscles that send feedback to our brain, telling it where the arm or leg is in relation to the rest of the body and its orientation in space (called proprioceptors). The feedback can be sharpened and amplified through training. Balance balls and balance boards can be incorporated into your usual

exercises to do double-duty for strength and balance.

At this point you might be saying, "Yikes, no way can I learn or find the time to do all that stuff". You can. You must because your life depends upon it. Many women hate to exercise because it seems so selfish to them, and it takes away time they could be devoting to their family, friends, church, neighbors, and job. Think of it this way, if you keep yourself in optimal health, you can do all of those other things for everyone else better and longer. Then, you realize, you are taking time to exercise *for all of them*. It is just the opposite of what you were thinking. *Not exercising is selfish.*

Part VI:
Combo Drives

This book has been written on an Apple computer. The computer has a single slot to read any type of disc, written data, photos, video, music, and probably other stuff we do not even know about. It is a combination optical drive referred to as a "combo drive". It is one thing that does everything. There are some exercises like that. You do not have to structure each workout to include a little of each of the phys-ed-5. Some exercises cover all or almost all of it. Take yoga, for instance. It is great for strength, balance, core, and flexibility. Yoga also has the advantage of incorporating relaxation training as a bonus. It is almost the perfect exercise all by itself. Just like a nice resort in Mexico; pilates, tai chi, kick boxing, standard aerobics classes, and others may be an "all inclusive" exercise routine. They are all convenient methods to exercise without having to put too much thought into what you should be doing. Like all exercise routines, they become stale after a while, and your body plateaus in development. Changing how you exercise at least every three months, or so, will stimulate new improvements. Remember, the only wrong exercise is no exercise.

Part VII:
Be a Nike Ad: "Just Do It"

Spending a penny a day more than is earned makes a person poor while saving just a penny over what is spent makes a person rich. Methodical and consistent exercise builds a healthful body, and it is never too late to start. It is possible to be healthier at 60 than you were at 40. In fact, aside from the physical upgrades an exercise plan bestows, most people need to be involved in an improvement plan of some sort to feel emotionally complete. It is not in the achievement of a goal that gives the deepest pleasure; it is the hard earned attempt that satisfies. Most beginning exercisers notice the more complete their written exercise plan is, the more unexpected time they find to do all the other stuff.

Find someone to workout with. Being held accountable to someone else is a powerful motivator to keep going. Besides, then you can return the favor and encourage your exercise partner too.

Invariably, women want to know, when in the day is the best time to exercise? The answer is easy, any time, just do it. There may be a few advantages to exercising first thing in the morning. First, early morning is the most controllable time slot of the entire day. As the day progresses, things get away from us. To-do lists get piled-up, reorganized, deleted, modified, and forgotten. This is least likely to happen first thing in the morning because all those people who might otherwise distract you are sleeping.

Second, usually the only thing keeping you from exercising in the morning would have to be attributed to laziness, and there is no way you can accept that. Third, there may be some hormonal considerations that make exercising in the morning more efficient, but that is kind of a fine point in the big scheme of things. Wouldn't you rather start your day with an exercise high and a feeling of accomplishment before most have even had their first cup of coffee?

Exercise in excess is as bad as gambling in excess, drinking milk in excess, or any thing else done in excess. There is a time and a place for everything under heaven. Twenty to sixty minutes of high intensity exercise five or six times a week is sufficient. If it is completed for four weeks, noticeable physical changes are guaranteed. If it is continued for life, then that life will be fuller and longer.

Exercising is only one part of a whole lifestyle decision. If one of your main goals is to trim down and to look your best, it may be tempting to put all your eggs into the exercise basket. That would be a mistake. Exercising without carefully managing your diet is futile. Remember this too; being your best is a lot more than just looking your best.

Maggi B.

Maggi was "giving-up and saying uncle". She could no longer stand the hot flashes. She worked for the State Natural Resources Department for 25 years. She had reached menopause ten years ago and had taken Premarin 0.625 mg a day for two years with no difficulties but stopped when her husband insisted hormones were going to give her breast cancer. She remembers the date well; it was the summer of 2002, just before they went on a camping trip to Vancouver Island. She had Hot Dreads for three days in the van coming and going and Hot Dreads all week long in a tent in the rain. She said she would never forget that trip. She commented drily, "At least I didn't get breast cancer and die on the trip."

Her hot flashes calmed down somewhat over the next few years, but they never went away completely. They had made a strange come-back this past year, and now they were intolerable again. She made an office visit with a menopause specialist to see if there were any other options.

Maggi, at age 60, was a full figured married mother of one "high maintenance daughter" who had moved back home at age 32 with her three children. Maggi felt a little guilty about wishing the grandkids would stay and her daughter would go.

Maggi's husband Bob seemed to like the arrangement just fine, probably because he never had to do any of the cooking, cleaning, or laundry.

Maggi's BMI was 30, and her wScore was 29 W with high values in Hot Flash Fever, Mood Matters, and Insomnia Queen. She reported 12 hot flashes a day, feeling blue, and frequent "brain-locks" when she could not remember the name of common objects. She had undergone a hysterectomy over 20 years ago but still had her tubes and ovaries. She was on no prescription or over-the-counter medicines. She had regular appointments with her family doctor but never brought up the hot flashes and memory problems because she did not think it was the time to discuss non-medical issues. She had obtained a bone density test three years ago. Her T score was minus 1.1 (Chapter 26).

There is no controversy about the effectiveness of MHT in treating the major estrogen withdrawal symptoms common in menopause. There is some controversy concerning the optimal age at which to initiate MHT. There is very low risk and many medical advantages for women initiating hormones within ten years of reaching menopause (wFriday women) and a slightly higher risk for wSaturday women. Maggi would, therefore, still be considered very low risk. She was informed about all the potential benefits and risks. In addition, she received information about the Womenopause Challenge, and she accepted it. She began treatment with Femring 0.05 mg, a vaginally inserted small soft ring that releases wBodyIdentical 17beta-estradiol systemically through the vaginal mucosa. The Femring is convenient and needs to be changed only once every three months.

Four weeks later Maggi reported some improvement. Her hot flashes were definitely better, but she still had a couple at night. She continued to feel tired and moody and wondered if there was a higher dose to use. Her new bone density T score was minus 2.0. Her mammogram, Pap test, cultures, and blood work were all normal.

After a discussion, Maggi admitted she had not started exercising or taking vitamin D and calcium yet. She was given the recommendation of, simply, instituting all of the Womenopause challenge steps first. She could go up on the dose of the Femring for her hot flashes, begin an antidepressant for her mood, and add a bisphosphonate for the prevention of osteoporosis, later, if still necessary. She agreed to join the health club and start taking the recommended supplements instead of taking all those medicines.

After another four weeks Maggi had really good news. Her hot flashes were gone; her sleep was great; her memory was restored; and her *daughter's* mood had improved (but maybe it was her own mood that was better).

Maggi's BMI had dropped a full point from 30 to 29. Her *w*Score improved from 29 W to 7 W. She had started an aerobics class that met three times a week and had advanced her walking to 15,000 steps a day. She produced a month long logbook that documented all of her hard work. She pulled a small pedometer out of her bra and showed she had already taken 9,243 steps that day. She had taken vitamin D 4,000 IU a day, along with her calcium citrate 1,500 mg a day and converted to eating only real food.

Every three months for the next year Maggi made verifiable improvements. Her BMI dropped one to two points every three months, and at the end of the year her BMI had gone from 30 to 24, and she had dropped two dress sizes. She now was a substitute aerobics instructor on weekends. Her daughter had remarried and moved into a house down the street, and they all could still see each other every day. Maggi's bone mineral density had improved to a T score of -1.0.

Who is to say what made the improvement? Was it the exercise, the estrogen, the vitamin D? All of them improve quality of life. They all help hot flashes, insomnia, and mood matters. They all work better, together, than any one of them alone.

Part VIII:
The Womenopause Challenge: Sweat Equity

1. Get an "I can do this" notebook. On the left-side page, write down everything you eat that day. On the right-side page, write down all your exercise activities.
2. Set out your shorts, shoes, and socks before going to bed.
3. Set your alarm clock to go off 45 minutes earlier than normal.
4. Forget about Brad, just do it everyday for four weeks and feel (and see) the difference.

Chapter 17

Vitamins, Minerals, and CAMs, Oh My!

Part I:
What's All The Fuss?

There is an unspoken tension between doctor-types and everyday women. Doctor-types may be suspicious and somewhat fearful of Complementary and Alternative Medical (CAM) therapy. On the other hand, many women consider CAM products perfectly natural and safe. There is a distinct disconnect between them on this interesting subject. Why all the fuss? Because it matters. It matters medically, and it matters emotionally.

Complementary therapy means something that "complements" or goes along well with standard medical therapy, perhaps even enhances medical therapy. Like a great pair of shoes goes well with your dress, there is no intrinsic competition between the two fashion items; they complement each other. Alternative therapy means just that. It is an "alternative" to standard medical therapy or something done instead of conventional medical care. It makes no sense to wear boots over your sandals. They do not go well together, so it has to be one or the other. If you travel to another city to go shopping, you may take route 10, or you may take route 38 as an alternate, but you cannot travel down both at the same time.

Although the technical definitions of CAMs are clear, in a practical sense, almost everyone mixes and matches indiscriminately between complementary, alternative, and medical so the boundaries between the three therapies can easily get blurred. This chapter will sharpen the edges of the controversy and provide some guidance for menopausal women seeking relief from the common transitional troubles, as well as, those searching for their best health possible.

Part II:
Where Do Vitamins, Minerals and CAM Products Come From? A Store.

The food, nutrition, and supplement industry in North America, Australia, the UK, and around the world is a profit driven business like any other business. Also, like other businesses, they make products people want, or they make people want the products they make. Many consumers believe the supplement industry's purpose is to bring to the public's attention the marvels of a hidden science and sage knowledge, hitherto, unknown by western medical science. Sometimes the marketing strategy makes it look like they are doing us a big favor by bringing an exiled herb to our attention "in spite of what western medical experts say". Often, it appears the more obscure the original discovery and use is, the better. Invariably, supplements marketed as complementary or alternative therapies are touted as more natural, and therefore, safer than conventional medical therapy. These assertions are made in spite of the fact that nature produces thousands and thousands of known dangerous and poisonous plants and animals. Everything in life has its own risks.

Last year in the US, consumers spent over $25 billion on dietary supplements with the hopes of enhancing, or at least maintaining, their health. Only a few of these have documented safety trials and can be unequivocally recommended for their effectiveness by physicians. A healthcare professional is bound by science, expert opinions, and accepted conventional care because they are held responsible for the well-being of their patients with every recommendation they make. Individuals may choose to consume something and have to answer only to themselves. Once either one (the doctor or the patient) decides on a medicine, a complex rationalization builds up within her psyche to support that decision. Opinions about supplements thus become extraordinarily emotional. The constant bombardment of effective marketing clearly moves opinions toward acceptance of whatever claims may be made. No one is immune to compelling advertising.

Nutritional supplements come into and out of vogue. Responsible physicians are frequently caught off-guard when pressed for recommendations. Because they may not watch the same TV programs or read the same magazines where the latest natural discovery is marketed, they may have never heard of it. Patients may think it is a sign of arrogance when their healthcare provider dismisses their questions about obscure supplements, but in reality it is a defense mechanism against looking ignorant. Everyone should step back a little and take a deep breath.

Part III:
And In This Corner, The Undisputed CAM-pions Of The World (Almost)

The following is a compilation of supplements almost universally accepted as complementary to standard medical care. In this usage, complementary care means supplements that enhance standard medical care. Within this list are vitamins, minerals, fish oil, and aspirin. These supplements have solid science backing their use in the treatment and prevention of disease. There is also a fair amount of information about safety and predictable risks with these agents. In short, they fall into the "known-safe-helpful" category instead of the "unknown-possibly-unsafe" category that many of the others fall into. The latter category constitutes most of the controversial herbs and botanicals women are most curious about.

The evidence for supplementing the diet with **calcium** and **vitamin D** is rock solid. Menopausal women are at significant risk of developing osteoporosis, thin bones, particularly if they do not take Menopausal Hormone Therapy. Osteoporosis may result in debilitating fractures that could be the first domino that falls along a line that leads all the way to death.

Calcium and vitamin D prevent and treat osteopenia and osteoporosis (Chapter 26) if taken in the proper amounts. The recommended doses are *in addition* to what is consumed in a normal diet. The recommended daily amount of calcium citrate is 1500 mg. Calcium citrate may be easier on sensitive stomachs than calcium carbonate and can be taken with or without food. To assure proper absorption it should be divided into three doses. Calcium occurs naturally in dairy products: milk, cheese, and yogurt. Vitamin D3 should be supplemented daily at 4000 IU for any woman (or man) who wants to decrease her mortality rate. Unless you live in Rio and spend a lot of time in a bikini on the beach you are almost certainly deficient in vitamin D. In addition to the bone benefits of calcium, vitamin D has been reported to significantly decrease the following:

- Breast cancer by an astounding 80 percent
- Colon cancer also by an astounding 80 percent
- Prostate cancer
- Cancer deaths
- Leukemia
- Diabetes
- Hypertension
- Cardiovascular disease
- Swaying and falling by 50 percent
- Nail thinness
- Muscle loss and weakness
- Excess parathyroid hormone
- Psoriasis
- Parkinson's disease
- Rheumatoid arthritis
- Multiple sclerosis

- Respiratory infections
- Alzheimer's disease
- Mood matters
- Insomnia
- Frailty by 50 percent
- Mortality by 30 percent

Vitamin D is also known to reduce falls by reducing the swaying and balance problems frequently encountered in elderly women. Incidentally, Vitamin D also decreases prostate cancer; if you know anyone who has one, let him know. Because of these health benefits, all women should consider being screened annually for their vitamin D blood level (25(OH)D). Vitamin D occurs naturally by exposing skin to the sun and in wild oily fish like salmon.

The evidence favoring **fish oil** supplementation is strong, and the recommended dose is 2 grams to 3 grams a day. Fish oil (omega three fatty acid) is deficient in the majority of western-style diets and is readily available as a supplement. Like all supplements, fish oil manufacturers are not regulated for quality or purity by the government. Therefore, it seems prudent to purchase quality supplements from established manufacturers. Ask your pharmacist for recommendations. Be careful not to rely on the advice of a teenager working part-time at a health food store. For omega three fatty acid there is also a prescription product available, Lovaza with documented science attesting to its ability to favorably effect blood lipids to reduce cardiovascular disease. Fish oil for menopause reduces Hot Flash Fevers and Vagina Sahara. There are many other unproven benefits that may come to light with more research. Look for fish oil that is "de-odorized" and try taking them with a meal. Burping a fishy smell is a distinct obstacle for some. Flax seed oil is another option.

A quality **multivitamin** delivers essential nutrients that could possibly be missing in a general American diet and poses very little risk. Women's One A Day is a good one for perimenopause because it contains iron; however, one a Day Women's 50 Plus Advantage for postmenopause or *any* woman without a uterus is recommended. If a diet consisting of whole real foods were substituted for the fast food-snack, food-junk, food-fake, food-like substances, diet supplements like a multivitamin would be unnecessary.

Many experts continue to recommend **vitamin C** at 1,000 mg daily because of reports that it decreases infections, cervical cancer, heart disease, and low sperm count. Vitamin C occurs naturally in citrus fruits, green vegetables, tomatoes, and potatoes.

Folic acid, also known as vitamin B9, is an underrated supplement, and women might consider supplementing their diets with 400 to 800 mcg every day, particularly if she is taking either cycle control pills (birth control pills) or menopause hormone therapy, or enjoys her wine. Eighty-eight percent of women in North America are believed to be relatively deficient in Folic Acid. It protects the breast from the possible harmful effects of alcohol and decreases the risk of metabolic syndrome. It also reduces the incidence of certain birth defects; any woman who could get pregnant should definitely take it on a regular basis. Folic acid occurs naturally in green leafy vegetables and whole grain breads.

There are several possible advantages of taking **vitamin B6** at 100 mg daily including control of Mood Matters, bloating, PMS, nausea, and hair loss. Vitamin B6 occurs naturally in whole grains and organ meats (euuuw).

Vitamin E has gone from superstar to an average Joe supplement in the past few years. Much of the hype about anti-oxidants has not panned-out in the real world. The body regulates the amount of oxidation/anti-oxidation very tightly, the same way it regulates pH; therefore, trying to control it from the outside just screws-up the system. For instance, relatively high doses of vitamin E (more than 800 mg daily) supplementation were associated with a higher all-cause mortality compared to low vitamin E supplementation. Most experts still recommend vitamin E at the level of 200 IU to as much as 400 IU daily. For menopause, vitamin E decreases hot flashes, breast tenderness, and treats the skin. Vitamin E occurs naturally in nuts, seeds, whole grains, and vegetable oils.

Low dose **aspirin**, in the opinion of most experts, is a conventional medical therapy. Because it is sold over-the-counter, it is included here for completeness. Low dose aspirin reduces the risks of heart attack and thrombotic stroke and should be considered for all perimenopausal women and beyond. There are well-defined risks like GI bleeding and side effects of even low dose aspirin; therefore, consultation with a healthcare provider is recommended before initiation.

Part IV:
Ho-Humm CAMs

Many CAMs fall into the ho-humm category because they have little or no proven medical benefits compared to placebo; and yet, they pose no potential harm. To be fair, an important scientific point should be made. Science is an experimental field dependent upon systematic study, observation, tests, documentation, logic, and reason. The ability to prove scientifically that a substance is more effective than an alternate therapy or even more effective than a placebo requires a lot of effort, time, and most of all, money. Generally speaking, research money is invested only into substances that can be patented because the motive for the investment is, of course, a return on investment. Because supplements are often "naturally occurring", they cannot be patented; therefore, who wants to invest money to study them: individuals, companies, universities, the government?

We are left with marginal hard science and a lot of personal opinions based upon "soft science". It is entirely possible one day in the near future, someone will investigate some of these CAM products and prove once and for all some do provide a benefit (or not). The FDA does not regulate supplements; and from time to time, manufacturers and retailers may make assertions about the benefits of certain products. Internet experts, entertainment personalities, and popular TV shows do not represent unbiased information either. As a rule, it is best to double check with your doctor and reliable online medical resources like the Mayo Clinic, North American Menopause Society, and WebMD before consuming any supplement.

If only 10 percent of the positive things attributed to **soy** supplements were true, it would be a true wonder drug. Soybeans are ubiquitous, nutritious, and cheap. Among other possible benefits, soybeans contain organic compounds that act like weak estrogens in women and are termed phytoestrogens. Those substances are not hormones, neither human nor plant, but by a quirk of nature, they have some affinity for the human estradiol receptor. They may slightly reduce, but not eliminate, hot flashes in women who suffer from mild vasomotor symptoms short term, from three to twelve weeks, but are not proven to be more effective than placebo long term. There are no known benefits to bone, heart, and vagina. There are some promising preliminary studies with soy on maintaining cognitive function and a small positive effect in treating mild hot flashes short term without known risks of breast and uterus stimulation.

At least soy is believed to be safe. As a caution, it is important to note if soy phytoestrogens are working to relieve vasomotor symptoms through activation of the estrogen receptor then they may possess some of the same risks as prescription estrogen plus the added risk of uncertain dose and purity. Phytoestrogens are promoted, by many, as the "natural" way to treat hot flashes, but what is not told is that they may have similar risks and side effects as prescriptions without any of the Government approved status. Wouldn't everyone prefer to take, for instance, an apple for a sinus infection rather than Keflex because it is more natural? Sure. But does it work; does it have pesticides on it; and how many have to be taken.

Homeopathic medicine theories contend that a poison causing certain harmful symptoms can be diluted down to an ultra low dose and given to eliminate those types of symptoms. It is a fascinating theory with a much wider acceptance in Europe than in North America. Several noted conventional biochemists have mathematically calculated that for many homeopathic recipes, the number of active molecules in the treatment is zero. Although that would certainly make it safe, it is a stretch of the imagination to understand how it could help. There are none known to be effective in the treatment of menopausal symptoms.

Skin surface **magnets** were quite the rage in the last decade as a treatment for a variety of ailments, but all formal studies have failed to identify any advantage of real magnets over sham metal plates. No harm would be expected.

All the items in this category share a common recommendation. If you want to try it and it seems to work for you, and you can afford it; then, by all means give it a try. As mentioned earlier, science does not have all the answers to these products and is not likely to any time soon.

Acupuncture has steadily gained support for use in a few specific circumstances such as nausea after surgery, menstrual cramps, fibromyalgia pain, and addiction. It has not been found to be helpful with menopausal symptoms like hot flashes, night sweats, vaginal dryness, or mood swings. In the hands of a well-trained professional, acupuncture is safe; however, acupuncture is not recommended as a treatment for menopausal symptoms.

After years of studies, **Glucosamine and Chondroitin** are still not conclusively known to have any lasting benefit for arthritis pain. That said, everyone knows someone for whom glucosamine changed her life: from near bed-ridden cripple to marathon runner. Perhaps, some day it will be known why certain individuals respond to certain supplements more than others. If you have the money, and it works for you, it might be worth it for you.

Traditional Chinese Medicine (TCM) is a combination of therapies. Some parts are similar to standard medical recommendations. Many women obtain some menopause symptom amelioration with meditation, breathing exercises, massage, and diet controls which are all included in forms of traditional Chinese medicine practice. Most people think of TCM as primarily herbs and special teas that have been perfected through centuries of use. There is not a great body of evidence regarding the benefits of the use of Chinese herbs in the treatment of menopausal symptoms, but since some of the teas taste great, try green tea for hair loss and chamomile tea for sleep.

Biofeedback is a technologically advanced technique to help women achieve a primitive psychological realm: relaxation. Who couldn't use a little of that? There is no harm being hooked-up to the monitors, and some women report menopause improvements after training. Any form of relaxation gets the brain into a similar brain wave state, whether it is biofeedback, progressive muscle relaxation, deep breathing, guided imagery, yoga, or meditative prayer. All forms have shown documented improvements in mood, sleep, pain, and feelings of well-being.

Cranberry juice is recommended as a temporizing treatment for lower urinary tract infections (UTI, cystitis). Cranberry juice works by preventing bacteria from adhering to the wall of the urinary tract. It has a role in the prevention of chronic UTIs, but its effect in treating an acute UTI is somewhat controversial. It is red and tastes great. Help yourself to a glass if you are not taking blood thinners, but take an antibiotic if you have an infection.

Licorice candy is fine for consuming at the movies, but concentrated licorice supplements have no effectiveness for treating menopausal symptoms and may increase blood pressure.

Part V:
Buyer Beware

Everyone has heard the saying, "There is no such thing as a free lunch". That means whoever offers you a "free" lunch is probably expecting to get something else out of you that you value and do not really want to give up. As far as herbs and other supplements for menopause symptoms are concerned, there is no such thing as a product that is effective without having some side effects and consequences.

There is tremendous interest among women to go through menopause without hormones and to treat the natural symptoms "naturally" with natural products instead of prescription products, but natural does not mean safer. The term "natural" is so complicated it will be discussed more fully later. Use of the following products by menopausal women may be as high as 40 percent. It might be fair to mention here that whole food and water are perfectly natural items to consume, but what is natural about consuming a concentrated extract from a plant you would never eat?

The most commonly used herb by menopausal women for the self-treatment of hot flashes is: **black cohosh** (Actaea racemosa). Studies of black cohosh are contradictory. Slight short-term effectiveness has been shown for the management of mild vasomotor symptoms. Reports of serious liver damage have surfaced, as well as, some milder GI problems. It may be tried for mild vasomotor symptoms for less than three months if liver function is concurrently monitored. This product suffers the same problems as all the other CAMs, lack of sophisticated systematic research. It is very hard to recommend products without knowing their risks. Asking only whether they may be helpful is only half of the real question. Are they safe is the important other half of the question. For example, many women have an unwarranted fear of hormones causing breast cancer, so they take black cohosh for their debilitating Hot Dreads. What are the risks of black cohosh?

Ginkgo Biloba has been promoted for the prevention and treatment of dementia, ringing in the ears, and peripheral vascular disease. There are a few positive studies supporting its claims for dementia. It causes bleeding disorders and should be used cautiously. It has no known benefit for menopause.

Red Clover (Trifolium pratense) has been tried for the same reasons that women try black cohosh: Hot Flash Fever. Studies are inconsistent, but as with black cohosh, some women insist they experience some improvement on Red Clover. It is fairly safe but might have harmful effects on hormone-sensitive tissues.

St John's Wort (Hyperricum perforatum) may be considered for the treatment of mild depression. It probably has a positive effect short-term but has not undergone long-term safety or effectiveness trials. St John's Wort has many drug interactions, so a complete pharmacological drug interaction report should be performed before using this product. Break through vaginal bleeding has occurred when used with cycle control pills (birth control pills), and it may cause irritability, insomnia, and light sensitivity.

Dong Quai (Angelica Sinensis) is another TCM botanical often tried by menopausal women for the relief of hot flashes. There are essentially no studies to support its use. In addition, Dong quai may have serious bleeding side effects.

Ginseng (Panax spp.) has traditionally been used in Chinese medicine for diabetes and fatigue, but the evidence for its use is insufficient. It may have an effect in reducing mild mood matters in menopausal women. It has no known effect on hot flashes, and like many other herbs, it may affect bleeding parameters.

Evening Primrose Oil (Oenothera Biennis) has been heavily marketed for the relief of hot flashes, and along with Dong Quai is a component of virtually every health food store combination menopause product. There is no evidence that it is more effective in relieving hot flashes than a placebo. Unlike the placebo, however, it has significant risks and side effects such as nausea, inflammation, seizures, and bleeding disorders.

Kava kava (Piper methysticum) is another TCM that has been frequently mentioned as a treatment for anxiety and hot flashes. There is some weak evidence that it calms anxiety at the risk of causing liver failure, sedation, and rash. It has no known benefit for relieving hot flashes.

Coenzyme Q10 (Co-Q-10) is promoted for heart failure, hypertension, angina, and Parkinson's Disease. It is generally well tolerated but may cause some bleeding problems. There is inconclusive evidence to support its effectiveness. It has no known benefit in treating any menopausal symptoms.

DHEA is a pro-hormone touted by some as a safer and more effective treatment for menopause. In truth, this is a compound with unknown risks. Why is it some people want to believe that unknown risks are presumed to be less risk than known risks? DHEA has no known receptor and uncertain target tissue. The risk for the uterus and breast are completely unknown. Beware.

Sorry if this all sounds a bit like a broken record. There may be some honest differences of opinion about some of the research; but on the whole, with the exception of vitamins, minerals, and fish oil, hardly any of the CAM products are very effective in relieving the symptoms they are purported to relieve. Particularly when it comes to relieving hot flashes, night sweats, mood swings, and vaginal dryness, CAM products just don't do much. There remain many women who, by personal experience, believe otherwise; but so far, the studies just don't support their use. They come with undetermined risks and side effects of which the consumer may be unaware. The North American Menopause Society (NAMS) states that evidence for safety and/or effectiveness is lacking for topical progesterone cream, dong quai, evening primrose oil, ginkgo, ginseng, licorice, Chinese herb mixtures, acupuncture, and magnet therapy. For that reason, NAMS does not recommend their use for the symptomatic relief of hot flashes.

Part VI:
When All The Dust Has Settled

The advantages of taking a botanical herb for health problems fall into one of four categories:

1. Consumption of an herb or botanical supplement is a self-directed affirmation of independence from the medical establishment. Taking responsibility for your own health is a *very* good thing. Almost everyone, at some point, wants to take charge of her own matters and not be required to rely on someone else (like a healthcare provider) to dictate or approve of what she does. In this regard, taking supplements is logical.

2. There is no point denying the enormous market pressure to buy stuff that is advertized and bought by everyone else, and it's fun to try something new. Falling victim to marketing is normal, welcome to the human race.

3. Standard medical care is expensive for unknown reasons. Standard medical care is often impersonal at the most inopportune times (like when getting a pelvic). Standard medical care puts up an invisible shield that pretends to know everything, when everyone knows it doesn't. Rejecting standard medical care has its points. It does not have to be that way. (CAM products are usually expensive too.)

4. The allure of "natural" is powerful. We all believe doing something natural is probably doing something the way "it is supposed to be", but supposed to be where, the Garden of Eden? We believe in natural childbirth, until we realize

that during natural childbirth, up until the 1950s, mothers and newborns died at alarming rates. Medical intervention in childbirth prevents thousands of deaths a year. Humans were endowed with the intelligence to figure things out for a good reason. At this point, the term "natural" has been co-opted by marketing gurus until it has lost all true meaning.

When all the dust has settled, there remains only one treatment known to be both safe and effective for all of the moderate or severe menopausal symptoms. There is only one treatment that restores the substance that is lacking in menopausal problems. There is only one treatment that the government-backed FDA has approved for the treatment of moderate to severe Hot Flash Fever, Vagina Sahara, and the prevention of osteoporosis: Menopausal Hormone Therapy, MHT. Currently, there are no other pharmacological or non-pharmacological treatments available that control the symptoms of perimenopause and the menopause as effectively and safely as menopause hormone therapy.

Part VII:
The Womenopause Challenge: You CAM Do These Two Too

1. Take the recommended supplements everyday: vitamin D 4000 IU, calcium citrate 1500 mg, a multivitamin, fish oil 2 g, vitamin C 1000 mg, vitamin E 400 IU, folic acid 800 mcg.
2. If you are experiencing moderate or severe hot flashes, night sweats, or osteoporosis, ask your health care provider about MHT.

Chapter 18

Sexercise: Romantic Aerobics For Outercourse and Innercourse

Part I:
Welcome

For those readers who glanced through the table of contents, skipped all the other stuff, and opened straight to the sex chapter: welcome. You will not be disappointed. As memorialized by Grocho Marx, "Sex is here to stay." He is right, of course: sex is not going away.

Sex will always be an important aspect of well-being for almost everyone, and sex will forever be a mysteriously essential ingredient of love. Intimacy promotes physical well-being. Sexual intercourse, that leads to physical and emotional satisfaction, complements intimacy but is not the object of it. During perimenopause and the wUpSide, physical, emotional, and relationship factors may impact intimacy. Real love is the gift of physical, emotional, and communal attraction, wrapped in mature commitment, tied with a bow of intimacy.

When the space shuttle takes off, there are millions of mechanical and electrical parts working flawlessly together. The captain pushes a switch and brings to life all the work and rehearsals of preparation. *Every* component has a critical role. A good sex life is similar, only more complicated. An examination of the elements of the sexual response make it seem miraculous it could ever all work together, for two people at the same time. In fact, it is a miracle.

Part II:
The Lamenting Facts

Sex is more important than sports. Why would that even need to be said? Because if a survey of standard medical textbooks were performed, it would be obvious that sports matter in medicine, but sex is inconsequential. There are whole chapters about sprained ankles in every single medical textbook, but a recent quick survey of textbooks for gynecologists, doctors who specialize in the care of women's female health, did not find a single chapter about sexual disorders. Astounding. If the average healthcare provider was only 10 percent as proficient with sex disorders as she was with sprained ankles, there would be a lot more sexually fulfilled couples. That is not to say sports injuries are unimportant because nearly 8 percent of Americans have a current sports related problem. In contrast to this, 50 percent of adult Americans of all ages are reported to have a sexual problem. Humm... 8 percent verses 50 percent. Sex needs to taken more seriously by physicians and couples.

Physicians and other healthcare providers, as a rule, do not deal with sex problems for two simple reasons:

1. 70 percent of women believe their doctor would be too embarrassed to discuss sex with them.
2. 75 percent of women believe even if they did bring up a sex problem, it would be a waste of time because they assume there are no treatments available for sex problems anyway.

The first reason probably has some merit, but the second one is absolutely wrong. It's time for a menopausal sex makeover.

Part III:
Sexual Outercourse

Sexual activity is based upon things that exist inside and

outside the body. External factors are the usual suspects accused of any and all sex problems. The standard joke about sexual problems draws from a different analogy pertaining to real estate values: it's relationship, relationship, relationship. The relationship dysfunction often harkens back to the notion that a good marriage is based on give and take. It is not. Successful marriage is based upon giving and giving. Sexual partners may have their own sexual dysfunctions. Identifying problems, then working around them or getting them treated may result in

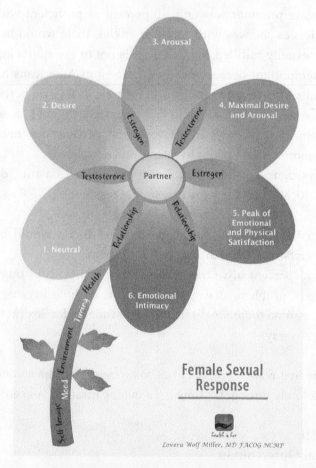

Figure 18-1 Female Sexual Response

improvements, but concentrating exclusively on partner problems is shortsighted.

Outercourse norms are the subjective ideas society seems to endorse about sex patterns for women. Those expectations may exert enormous pressure upon women and are frequently overlooked. Social conventions may vary significantly depending upon gender, age, and ethnicity.

Part IV:
Sexual Innercourse

Interior factors that govern sexual activity include psychological, interpersonal, and biological. Mood disorders such as depression, have a complicated and dramatic effect on sexual functioning. In addition to that, some standard medical treatments for depression actually worsen sexual function while it improves mood: more on that later. Interpersonal relationships are a two-way street. Some relationships are eight-lane super highways, while others are impassable, narrow dirt rutted lanes. How your partner acts is external, but how you act is internal.

For the best sex life possible, focusing on the parts of the relationship that come under your control instead of concentrating on finding fault in your partner, is more likely to yield improvement.

Biological factors play a bigger role in the sexual response than many women and their doctors realize. In perimenopause, women may experience progressive vaginal dryness. In truth, vaginal dryness is only a small part of what is going on. The entire external and internal sex organs may become desensitized resulting in both lack of pleasure with sex and dyspareunia, pain with sex. Repeated unpleasant sexual experiences prod the psyche away from sexual desire. It can be a vicious circle: much more on that later.

Genuine sexual intercourse satisfaction is possible only when the sexual innercourse and outercourse are optimally healthy.

Part V:
Sex Dissection

Unfortunately, many women shy away from a discussion about sex as if keeping sex shrouded in mystery might help it remain mysterious. Imagine what it would be like if we left the rest of our body functions mysterious. In times past, people dropped like flies from heart attacks. Somewhere along the line a free thinker took out a knife, cut open a chest, and sliced open a coronary artery. They found the artery was clogged with gunk. Today we have lifestyle options, lipid lowering drugs, stents, and bypasses that would never have existed except for a brave dissection. The female sexual response should be dissected, and the parts identified so solutions can be found.

The female sexual response (Figure 18-1) charts a formal evaluation of sexual function. Beginning on the lower left side of the flower, find the first petal, **Neutral**. All women will have periods of sexual neutrality when there are no apparent sexual thoughts. The duration of these times is highly variable within a person and from one person to another. To move from **Neutral** to the next petal there needs to be either an internal motivation or an external force such as a partner's initiation. If the input is sufficient and facilitated with some hormones, there is an advance to **Desire**. With additional input from partner and hormones, development of **Arousal** is achieved, and physical changes begin to be noticeable with increased blood flow to the genitals and the creation of vaginal lubrication. As the sexual response progresses, there is a confluence of **Desire** and **Arousal**, a positive emotional—physical feedback loop that drives the response to **Maximal Desire and Arousal**. Encouraged by the hormone helpers, this leads to the **Peak of Emotional and Physical Satisfaction** (with or without orgasm). There is significant variability all along this response cycle. The complementary interaction of the physical, emotional, and relationship factors produces a state of enhanced **Emotional Intimacy**. It is believed repeated satisfying intimate experiences raises the baseline level of sexual neutrality, which positively inspires future sexual experiences to continue to reinforce the process. What a miracle!

Part VI:
What Can Go Wrong

It always seems a little perverse to understand what is great about something by looking first at its problems. An intimate sexual relationship, for most women, is one of the most wonderful part of their lives. When their sex life suffers, their whole life may be thrown off. The following list shows some of the things that may go awry. The next section will outline some sex solutions.

1. **Low Estrogen:** The most common, the most overlooked, and the easiest to treat female sexual dysfunction is Vagina Sahara. Although uncommon during the reproductive years, wMonday and wTuesday, vaginal dryness may affect 75 percent of women wFriday and beyond, the wUpSide. The first sign of the problem appearing during perimenopause may be reduced vaginal lubrication. For many women, vaginal dryness progresses to impaired sexual pleasure. The vagina and the external female organs, called the vulva, are strongly influenced by circulating 17beta-estradiol. The estrogen hormone exerts essential growth stimulation to all the involved tissues. When estrogen production becomes erratic during the ovaries' declining function of perimenopause, the tissues of the sex organs begin to suffer. There are gradual changes in the thickness and texture of the labia and vagina, resulting in loss of lubrication and thinning of the mucosa. There develops a change in the sensory nerves imbedded within the atrophying mucosa internally and externally; they cannot give as much positive feedback

during sexual stimulation. Thus, there develops reduced sexual arousal with less blood flow engorgement of the sex organs, which in turn leads to diminished sexual desire. Reduction of arousal often leads to impaired ability to achieve sexual satisfaction or orgasm. No stretch, no lube, no arousal, and no desire may add up to "no go" for some women. Even though a woman may start out with a normal sexual desire, repeated unpleasant sexual experiences may curb that desire (Figure 18-1) and shift her baseline **Neutral** down a couple notches. When the problem of painful sex, dyspareunia, comes to the forefront, **Emotional Intimacy** problems might be expected to follow close behind. In addition to the obvious and direct effects on the vagina and the vulva, diminished estrogen exerts a major influence on the brain and cardiovascular system (by impairing arterial blood flow). Sexual desire, arousal, and orgasm are all modulated by centrally acting, as well as, peripherally acting estrogen.

2. **Low Testosterone**: Women and men have both estrogen and testosterone. Women have a lot more estrogen than testosterone (one-tenth as much as men), and men have a lot more testosterone than estrogen, but both are important. The small amount of testosterone women do have plays an important role in their sexual **Desire**, and **Peak of Emotional and Physical Satisfaction**. The ovary is the primary source of female testosterone production. It is not from the eggs or follicles of the ovary but from stromal support tissue within the ovary. There is not an abrupt change of testosterone at menopause such as seen with estrogen. Testosterone just naturally, slightly declines over time, and it may begin, for some women, in their thirties and then stay relatively stable for decades. Sexual desire can be approximated by consideration of the frequency with which a woman has sexual thoughts and fantasies

compared to prior times in her life. Low testosterone may result in diminished motivation and desire for sex, as well as impaired sexual sensitization. Hypoactive Sexual Desire Disorder (HSDD) is a medical diagnosis that encompasses low sexual desire when it is accompanied with personal distress. Some women, particularly after menopause, may become less interested in sex for a number of reasons, but if it does not bother them, it is definitely not a "disorder". Induced menopause after hysterectomy and oophorectomy (removal of the uterus and ovaries) may incite a dramatic immediate change in estrogen and testosterone with predictable negative effects on sexual function. This is true for testosterone even if the surgery is during the wUpSide because postmenopausal ovaries continue to secrete small amounts of testosterone. Removing the ovaries will reduce the testosterone level by 50 percent.

3. **High SHBG:** Okay, this part is going to be a little technical but, in the end, will be clearly important. Both estrogen and testosterone are transported through the blood stream to the target tissues by being bound to Sex Hormone Binding Globulin (SHBG). Think of SHBG as the hormone "bus" picking up kids (estrogen and testosterone) at school (ovary) and dropping them off at their homes (target tissues). The only kids that can get off the bus are the ones closest to the door. SHBG holds estrogen and testosterone tightly, and only a very small percentage gets "free" and able to exert it's influence by getting off the bus. *Oral hormones* (but not transdermal hormones), both cycle control pills (birth control pills) and menopause hormone therapy (MHT), have a tendency to increase the amount of SHBG resulting in lower "free" (active) testosterone. More on this in Chapter 21. Analogous to making the bus much bigger, the kids cannot find their way to the door in order to exit. In this way oral but not transdermal hormone

therapy may interfere with sexual response by reducing the amount of free active testosterone. It is one of the strangest medical ironies: birth control pills may free some women to potentially enjoy sexual encounters more, but may at the same time, reduce the desire to have them. Lowered SHBG levels develop in 20 percent of wUpSide women, elevating the amount of "free" active testosterone, and they may experience a spontaneous increase in sexual desire, described as the menopausal zest. Forty percent experience no change, and 40 percent have reduction in their "free" active testosterone. Women in their sixties may have about one-half of the amount of total testosterone than women in their twenties, but the "free" active testosterone level (only 1 to 2 percent of the total testosterone) may remain relatively stable. Continuing sexual activity is a realistic and expected part of the wUpSide.

4. **Mood disorders**: Major Depressive Disorder (MDD) is a serious health problem and warrants expert medical/psychiatric care. More prevalent is its well-known cousin, depression. Depression is common among women of all ages and may contribute to impaired sexual function. Neurotransmitters in the brain that are involved with mood production are also involved in aspects of normal brain sexual response.

5. **Medications:** There are many prescription medications with known negative effects on women's sexual function. As mentioned above, SHBG might rise with treatment with any oral hormone therapy (oral contraceptives, or oral MHT)) with a resulting decline in free testosterone. Lower testosterone in women is correlated with impaired desire and arousal. Some antidepressants may interfere with normal sexual desire by causing alterations of brain neurotransmitters. The classic antidepressants in the class called **SSRI's** (Serotonin Specific Reuptake Inhibitors) may result

in impaired sexual function for some women. It is an interesting dilemma because depression by itself has a tremendous negative effect on sexual function and treatment for the depression with an SSRI reliably helps mood but not the sexual function. Antidepressant-induced sexual dysfunction is often underestimated. Typical product names of SSRI's are Prozac, Zoloft, Celexa, Lexapro, and Paxil. **SNRI** (Serotonin Norepinephrine Reuptake Inhibitors), a slightly different group of antidepressants have less effect on sexual function. Typical products of the SNRI are: Effexor, Cymbalta, and Pristiq. Wellbutrin, a **DNRI** (Dopamine Norepinephrine Reuptake Inhibitors) antidepressant, may improve both mood and sexual function (Chapter 12). Certain antihypertensive medications may interfere with the female sexual response. Corticosteroids used to treat severe asthma or arthritis, may interfere with sexual function. All illicit drugs, especially marijuana, impede arousal, delay orgasm, and diminish sexual pleasure. Progestins are not wBodyIdentical progesterone and may interfere with sex.

6. **Dyspareunia:** Genital pain with intercourse interferes with female sexual health. The three common types are: 1) **Vulvodynia:** Pain and chronic discomfort in the vulva, often described as a burning pain without objective findings or specific signs of a neurological disorder, may represent Vulvodynia. It may be present, to a degree, in 7 percent of sexually active women. It has no known cause, but there are treatments available. 2) **Vaginismus:** Involuntary painful muscle spasm of the vagina may make penetration difficult or impossible. It may be present in a small minority of women. 3) **Pelvic Pain:** There are numerous causes for pain arising from structures located in the pelvis and lower abdomen. This is rarely found in wUpSide women.

7. **Serious Health Problems**: Cardiovascular disease, Diabetes, and the Metabolic Syndrome are insidious saboteurs of normal sexual health. They undermine the neurovascular response to arousal and impede the Peak of Emotional and Physical Satisfaction. In a roundabout way, being full or fulsome figured, with a BMI over 30, reduces sexual enjoyment. Sexperts believe that a deterioration of body image negatively effects sexual desire by reducing a woman's confidence in her "attractiveness". Women who smoke have significantly more problems with sex than non-smokers (another reason to quit smoking). Lower urinary track dysfunction interferes with sexual function. It may be related to relative lack of estrogen needed to stimulate normal health of the urethra and bladder.

8. **Relationship Dysfunction**: It takes two to tango. Partner problems quickly become "couple" problems. Many mistakenly dismiss male sexual disorders as simply erectile dysfunction. Men are people too! They participate in approximately the same sexual response cycle as women. There are as many places along the way where men can have the same malfunction as women can. Being open to an evaluation of sexual disorders is socially harder for men to accept than for women. It is relatively painless for men to focus on erections and order Viagra over the Internet. That rarely fixes a relationship disorder. It does little to improve a couple's sexual health to focus exclusively upon the woman's problem and to ignore the man's, and vice versa. It is now recognized that men experience a gradual decline in testosterone production with age. By age 50, forty percent of men may have a measurable deficiency in testosterone (Chapter 25: *Man*opause). Partner health problems, mood disorders, problems with intimacy, and lack of general knowledge about sex also put up roadblocks to a satisfactory sexual relationship.

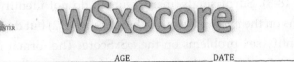

NAME_____AGE_____DATE_____

Instructions: Please circle one answer on the right for each question.

	o	S	E	X
#1 How often do you have sex thoughts or fantasies? 0) once or more a day S) a few times a week E) a few times, or so, a month X) a few times, or less, a year	*o*	*S*	*E*	*X*
#2 How often do you have sex? 0) more than once a week S) a few times a month E) about once, or so, a month X) a few times, or less, a year	*o*	*S*	*E*	*X*
#3 How often do you experience an orgasm? 0) most of the time S) about half of the time E) occasionally X) never, or almost never	*o*	*S*	*E*	*X*

Please indicate (by circling 0, S, E, or X) how much of a problem you view the following to be

0) not a problem S) minor problem E) moderate problem X) major problem

	0	S	E	X
#4 a feeling of well-being	0	S	E	X
#5 a stable relationship with your partner	0	S	E	X
#6 intimacy with your partner	0	S	E	X
#7 your desire for sex	0	S	E	X
#8 your arousal during sex (turned-on)	0	S	E	X
#9 partner's erection	0	S	E	X
#10 lubrication during with sex	0	S	E	X
#11 pain associated with sex	0	S	E	X
#12 medical or physical issues that interfere with sex	0	S	E	X
#13 distressed about your sex life	0	S	E	X
#14 depressed mood	0	S	E	X
#15 satisfaction with your sex life	0	S	E	X
#16 your partners satisfaction with his sex life	0	S	E	X

Number_____   wSxScore: _____

Figure 18-2 *w*SxScore

Part VII:
*w*SxScore: Measuring Love Making

The *w*SxScore (Figure 18-2) is a simple tool to gauge sexual function in women. There is a corresponding *m*SxScore for men

(Figure 18-3). Surprisingly, many women do not identify sexual problems on the *w*Score Sexercise box (Figure 1-2) but do open up and identify sex problems on the *w*SxScore. The format is much like the *w*Score, and the scoring is done by adding up the

Pain CENTER

mSxScore

NAME_____AGE_____DATE_____

Instructions: *Please circle one answer on the right for each question.*

	a	b	c	d
#1 How often do you have sex thoughts or fantasies? a) once or more a day b) a few times a week c) a few times, or so, a month d) a few times, or less, a year	*a*	*b*	*c*	*d*
#2 How often do you have sex? a) more than once a week b) a few times a month c) about once, or so, a month d) a few times, or less, a year	*a*	*b*	*c*	*d*
#3 How often do you experience an orgasm? a) most of the time b) about half of the time c) occasionally d) never, or almost never	*a*	*b*	*c*	*d*

Instructions: *Please circle one answer for each question to indicate how much of a problem each of the following are :   a) no problem b) mild problem c) moderate problem d) major problem*

	a	b	c	d
#4 a feeling of well-being	*a*	*b*	*c*	*d*
#5 a stable relationship with your partner (spouse)	*a*	*b*	*c*	*d*
#6 intimacy with your partner	*a*	*b*	*c*	*d*
#7 desire for sex	*a*	*b*	*c*	*d*
#8 arousal during sex (get turned-on)	*a*	*b*	*c*	*d*
#9 get and maintain an erection	*a*	*b*	*c*	*d*
#10 your partner gets aroused (wet) with sex	*a*	*b*	*c*	*d*
#11 pain associated with sex	*a*	*b*	*c*	*d*
#12 medical or physical problems that interfere with sex	*a*	*b*	*c*	*d*
#13 distressed about your sex life	*a*	*b*	*c*	*d*
#14 depressed mood	*a*	*b*	*c*	*d*
#15 your personal overall satisfaction with your sex life	*a*	*b*	*c*	*d*
#16 your partners overall satisfaction with her sex life	*a*	*b*	*c*	*d*

Number_____   mSxScore_____

Figure 18-3 *m*SxScore

"points" for each question. For example, question #1 asks, "How often do you have sexual thoughts or fantasies?" Answers are "0" for once or more a day, "S" a few times a week, "E" a few times, or so, a month, and "X" a few times, or less, a year. Simply circle the correct response. The "0" counts for zero points, the "S" counts for one point, the "E" counts for two points, and the "X" counts for three points. (Notice that the answers are completely subjective, and only you would know the correct answer, and yes, it is true, the answers spell-out "Oh sex" and corresponds to zero, one, two, or three points). Add all the points for the 16 questions and place the total on the line at the bottom. The wSxScore is useful for comparisons between before and after treatment for sexual disorders (if present). It also serves as an icebreaker to allow a more thorough discussion about sex and sexual relationships. The wSxScore brings into focus the components of the sexual response cycle that may be misfiring such as low desire, poor arousal, problems with orgasm, problems with pain, and relationship complications.

For many women, the Womenopause Challenge renews their interest in all aspects of their health and well-being. Improvement in their sex lives often occurs as a bonus without specific sex therapy.

Maryjane J.

Maryjane, age 50, was considered to be the smartest OR nurse among many talented nurses at the Regional Medical Center. With 25 years of experience she never quit learning. Frank, her husband of 28 years, farmed 700 acres of family land mostly in beans and corn. At age 52, he was a kind and humble "Adonis-in-overalls".

One was as intense as the other, and they proved the saying, "If you want to get anything done, ask a busy person to do it." Frank and Maryjane were givers: active in family, with neighbors, at church, and involved in many community projects.

Their three kids had completed school. Two were married, and the prospects for the third were looking up. The two of them rattled around inside the large farm home and had a happy respectful marriage.

For Maryjane's first gynecology visit in four years, there was a lot to "catch up on". She weighed 165 pounds and was 5'5" tall with a calculated BMI=27. Her total wScore (Figure 1-2) was a modest 22 W with evidence for hot flashes and vaginal dryness. She reported the date of her last menstrual period was difficult to pinpoint exactly because she had become so irregular there had been months without one. Mammogram, Pap test, and Blood work were ordered and later were confirmed to be normal. Her physical examination revealed a contracted dry vagina without evidence of any other pathology.

Maryjane's mood was uncharacteristically withdrawn during the history and exam part of her appointment. Maryjane was asked if there was anything bothering her she wanted to discuss. Then she dropped the "D-word", divorce. At first she lamented she and Frank had "just drifted apart" but soon changed it to "He does not find me attractive any more." She was fearful of anyone else finding out and was reassured anything said in the doctor's office was held strictly confidential. Maryjane's Carroll Rating Scale (CR) for measuring depression was 18, suggesting moderate depressive symptoms, and she confirmed she had lost interest in her clubs and just sat at home and ate all evening. After a few general questions about their relationship, Maryjane was asked if their sexual relationship had been suffering; and if so, for how long.

Frank and Maryjane's sex life had been on the decline since the birth of their last child. Their three times a week frequency spread out to three times a month; and before they knew it, it was three times a year, or less. The last two years had produced two huge fights about sex, and neither one felt that the other was concerned about the "real problem".

Maryjane filled out the wSxScore (Figure 18-2) to help identify any problems that might be concerning. Her score was 33 indicating significant sexual problems. By her responses it was obvious that she had potential malfunctions in several points along the Female Sexual Response cycle (Figure 18-1). Maryjane indicated that she was very distressed about her sex life. She reported zero desire, absent arousal, no orgasms, and severe relationship intimacy discord. She said that getting a divorce was the last thing she wanted to do and regretted screaming it at Frank last night.

Maryjane was advised relationships are complicated, and only the people within the relationship could know how happy or hurtful it can be. Maryjane said she wanted any and all help she could get to improve her situation and blamed herself for "most of it."

She accepted the Womenopause Challenge and agreed to start by beginning to control her nutritional supplements, diet, sleep, and mood. Maryjane was advised some of her symptoms were hormone related menopausal problems that might be alleviated by trying MHT. As an alternative she could consider counseling, antidepressants, Neurontin, and vaginal moisturizers. She opted for beginning wBodyIdentical 17beta-estradiol transdermal gel (Divigel) in the morning coupled with oral progesterone (Prometrium) in the evening, for the next 4 weeks.

Upon return, Maryjane laughed about how her husband quipped, "She stopped yellin, when she started gellin". Her wScore improved from 22 W to 6 W and her CR was down to 8. Her hot flashes were under control. She reported she and Frank had taken it slowly with sex and tried once just this past week. Although it was Frank's idea, she enjoyed sex more than she had in a long time. She thought she "got wet" after a few minutes and her "tensions melted away". She did not experience an orgasm but found the experience very rewarding. Her wSxScore lowered a few notches down to 21 (from 33).

She was advised about how different hormones interact with the Female Sexual Response cycle, and it appeared estrogen had helped with her arousal but that her desire and satisfaction functions may require the addition of another topical hormone to complement the estrogen, transdermal testosterone. Maryjane began treatment with Testim by applying one drop to the inside of her wrist daily for two weeks, and if no problems were noted, she would go up to two drops daily, thereafter. Testim is topical testosterone that is used "off label" in the U.S. for the treatment of Hypoactive Sexual Desire Disorder (HSDD). Maryjane was given extensive information about the rare potential side effects of low dose testosterone in women including oily skin, pimples, breast tenderness, and rarely, unwanted hair growth. These remit with lowering the dose. Long-term safety data about testosterone therapy for women is lacking but is currently under research.

Four weeks later Maryjane returned in a rush because she had six other things to go to that day. She and Frank had had sex once a week, and she had had two orgasms, the first she had had in more than a decade. Somewhere along the way she also realized how cute Frank's tuft of grey hair looked when he wore a ball-cap.

Part VIII:
Sex Solutions: What We've All Been Waiting For

Every problem has a solution; otherwise, it would not be a problem; it would be an enigma. For instance, the concept of time is not a "problem" because there is no solving or fixing time. Time is an enigma. Sex problems are real problems with real solutions. Therefore, the sexual problems of **Desire, Arousal, Maximal Desire and Arousal, Peak of Emotional and Physical Satisfaction,** and **Emotional Intimacy** have some known solutions. For sure, some solutions are more satisfying than others.

At the risk of sounding like a broken record, everything about menopausal health is connected. Good health is connected to good exercise, and good exercise is connected to good nutrition, and good nutrition is connected to good sleep, and good sleep is connected to good mood, and good mood is... and so on, until you connect all the way to good sex. It is all connected and important. A complex psychobiological function like sex will improve in conjunction with improvements of your biological-body and your psychological-mind. It is impossible to have a good sex life without ALL the other stuff. Accept the Womenopause Challenge, and transform your life in four weeks. Most of what can be accomplished depends upon you, not your doctor.

For women in perimenopause and wUpSide, the solution of a sexual disorder (we hope you know by now) does not involve dumping your partner straightaway.

Examine Figure 18-1 to determine possible places of inter-ference. Many women will have an element of Vagina Sahara as a jumping-off point for a menopausal disorder. Vaginal dryness is the tip of the iceberg so-to-speak. Below the surface, estrogen deficiency results in impaired touch sensation, impaired vibration sense, delayed or absent lubrication, delayed or absent orgasm, reduced sexual satisfaction, and increased discomfort and pain. Chapter 10 details the current recommendations for the relief of vaginal dryness including moisturizers and lubri-cants. A novel product, Zestra Feminine Arousal Fluid, assists some women with vaginal dryness by producing a pleasant tingling feeling in the vagina and on the labia. For any advanced form of the condition resulting in significant loss of tissue elasticity, thinning, internal and external de-sensitization, loss of spontaneous and arousal lubrication, absent labia, and pain; the best and most direct treatment is estrogen therapy. Topical and systemic estrogen cures vaginal dryness with close to 100 percent results; when used together, better results can often be obtained. Estrogen even re-grows atrophied labia. So far, research does not find medications such as Viagra to help women, like they do for men.

The female sexual response requires the coordinated activities of three distinct biological systems: the autonomic nervous system, the circulation system, and the pelvic floor muscle system. Pelvic floor muscle strength and condition can be improved through specific exercises called Kegel exercises. Here is an example of one. Imagine you are in the middle of urinating, and you are told to stop before your bladder is empty. That squeezing of the muscles around the vagina, urethra, and rectum is a contraction of the pelvic floor muscles. Practice holding that muscle contraction for ten seconds, twenty times, three times a day. It can be done almost anywhere, anytime; and the best part is, no one around you would ever guess you are working out for intercourse (and improving bladder control.)

Many women overlook the importance of a planned conducive environment for sex. In a way, perhaps, many are waiting for that spontaneous magic to overwhelm her partner (like sometime in the distant past?) and have him sweep her away in uncontrollable mad passion. Guess what, your partner is probably hoping for the same thing. There is nothing wrong with a little preparation, like having the bedroom lighted with candles, soft music playing, an opened bottle of wine, a warm shower or bath together, and most importantly, time set aside with the schedules clear and the phones and the TV off. Your partner will appreciate the gesture more than might be expressed. Talk about sex together. Reminisce about past experiences and plan future ones. Love is a sensitive and fragile thing. Some bridges take a lot of time to build (or mend). Rivers are crossed by creative bridge workers who show-up, day-in and day-out, and who stick to it.

Low sex drive, Hypoactive Sexual Desire Disorder (HSDD), is finally receiving interest as a research area for women's health. There are now accepted biological explanations for low sex drive, and it is not all attributable to "just changing and getting cranky".

The role of testosterone in generating women's sexual desire is established, but the solution to the problem remains somewhat controversial. Part of the problem involves the technical difficulties of measuring testosterone because most of it, 99 percent, is bound to SHBG. Another part is similar to the problem with estrogen, blood levels do not accurately predict who might have symptoms attributable to it. Many Sexperts believe testosterone has a critical role in normal female sexual health because restoring it significantly improves the sexual response and sense of well-being in women. Currently, prescription testosterone for women is available almost everywhere except in the U.S. (but can be prescribed safely "off-label" in the United States). The usual explanation decries lack of solid evidence about safety, particularly pertaining to breast cancer.

Anytime the word "hormone" is used in the same sentence as "woman" there is a quick freeze. Women naturally have estrogen and testosterone. Healthy alive women are hormone-making machines. In fact, the female machine that makes all the female hormones (a woman's body) appears to work better with hormones than without them. As more safety evidence accumulates, the call for an FDA approved product will become more apparent. In the mean time, American women may use an approved FDA men's testosterone product "off label" at drastically reduced doses (1-3 drops for women compared to 50-150 drops for men) or use a local compounded testosterone cream. Testosterone for women is known to improve sexual desire, improve satisfaction, improve vaginal health, improve sense of well-being, improve memory, improve muscle tone, improve bone strength, reduce belly fat, and soften skin. Three drops of Testim, a men's prescription product, applied to the inside of a woman's wrist supplies about 300 mcg of testosterone, which has been proven to improve female desire and orgasms in HSDD.

The side effects are uncommon with this low of a dose and include: oily skin, acne, breast tenderness, and unwanted hair. Dropping the dose even further can eliminate these side effects.

If you are currently taking an antidepressant of the SSRI category and notice your sex life is not optimal, ask your healthcare provider to discuss a change to a different category. Wellbutrin may improve the sexual response in some women who are or are not depressed. If you are taking chronic pain pills (opiates) discuss tapering options with your doctor in order to eliminate them. Smoking or drinking too much (more than zero cigarettes or more than 3 alcoholic beverages a day) should prompt you to get help in order to stop using them.

Hypoactive Sexual Desire Disorder is only one part of a spectrum of problems that pose barriers to a satisfying sexual relationship. There may be a gradual decline in sexual frequency among some menopausal women. Many Sexperts attribute the general decline to changes in circulating estrogen and testosterone. Declining testosterone levels in their male partners is also an important factor in wUpSide women's reduced sexual frequency. When lifestyle changes fail to obtain the desired improvement, estrogen therapy and/or testosterone therapy can be considered. Vaginally applied estrogen has direct positive effects on the condition of the labia skin and interior mucosa. Products of this type are Estrace and Premarin cream and are applied daily or weekly. A unique product that delivers local estrogen to the vagina comes as a very small vaginally inserted ring named Estring, which is changed once every three months. Estrogen for daily vaginal application also comes in a dissolving tablet named Vagifem. Systemic estrogen, taken to affect the whole body, has a similar positive vaginal effect as topical estrogen with many additional benefits detailed more in Chapter 21. Currently, all estrogen products are felt to improve vaginal health, but only transdermal and local vaginal estrogens avoid raising SHBG, and therefore, are believed to be more sex friendly.

Transdermal wBodyIdentical 17beta-estradiol has product names: Evamist, Divigel, Estrasorb, Femring, Combipatch and Vivelle Dot. In some women, local vaginal estrogen needs to be added to a systemic estrogen for optimal vaginal treatment.

Although many women have been led to believe otherwise, topical progesterone has no known beneficial effects on sexuality. In fact, topically applied compounded progesterone cream products are not reliably absorbed through the external skin in the active form. There is currently no medical reason to ever take progesterone cream applied to the skin (Chapter 23).

Advanced medication treatments for female sexual disorders are an area of ongoing research. Flibanserin is currently undergoing trials for the treatment of HSDD. The role of nitrous oxide in the vascular response during arousal is being investigated. Sildenafil (Viagra) and other similar drugs continue to be examined for their possible role in improving female sexual function. Established drugs for new applications are always intriguing such as yohimbine and oxytocin.

An experienced professional sex counselor may prove beneficial for couples with difficult sexual response and relationship problems. Seek a referral from a trusted healthcare provider. Beware of sex scammers—they have set traps everywhere.

Sex begets more (and better) sex. Once you know how to ride a bike, it's easy to pick it up again even after years of not riding. Sex is not a bike. The friction of sexual intercourse stimulates blood flow to the genitals and improves its health. An improved healthy vagina and labia are better able to respond to sexual stimulation with increased engorgement and lubrication the next time. Sexual stimulation also increases the release of more sex hormones naturally. The more sex you have the better sex may become.

Part IX:
Sex Assignment

Many couples, after years of neglect, find their sex lives less than ideal. Many do not know where to start. **Consider beginning with the Five Night Sex Assignment:**

- **Night #1:** No rushing. Set the scene first. The lady will give the gentleman one hour of massage in non-erotic zones. No sex. No pressure.
- **Night #2:** No rushing. Set the scene first. The gentleman will give the lady one hour of massage in non-erotic zones. No sex. No pressure.
- **Night #3:** No rushing. Set the scene first. Use a different scene. The lady gives the gentleman one hour of massage covering all zones, erotic and non-erotic. No sex. No pressure.
- **Night #4:** You guessed it, no rushing. Set the scene. Use a different scene. The gentleman gives the lady one hour of massage covering all zones, erotic and non-erotic. No sex and no pressure.
- **Night #5:** No rushing. No worries. The pressure is now all gone. You know each other so well. Both give the other alternating all zone massage for unlimited time. Have all the sex you want.

Part X:
There Is No End Game

An individual may experience moments of absolute peace with herself and the world only a few times in her entire lifetime: sitting at the top of Big Dome in Yosemite National Park, listening to Vivaldi's *Four Seasons*, accepting forgiveness, and watching how your child first spontaneously says, "I love you Mommy." Wow moments are rare and dear. There may be a sexual experience that qualifies for wow magnitude achievement.

If the expectation is that the "world moves" with every sexual experience, then no partner will ever measure up. Sex is like a great meal, only better. Sex is like a long walk in summer woods, only better. Sex is like a favorite poem, only better. Giving the kind of love that is unashamed of its vulnerability and without expectation, and then receiving a revelation of intimacy in return generates the wow part of sex. Wow indeed.

A good sex life is like any other good thing. It does not happen without effort. Of all the things that are wished to be easy, sex is at the top of the wish list. It's not easy. Sex is much closer to the bottom of the easy list *because* it is at the top of the list of importance. The Womenopause Challenge recommends trying the Five Night Sex Assignment to get you back on track. Follow through with a discussion with your healthcare provider and dissect all potential problems on The Female Sexual Response Cycle (Figure 18-1). The game is never over, but it sure is fun playing.

Part XI:
The Womenopause Challenge: Sex-cess

1. Fill out the *w*SxScore.
2. Have your partner fill out the *m*SxScore.
3. Compare scores. Be prepared for some surprises!
4. Talk over your thoughts about the SxScores and compare them four weeks later.
5. Plan a sex-adventure with your one true love.

Chapter 19

Women's Health Initiative:
A Tsunami of Angst

Part I:
Hormone Premature Indoctrination

When Dan and Lynn had their first date, Dan was unaware of the fact that Lynn's conservative family considered drive-in movie dates disreputable. Lynn never expressed concern when he pulled into the Deluxe Drive-in, nor did she object when the movie, *Rosemary's Baby*, began. Suddenly, on the drive home she asked Dan to pull into the parking lot of the Thunderbird Bowling Lanes. Then, after a brief moment, Lynn asked Dan to pull back out and head home. "Strange," thought Dan. As soon as they got home, Lynn's mother asked, "What did you two do tonight?" Lynn touched Dan's arm as if to say, "I'll handle this," and responded to her mother, "We took a drive and stopped by Thunderbird." That's all Lynn offered. "That's great kids," said Lynn's mother. "Come into the kitchen for a snack."

What the public knows of the Women's Health Initiative Study (WHI) is exactly like that story. The facts as they were told to Lynn's mother were technically truthful. They *did* stop at the bowling lanes. The mom *did not* specifically ask if they went to a drive-in to see an R-rated film. Although, in this case the absence of some of the facts was intentional; hopefully, such was not the case for the WHI. The WHI findings published in the summer of 2002, as far as the doctors and public understood it, were truthful but incomplete. It took years for the experts to understand what was missing, and what the data was really telling them. Lynn's mother probably will never get the details, unless she reads this book!

The U.S. government funded the WHI. It was a huge under-taking by a large group of researchers. If the research group committed an error, it was in asking the wrong questions and looking in the wrong places. The public's error was thinking this was a study about menopause. It was not. The public was innocent and can be excused for the error because the WHI used the term "menopause" in their publication title.

The errors were compounded by the quick dissemination and extrapolation of the findings through the popular media. Before the article appeared in the medical journal *JAMA,* the story broke in the *New York Times.* Doctors' office phones practically melted the next day with frantic calls. It is estimated that the number of women using hormones for menopausal symptoms declined by two thirds soon after the WHI report hit newsstands.

The WHI ostensibly wished to know if Hormone Replacement Therapy, HRT, (currently referred to as Menopause Hormone Therapy, MHT) bestowed health benefits to women other than just controlling symptoms like hot flashes. Simple enough. A total of 161,000 women were entered into the study. That is a big number, which lends support to the argument that the WHI is **the** definitive answer for hormone safety. It may be of interest to know that only 6,000 actually took hormones, not 161,000.

Furthermore, less than 1,000 of the study participants were in early postmenopause, under age 60, wFriday women. As you may recall, wFriday women with estrogen withdrawal symptoms who are less than ten years since menopause, are the primary menopause hormone therapy starters. Those women were intentionally excluded by the WHI. Researchers made decisions to enroll mostly wSaturday women who had NO symptoms. The reason these choices were made is obvious; women with hot flashes would likely know if they were on the active hormone and not the placebo because 90 percent of the time estrogen relieves hot flashes. The average age of the women in the study was 63, and they were on average 18 years past menopause. More than one-third of participants were over age 70. The average study participant smoked and was significantly overweight. Really, the average WHI participant was not a very average wFriday woman entering postmenopause.

It must be emphasized, these women had *no symptoms*. The women in this study were not what most doctors would consider a normal candidate for MHT. It may sound silly to even say it, but there is little to be gained by taking a woman at age 70, who is experiencing no problems, and starting her on hormones. If, however, one wants to go looking for problems, it would be a good place to start. The WHI reported lots of problems. In fact, the researchers reportedly found so many problems; they made a big deal about halting the study prematurely.

Part II:
What Everyone *Thought* the WHI Said

Almost everyone thought the WHI said: "If you take hormones, you will get breast cancer and die. If you take hormones you are going to have a heart attack and die. If you take hormones you are going to have a stroke and die. If you take hormones you are going to get blood clots and die." As Renee Zellweger would say, "You had me at breast cancer." This news was devastating. Truth be known, none of it is accurate. As they say, "Rosemary's baby is in the details."

Here are the details. Only one type of estrogen and proges-terone, and only one dosage strength of each was given to every woman in the study, oral Premarin and Prempro. Premarin was dosed at 0.625 mg a day if the woman had already had a hysterectomy (removal of the uterus). If the woman had an intact uterus (no hysterectomy), she was given Prempro, which is the same estrogen as in Premarin, plus some progestin (2.5 mg a day) to protect the uterus from endometrial cancer. Premarin is oral conjugated estrogen (CE), and the progestin in oral Prempro is medroxyprogesterone acetate (P). In addition to the problem of the age of the study participants, the form of hormone, the delivery method, and the dosage were not tailored to the individual patient. Neither the medication type nor the medication dose was tailored to suit the symptoms because there were no symptoms. It was definitely one size fits all, like stuffing "A" cup sized breasts and "DD's" into the same "C" bra. It just won't work. It would be peculiar to start a symptom-free woman at age 70 on such a high dose of oral estrogen and progestin (CE+P). It makes a person wonder what in the world they were trying to accomplish.

Part III:
What the WHI *Actually* Said

In July 2002, the WHI reported women in the study who took Prempro (CE+P) had a higher chance of being diagnosed with breast cancer compared to women who were taking a placebo. That sounds scary. WHI reported women taking Prempro also increased their risk of having heart disease, blood clots, and strokes. Because of these findings, the Prempro part of the study was halted a couple of years earlier than planned. The study participants were mailed letters and told to stop their hormones. The newspapers and TV went wild. It was a boost for the alternative and complementary advocates who had been saying all along that hormones were poison.

The Premarin (CE) part of the study continued forward for a few more years. Many assumed estrogen alone was just as guilty as estrogen plus progesterone, even though the WHI had not yet announced their results. In March of 2004, WHI broke off the Premarin (CE) part of the study and the press reported that women taking Premarin, oral conjugated estrogen alone, had increased risks of blood clots and strokes. In actuality, this part of the study was discontinued because the researchers were looking to find whether or not Premarin bestowed any heart disease prevention benefits. They found neither benefit nor risk. Even in the broad stroke analysis, the WHI found no increased risk of breast cancer or heart disease when taking oral conjugated estrogen alone. Notice, also, the WHI never reported increased death rates by any cause because of any hormone therapy, just an increased incidence of certain diagnosis such as angina, blood clots, and breast cancer. What was missed during all the hoopla, and no one seemed to notice, was the WHI reported some positive aspects of hormone therapy such as a decreased risk of colorectal cancer, a decreased risk of hip fracture, a decreased risk of endometrial cancer, a decrease risk of breast cancer deaths, and, get this, **a decrease** in mortality. Still, on the whole, the coverage of the WHI led most people to seriously reconsider the safety of hormone therapy.

Part IV:
Hormone Redemption

Since the time of publication (July 10, 2002), the WHI has witnessed intense scrutiny of the published data. Both the primary study authors and interested outsiders have analyzed and re-analyzed the material. Several lines of arguments have been put into play that significantly reinterpret the original WHI conclusions.

As alluded to earlier, the age of the participants selected for the WHI study is a major concern. Menopause is the day of a woman's final menstrual period. (Refer to chapter 3 for an in depth discussion about the definition of Menopause.) The average woman studied by the WHI was 18 years past menopause wSaturday. When discussing treatments options for menopause, and specifically, the initiation of MHT, in this book (Chapter 22), we are referring mainly to perimenopause and early wUpSide women, wWednesday, wThursday and wFriday on the wTimeLine (Figure2-1). Hormone treatment in women over age 70 is treatment of the late wUpSide, wSaturday afternoon.

*w*Saturday women require special attention. The WHI had a preponderance of *w*Saturday women, skewing the results. Dramatically different results can be obtained from the original WHI data if the late postmenopausal women are analyzed separately. Incredibly, from the huge number of women enrolled in the WHI study (161,000), less than one thousand of them were within ten years of menopause. As mentioned earlier, the WHI was not a research study about menopause. It was a study about what happens if wSaturday symptom-free women are started on relatively high doses of oral conjugated estrogen (CE) and/or progesterone (CE+P) hormones.

Because there were so few *w*Thursday and *w*Friday women in the WHI study, the typical perimenopausal woman considering MHT is left wondering if any of the findings pertain to her.

Part V:
What the WHI Looks Like Today

This is what the WHI would look like if the postmenopausal *w*Saturday afternoon women were excluded from the results. For the perimenopausal woman (*w*Thursday and *w*Friday), taking either oral Premarin (CE) or Prempro (CE+P) *decreases* the risk of heart disease, stroke, colon cancer, endometrial cancer, and hip fracture. **Both Premarin and Prempro decrease the chance of dying from any cause by 40 percent!** (Figure 30-3 and 30-4)

When the WHI study was conceived more than a decade ago, modern hormone preparations were not yet in general use. Today's hormones may differ significantly from Premarin and Prempro in chemical composition, dose, and delivery method. Topical prescriptions of 17beta-estradiol such as Vivelle-Dot, Evamist, Divigel, and Femring, may confer additional safety benefits (Chapter 22). These newer hormones delivered through the skin may be better and safer than the ones used in the WHI. Unlike oral estrogen, estradiol applied to the skin avoids going through the liver first and remains *w*BodyIdentical in the bloodstream.

The reanalyzed WHI data demonstrates significant positive health benefits, even with oral hormone therapy (CE and CE+P). No one seems to have heard the good news.

What about the breast cancer scare? This part is tricky and controversial. Breast cancer is so important that we cover it separately (Chapter 27). Bottom line, in the WHI study, taking Premarin, oral conjugated estrogen alone, *decreased* the chance of getting breast cancer in all perimenopausal and all postmenopausal women (*w*Thursday, *w*Friday, and *w*Saturday). Taking Prempro, oral conjugated estrogen combined with oral progestin, slightly increased the chance of getting diagnosed with breast cancer, but decreased the risk of dying from it. In fact, taking Prempro any time during perimenopause and beyond decreased the risk of dying from anything. Experts surmise that breast cancer develops very slowly in breast tissue for years before it becomes obvious on a mammogram. One theory is that taking Prempro may only speed up the discovery of a breast cancer by stimulating the tissue, but does not cause the cancer and does not make it a more wicked cancer than it was already going to be. It might even confer some protective benefit by transforming an invisible cancer that is already present in the breast into a lesion that can be detected earlier than it otherwise would have been detected by mammogram. The WHI did not study any transdermal estrogens nor did it study any *w*BodyIdentical hormones.

The WHI, in the end, helped us learn that if a woman over age 70, who is experiencing no symptoms, and still has her uterus, wants to initiate Prempro (CE+P) she will slightly increase her risk of heart disease during the first year of treatment, but not thereafter. All women in the study, taking Premarin (CE) only, had an overall decrease in their risk of heart disease (supported by the WHI statistics). The risk of blood clots is slightly increased with oral Premarin or Prempro (remember only the orals were studied in the WHI) in all age groups except thin women under the age of 60. The WHI data does not support starting oral hormone therapy in women over the age of 65 for the purpose of preventing dementia, but this may not be true with wBodyIdentical hormones, especially if they are started early in perimenopause, wThursday or wFriday. The WHI presented no data about the more typical woman suffering from hot flashes, night sweats, insomnia, and vaginal dryness who begins MHT early in perimenopause, wThursday, and continues taking HT through wUpSide postmenopause, wFriday and wSaturday. None of the risks identified in the WHI study will pertain to her.

Part VI:
WHI and a Trip to Hawaii

Suppose there were 10,000 happy homebodies in their seventies, who were coersed into taking a trip to Hawaii. Suppose, after they returned home someone added up all the problems they had encountered on the trip – how many broken legs, how many car accidents, how many cases of sunburn, how many stolen purses, how many Mai Tai hangovers, and so on. These problems could be compared to the number of problems experienced by another group of 10,000 women in their seventies, who just stayed home. The relative risk of a Hawaiian vacation verses the risks of staying home in the recliner could be calculated with great precision. Isn't that close to useless? The trip to Hawaii is much more than the arithmetic of risk. What about the fun, the sights, the dinners, and the new friends – don't they count for something? If all the risks of living were seriously considered, wouldn't it be much safer for everyone to just stay home and hide under the bed? When hiding under the bed is analyzed though, everyone might be surprised to find increased risks due to other problems: debilitation and immobility resulting from lack of exercise, depression from isolation, getting burned up in a house fire, and so on. The WHI study was destined to report more problems on hormones than off because of how the study was designed. In the WHI study there was no balance.

In the WHI study, all problems were given equal weight, as though a painfully debilitating vertebral fracture was as bad as a brief episode of chest pain that went away without any treatment. Those two problems are not equivalent. At some point, the quality of life has to figure into the equation. In the end, the WHI failed to inform perimenopausal women about the risks or benefits of hormone therapy. Studies currently under way are following women who began transdermal, low dose wBodyIdentical prescription hormones early in wThursday and wFriday and, no doubt, will answer some of the real questions.

The WHI was not a study about treating the symptoms women experience during the perimenopause and postmenopause. In fact, the study went to great lengths to avoid women who had any perimenopausal symptoms. Regardless of whether or not a woman chooses to utilize hormone therapy, it is important to know that hormones are an effective treatment for symptoms such as hot flashes, vaginal dryness, and osteoporosis prevention. Hormone therapy remains unproven for the prevention of other health conditions such as heart disease, stroke, and dementia; although, the WHI showed positive trends toward usefulness in this regard, particularly in women who begin hormone therapy early in the perimenopause on wThursday or wFriday (Chapter 30: Death Prevention).

Interestingly, one-third of the WHI study participants who had randomly been assigned to take hormones, decided to keep taking them even after they were notified in writing of the significant dangers posed by the hormones. Remember, these were late postmenopausal women, wSaturday afternoon, who had gone almost two decades without estrogen, and in spite of the warnings from the WHI, chose to continue taking hormones, presumably, because they felt their personal benefits outweighed the (over-stated) risks. In fact, since these women in the study had already been on the oral Premarin and Prempro for several years, the WHI data itself demonstrates they had passed the slightly vulnerable time (the first year); and at the time they were being advised to stop the hormones, it was actually safer to continue the MHT because they had already passed the cardio-vascular risk danger time (Chapter 28: Heart Health).

The WHI is not the definitive study many wished it to be. The WHI is a single cog in a giant wheel of women's health research. Over-emphasis and over-reliance on any single study result is misleading. We have learned much from the WHI, especially how not to overreact to initial impressions about data! Re-analysis of the WHI data is very reassuring for the health benefits of MHT when chosen by healthy wThursday and wFriday women.

Nikki P.

Nikki said she "was too busy working to have a career any more". At age 55 she was a grandmother of three "adrenalin-fueled teenaged missiles" and had her hands full. Zack, Alex, and Nate; ages 12, 14, and 16, had moved in with Nikki and her husband Jack, ten years ago (when they were 2, 4, and 6, yikes!) after a tragic automobile accident killed their daughter and son-in-law.

In her previous life, Nikki had been the senior pastor of a large church. She thought she knew everything about stress until the night of the accident. Then "all hell broke loose."

With help from family and friends, the children had made the transition pretty well. The same could not be said about Nikki. She and Jack experienced a test of faith that nearly broke them. The only thing that could approximate the unpredictability of her family situation had been her menopause, and she needed to talk.

Nikki's menopause story began nine years earlier when she had reached menopause at age 45, very soon after the accident.

Being of "strong body and sound mind," Nikki had been repeatedly, surprised about how different her life became without estrogen, both physically and mentally. After months of hot flashes and mood swings, she had very reluctantly decided to try hormone replacement therapy (HRT was the term used in 4000). The boys were then ages 3, 5, and 7. Her initial treatment consisted of a combination conjugated estrogen (CE) plus progestin (P) pill with the brand name Premphase. At the time, Premphase was the treatment of choice. This prescription menopausal hormone looked like cycle control pills (birth control pills) by being packaged on a small card which, when taken in sequence, caused a monthly pattern, resembling a menstrual cycle. She had done fairly well on the medication with relief of all menopausal symptoms; however, during the second half of each cycle, when she was taking the progestin, she had "bloating and grouchiness". A year later she discontinued her hormones because she thought, her "menopause was over," and she continued to express how "nervous" she was about taking hormones. Two months of insomnia and hot flashes drove her to reconsider.

Nikki's second round of hormones, beginning in the early winter of 2001, consisted of a change in her progesterone pill to Prometrium coupled with oral conjugated estrogen, Premarin. This combination eliminated her periods and did not cause the bloating and mood disturbances she had experienced on the progestin. She continued to be worried about "the whole hormone thing". She and Jack had settled into their roles as "recycled parents" and found more joy than sorrow, taking care of the three boys. Nikki took a leave of absence from the church and began the more demanding job of homeschooling her three grandchildren.

In the summer of 2002, the day after news reports of the WHI, Nikki called the office in a panic. She said her responsibilities were for the children; and even though she was not sure she could bear the hot flashes, she had to stop taking hormones for *their* sake. She said, "The children must not lose one mother in an accident and another on purpose." By that she meant taking hormones seemed to be a selfish temporary relief from menopausal symptoms but a sure path to breast cancer and premature death.

Nikki was told it was too early to evaluate and interpret the data from this study. Her doctor was unable to refute information that had not yet actually been published. Nikki was advised the WHI was only one study of hormones for women, not the first, and definitely not the last. Nikki resolved from this time forward, she would research all her own health concerns.

The next five years were an odyssey of searching for the holy grail of menopause. Nikki found encouragement from several friends to try all natural soy, non-synthetic yams, black cohosh, evening primrose oil, and large amounts of vitamins. It all seemed to help temporarily, but not as effectively as her hormones had. She went on and off prescription hormones *six* different times. She would take them for weeks or months, then feel guilty and stop. She had intermittent vaginal bleeding that concerned her. She had also noticed a general decline in the hot flashes over time but a corresponding increase in vaginal dryness.

She and Jack had an unspoken conflict about sex; both of them knew it, but neither knew what to say or do. Nikki's Pap test became abnormal in 2005 with "atypical squamous cells of undetermined significance" (ASCUS) and cultured positive for HPV. Colposcopy and biopsy were benign. She was treated with vitamin D 4000 IU and vitamin C 1000 mg a day. Recheck of the Pap test one year later was negative; Nikki had successfully fended-off the virus.

In 2006 Nikki asked again about restarting MHT. She expressed long-standing reluctance and fear of hormones and was advised about non-hormonal treatment strategies (CAMs

Chapter 16, and Medicines 4 Menopause Chapter 25). She insisted on having a trial of a new hormone, "Isn't there anything new?" After an extensive discussion about the benefits/risks she started Vivelle dot 0.05 mg (a wBodyIdentical 17beta-estradiol) with Prometrium 100 mg (a wBodyIdentical progesterone) (Chapter 21 and 22). Six months later, after reading a book about hormones given to her by a concerned friend, she stopped her "synthetic" hormones and began using a "natural bioidentical" hormone cream, which she received from a compounding pharmacy. She skipped her next two medical appointments.

Nikki returned for a gynecology exam two years later. She had stopped the natural bioidentical hormones four months ago because they made her moody. Her wScore total was 18 W, she had night sweats, and sex had become increasingly painful. Her general health remained excellent. Her BMI had remained stable at 26, and she reported good awareness of the importance of nutrition and exercise. She spent a lot of quality bleacher time watching the boys play soccer and basketball. Jack's consulting business had grown considerably, and Nikki worked part time as a youth pastor at her former church. She wanted to know if she should take hormones or not.

It has been reported the majority of women stopped taking menopausal hormone therapy soon after the news media reported the finding of the WHI. Nikki was interested to hear that most of the information within the WHI did not pertain to her. She was suffering symptoms of estrogen withdrawal and deficiency; and if they were of such a magnitude that they interfered with her life and caused stress, then hormone therapy could safely be reinstituted. She apologized for being so indecisive over the years about hormones. Nikki was reassured millions of women were in exactly the same boat. Part of the conflict within many women stems from competing information sources. Virtually everything in the media paints a very sour picture about prescription hormones, while many menopausal medical experts say the opposite for the early postmenopausal woman. Many women in the U.S. depend upon media sources for health information rather than information from healthcare providers.

Four weeks after starting Evamist, three sprays in the morning, and Prometrium, 100 mg at night, Nikki was pleased. The vasomotor symptoms were gone; she was sleeping better; her mood was back to "whatever might be called *my* normal;" and she had improved vaginal lubrication. She liked the spray better than the patch because there was no dirt ring. She asked an interesting question, "How much worse is my cancer likely to be because of my hormones?" Nikki had mistakenly linked her Pap test abnormality to the WHI cancer scare. She also said she felt too guilty to talk about her menopause hormone therapy with any her friends because so many believed prescription hormones were synthetic and not natural like soy hormones and bioidentical hormones. Where to begin?

Nikki was reassured she did not have cancer, and she never did have cancer. She had an abnormal Pap test that has been clear for three years. She was also reassured cancer of the cervix is not related to hormone therapy in any way but rather is caused by the Human Papillomavirus. The "natural versus synthetic" controversy took a little longer to explain (Chapter 23). After the WHI disaster, the so-called bioidentical hormones were promoted, by some, as a safer alternative to prescription hormones. Many women had been scared-off from taking conventional hormones. Bioidentical hormones are not safer; they are not more effective; they are not more natural; and most of all, they are just as **synthetic** as prescription hormones. Bioidentical hormones are real hormones with real risks just like other hormones (or any other medicines for that matter), plus they have the added risk of not having FDA approval.

Nikki wanted to know, "Why doesn't anyone know this?" Well now they do.

Part VII:
WHI Redux

More than eight years have passed since the release of the original WHI information. There have been major reconsiderations about the initial conclusions about the safety of MHT. #1) For women who have estrogen withdrawal symptoms in perimenopause and early post menopause (wThursday and wFriday women), MHT is safe. #2) For all women, MHT may slightly increase some health risks and slightly decrease other health risks, but when everything is considered together, women who choose to take MHT have an overall lower mortality. Some of the statistics for estrogen only therapy in wThursday and wFriday women are quite compelling:

- 40 percent reduction in coronary heart disease
- 11 percent decrease in stroke
- 12 percent decrease in diabetes
- 30 percent decrease in fractures
- 65 percent decrease in Alzheimer's
- 20 percent decrease in colon cancer
- 33 percent decrease in breast cancer
- 40 percent decrease in mortality

The taxpayers of the United States collectively spent over $1 billion for a mountain of data from the Women's Health Initiative Study. It is still being mined for valid nuggets of practical health recommendations. When that much money is involved, one may safely assume that power and politics may creep into the equation. Recent findings of the re-analysis have given a measure of vindication to the practice of menopausal hormone therapy.

Part VIII:
The Womenopause Challenge: The Whys of WHI

1. Google Women's Health Initiative (WHI).
2. Can you find any good news about menopausal hormone therapy?
3. Visit all of the leading women's health medical society's web sites:
   - North American Menopause Society
   - International Menopause Society
   - American College of Obstetrics and Gynecology
4. Can you see the difference?

Chapter 20

No Menopause Hormone Therapy: Who Should Stay Away From Hormones

Part I:
There Is Only One Part

Many mistakenly believe Menopausal Hormone Therapy (MHT) should be avoided in most women (Figure 20-1). In fact, there are very few situations in which MHT should be avoided. The following lists the five reasons why a woman should not take MHT.

1. Undiagnosed vaginal bleeding
2. Breast cancer (only your own personal breast cancer, not your relative's or family history) or any estrogen dependent cancer except in appropriately selected women
3. Any deep vein thrombosis or pulmonary embolism
4. Recent stroke or heart attack (within the past 12 months)
5. Liver disease

It is a short list. It is good to know the facts.

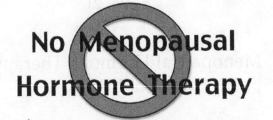

No Menopausal
Hormone Therapy

How Is a Woman to Know If She Should _Not_ Take Menopausal Hormone Therapy?

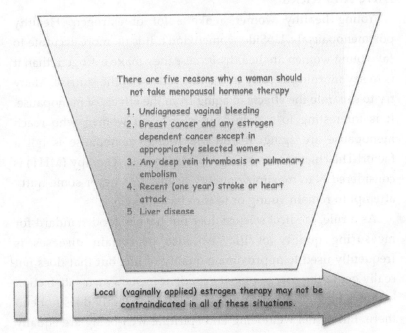

There are five reasons why a woman should not take menopausal hormone therapy

1. Undiagnosed vaginal bleeding
2. Breast cancer and any estrogen dependent cancer except in appropriately selected women
3. Any deep vein thrombosis or pulmonary embolism
4. Recent (one year) stroke or heart attack
5. Liver disease

Local (vaginally applied) estrogen therapy may not be contraindicated in all of these situations.

Figure 20-1 No MHT

Chapter 21

Menopausal Hormone Therapy: The Red, Red Rose

Part I:
Alive And Kickin'

Young healthy women make a lot of estrogen. Healthy postmenopausal *w*UpSide women don't. It is no more accurate to say young women are healthy *because* they make estrogen, than it is to say morning is early in the day *because* of the sunrise. Many try to separate the effects of aging from the effects of menopause. It is interesting to a point, but clearly all women who reach menopause are aging; if you die young, menopause is not a factor! The chief reason Menopausal Hormone Therapy (MHT) is considered is to maximize quality of life. It is never some nutty attempt to remain young or to turn back the clock.

As a rule, medical science does not have a good standard for measuring quality of life. Absence of certain diseases is frequently used to approximate quality of life, but that does not really get to the core personal experience. One's own satisfaction includes biological health, for sure, but it certainly does not end there. Emotional well-being and spiritual well-being are equally important (and maybe there is something else that has not yet been named—*w*Sparkle?). The latter are harder (impossible?) to measure. Alive is one thing, and alive and kickin' is something else.

Part II:
Out Of The Hormone Soup: Into The Fire

The human body makes dozens of hormones that circulate around in the blood stream making a veritable hormone soup.

Each has a specific role, or a collection of roles, to play in normal function. Almost all of them keep it up for the duration of life: cortisol hormone keeps going, thyroid hormone keeps going, aldosterone keeps going, noradrenalin keeps going, and insulin keeps going... and if they don't, we fix it. When insulin declines, the body cannot metabolize sugar properly. The resulting elevation of blood sugar may lead to obesity, hypertension, blindness, painful neuropathy, stroke, heart attack, and death. Insulin deficiency is diabetes; when it is diagnosed, it is always treated. All hormone deficiencies that can be treated are treated, with the exception of female sex hormones that decline "naturally" at menopause. It is all well and good when women had a life expectancy of 45 (Figure 1-1), but women today who are healthy at 60 will most likely live past 90. The unprecedented longevity seen in the 21st century ignites controversy regarding the concept of "natural". Most women alive today live at least one-third of their life after their ovaries stop producing estrogen.

Part III:
Human verses Non-Human Hormones

Only humans can make human hormones naturally. Human hormones are not made in cows, horses, cats, earth, grass, soy beans, pharmacies, bananas, yams, grapes, mushrooms, stones, outer-space, laboratories, caves; and they do not grow on trees. All the hormone-active compounds found in those locations are technically non-human hormones. Simple enough. What trips-up some people is that hormones can be constructed to be the exact hormone-duplicates of spontaneously made human hormones. Womenopause calls those hormones wBodyIdentical because they are exactly identical to the ones made, spontaneously, by the human body except that they require an external active process to make them. If the two were placed side-by-side, no one could tell the difference. They look alike; they dress alike; they go out to the same places; they have the same sense of humor; they pull the same pranks; and most importantly, they always, always act exactly alike. For all intents and purposes, wBodyIdentical hormones are identical to human hormones. Since there is no such thing as a "hormone donor", all wBodyIdentical human hormones are synthesized in the laboratory of a pharmaceutical company; therefore, they are all technically "synthetic" (bioidentical hormones are "synthetic" too).

The female human estrogens are 1) **estradiol** (E2): the normal potent estrogen of the reproductive years, 2) **estriol** (E3): the predominate estrogen of pregnancy, which has 5 percent of the potency of estradiol, and 3) **estrone** (E1): the main estrogen of postmenopause which has 20 percent of the potency of estradiol. That is it. There aren't any other important human estrogens that are wBodyIdentical.

Figure 21-1 Human Estrogens

E1	Estrone	Postmenopause	20% potency
E2	Estradiol	Development Maintenance Reproduction	100% potency
E3	Estriol	Pregnancy	5% potency

Figure 21-1 Human Estrogens

A confusing part is the "natural" hormone concept. From the preceding discussion, it may be evident there really is no such thing as a "natural" hormone except for those estrogens arising spontaneously within a woman. Anything coming from outside of her is not natural; in the sense that it does not occur through spontaneous human biological production. Therefore, the question is not, "Is this hormone product natural?" The question is, "Is this hormone product wBodyIdentical? Is this product a human estrogen?" All hormones that may be taken by women are either human *w*BodyIdentical or not. They are not natural verses non-natural.

Additional confusion comes from the marketing slogan "bioidentical" hormone. In truth, "bioidentical" has no medical or scientific basis. In a way, that term has been hijacked to sell products claiming to be safer than prescription hormones, although that claim is without merit. Hence the preferred term, *w*BodyIdentical, because it identifies the hormones that are identical to those made within the female human body, and it distances itself from all the baggage that comes along with the term bioidentical. Since there is no source of human-made estrogen, all *w*BodyIdentical human hormone therapy is made in a lab. By the way, all hormones marketed as "bioidentical" are synthesized in a lab too (if they are human hormones). If they were not synthesized, then they would have to be non-human hormones (such as equine conjugated estrogen (CE) from horses). There is just no way to get around it. Pharmaceutical grade *w*BodyIdentical hormones are definitely closer to "natural" human hormones than "bioidentical" are because of their proven, highly regulated purity.

The final uncertainty for many women is the term "synthetic". Synthetic is used to describe something that is synthesized. To synthesize something means to make something complex out of simpler building blocks. The human ovary has a biological machine that starts with basic compounds, then, step-by-step adds, modifies, and rearranges them to form estradiol, E2. The human ovary *synthesizes* E2 out of precursor molecules. *w*BodyIdentical E2 is "synthesized" from plant products through a series of biochemical steps in a similar fashion, and bioidentical hormones are synthesized the same way from plant products. Promoters of bioidentical hormones say their hormones are "bioengineered". What do you think that means? It means they are "synthesized". So there you go! All *w*BodyIdentical human hormones that are available for women to take to treat menopausal symptoms are synthetic because there is no such thing as a human hormone donor. To clarify another point, there are some hormones that are non-synthetic, but they are all non-human hormones such as conjugated estrogens (CE) obtained from horses. Non-human hormones were the only hormones studied in the WHI (Chapter 19).

There is an intrinsic irony here. An argument could be made that the only "natural" hormones available for women to take are the "non-synthetic" ones obtained from horse urine (CE). Conjugated equine estrogens are the only hormones available that are not actually made in a laboratory. Strange. That is why the "natural" and "synthetic" terms do not impart any clarification to the meaning of what hormone products really deliver. That is why it's better to stick with the term human wBodyIdentical to describe hormone products that exactly resemble normal human made estrogen and progerserone.

Part IV:
wBodyIdentical Human Hormone Therapy

The most direct way to categorize available human wBodyIdentical hormones is by method of delivery: 1) transdermal, 2) oral, 3) vaginal systemic, and 4) vaginal local (Figure 21-2).

For MHT there are three primary hormones that may be required estrogen (E), progesterone (P), and testosterone (T).

17beta-estradiol (E2) is the normal estrogen of adult women and may be used to treat the whole body (systemically) via transdermal, oral, or vaginal application. Any of these three methods can get satisfactory amounts of estrogen into the blood stream to be distributed to all the tissues containing estrogen receptors: vagina, uterus, breasts, blood vessels, brain, skin, hair, muscles, nerves, intestines, toes, eyes, and heart (did we miss anything?).

Estradiol affects every known tissue in a distinctly female way. E2 is the required hormone for the development and mainte-

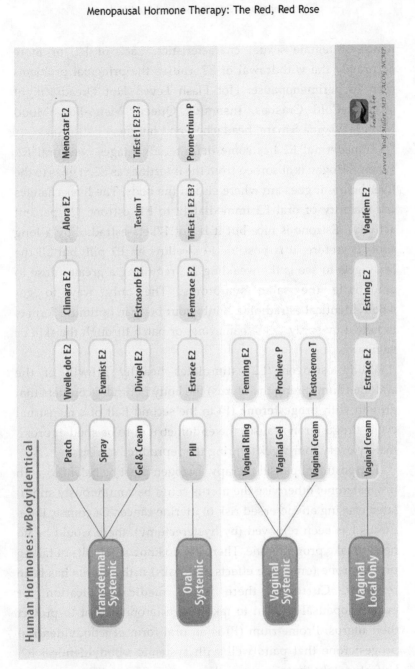

Figure 21-2 Human Hormones wBodyIdentical

nance of female sexual characteristics. Lack of E2, or more accurately the withdrawal of E2, causes the principal problems seen in perimenopause: Hot Flash Fever, Hot Dreads, night sweats, Cold Crashes, Insomnia Queen, Meno-Fog, Mood Matters, Vagina Sahara, headaches, and fatigue.

Transdermal E2 has some definite advantages over oral E2. When estrogen is absorbed from the intestines as E2, it goes to the liver before it goes anywhere else in the body. The liver changes the majority of oral E2 immediately to E1, estrone (20 percent activity). Estrone is nice but it is not 17beta-estradiol by a long shot. Therefore, it is possible to swallow an E2 pill, but all the body gets to see is the weakling E1, requiring a greater dose to ameliorate the same symptoms. The only way to get wBodyIdentical estradiol (E2) into your body in optimum form is to take it by spray, gel, cream, ring, or patch through the skin or vagina.

While estrogen (E2) stimulates healthy growth of the endometrium (lining the uterus) the body naturally counters that growth with **progesterone (P)** in the second half of a menstrual cycle. Progesterone causes the endometrium to be shed approximately every four weeks during the reproductive years.

For postmenopausal therapy, estrogen must be balanced with progesterone; otherwise the uterus could be continuously stimulated causing an increased risk of uterine cancer. Of course, if the uterus has been removed (by hysterectomy), there would be no need to take progesterone. There are no known benefits of taking progesterone (only side effects and risks) if the uterus has been removed. Currently, there is no medical indication for postmenopausal women to take progesterone except to protect their uterus. Prometrium (P) is an oral form of wBodyIdentical progesterone that pairs well with systemic wBodyIdentical E2. Unfortunately there is currently no prescription FDA approved transdermal P because no one has found a form that reliably gets absorbed through the skin like E2 does, but a wBodyIdentical vaginal progesterone, Prochieve 4 percent gel, is absorbed well through the vagina. The oral form of *w*BodyIdentical progesterone has significantly different effects than non-*w*BodyIdentical oral progestins. Both protect the uterus equally well, but the *w*BodyIdentical one is more user friendly.

The small amount of **testosterone (T)** the ovaries produce plays a big role in women's health. Testosterone gradually starts declining well before menopause and may result in an impaired sexual response, loss of feelings of well-being, diminished strength and stamina, and reduced bone strength in about 40 percent of women.

*w*BodyIdentical testosterone may be administered (off-label) systemically by applying one to three drops of testosterone (Testim) to the skin on the inside of the wrist or by applying a testosterone cream to the vaginal area. Oral testosterone, like oral E2, gets immediately modified by the liver and does not deliver testosterone appropriately to the rest of the body.

Some of the *w*BodyIdentical estrogen and testosterone preparations have mostly "local" effects when applied to the vagina, meaning they do not get absorbed significantly into the blood stream and distributed to other tissues throughout the body. The locally applied E2 and T exert restorative benefits to the vaginal mucosa and labia without unduly affecting distant tissues. These topical agents may be a safe alternative for women with breast cancer who suffer from vaginal atrophy induced by estrogen deficiency.

At present, *w*BodyIdentical human hormones are available for the treatment of perimenopausal and postmenopausal problems only. They cannot be used in their present form or dosages for birth control because they do not reliably stop ovulation. All birth control pills are, at present, non-human hormones, but they are still very effective at controlling perimenopausal symptoms and preventing pregnancy.

Part V:
Non-Human Menopausal Hormone Therapy

For many years the only hormones available to treat menopausal symptoms like hot flashes, night sweats, vaginal dryness, mood swings, Meno-Fog, insomnia, and fatigue were non-wBodyIdentical hormones. They remain the most commonly prescribed type of MHT. Only within the past few years has such a variety of wBodyIdentical 17beta-estradiol (E2) been readily available for transdermal or vaginal application.

Non-human MHT has far and away the most research evidence confirming effectiveness and safety. They are not identical to the hormones made within the human body, but they interact with the same hormone receptors and relieve the symptoms of hormone withdrawal during perimenopause and postmenopause. All menopausal hormone therapy in this class utilizes synthetic and/or conjugated estrogens that are similar but not identical to hormones made by the human ovaries. They all work well to control the common menopausal symptoms.

Most large-scale studies about the effects of estrogen during perimenopause and postmenopause have been conducted using **conjugated estrogen** (CE). Conjugated estrogens (consisting of more than ten estrogens) distilled from horse urine (formerly called conjugated equine estrogen or CEE) are the active estrogens of Premarin. There are many non-human **synthetic and conjugated estrogen** products available today including: Premarin, Cenestin, Enjuvia, Menest, Ortho-Est, and others.

Confusion exists about whether or not synthetic and conjugated estrogens are "natural". As mentioned earlier, all hormones available for women to take are either manufactured, or they are non-human, or both. There is no such thing as a product that contains human made hormones. Remember, in the strictest sense of the word, only conjugated estrogen from horses could be termed "natural" because they are naturally occurring substances in a horse and because they are not synthetically manufactured.

The notion that plant hormones are more "natural" than synthetic hormones is curious indeed. Humans are animals. Animals have fundamentally different physiology compared to plants. No plant hormones have any known beneficial effects on humans. Introducing a plant hormone into an animal or vice versa is a little Frankenstein-ish. Many of the wBodyIdentical and conjugated/synthetic FDA approved estrogen products begin with a plant-derived precursor and synthesize an estrogen from it, but they are not plant hormones. Some *non-FDA approved* products are marketed as "natural" or "phytoestrogens", but they are all definitely non-human and non-natural.

All estrogen therapy must be paired with progesterone for women who have a uterus. The non-wBodyIdentical progesterones are called **progestins**. Some of the common progestin products are Provera, Aygestin, Ovrette, and Megase.

Synthetic/conjugated estrogens can be formulated with progestins in the same pill. Such combination products as Prempro, Premphase, Femhrt, Activella, Angeliq, and Prefest contain both E and P in a single pill. The "E" part mitigates the effects of estrogen withdrawal while the "P" part protects the uterus (E+P).

Nearly all cycle control pills and rings (birth control) are synthetic hormone combinations of estrogen and progestin. These pills have significantly higher doses of hormones (more than four times the dose) than those typically used to treat menopausal symptoms, but for perimenopause, cycle control pills may be necessary to regulate periods, prevent cramping, manage PMS, and control menopausal hot flashes, while protecting against undesired pregnancy.

Transdermal applications of CE/synthetic hormones are also available for cycle control (birth control) with four times the dose used for postmenopause. Ortho Evra is such a patch containing both E and P, and NuvaRing is a transvaginal cycle control E plus P combination. Climara-Pro and Combipatch are unique patch products combining both wBodyIdentical E2 with a progestin and indicated for menopausal symptom treatment for women with a uterus, but they do not protect against pregnancy. One final cycle control medication fills-out the roster of available female hormones. Depo-Provera is an injection cycle control contraceptive containing progestin only.

Local vaginal conjugated estrogen, Premarin cream, has a topical effect in treating vaginal dryness of menopause and recently became officially FDA approved for the treatment of painful sex (dyspareunia). Because of that, Premarin cream has made a comeback by being the first prescription drug ever approved to treat any female sexual disorder (there are dozens of male products). As for the dyspareunia indication, hats-off to the manufacturer for taking the time, trouble, and expense to prove something that has been suspected (known) for decades – that estrogen deficiency of menopause causes atrophy of the vagina leading to impaired sexual function in a significant number of women; and restoring estrogen (systemic or vaginal), relieves vaginal dryness and atrophy and improves sex.

Lynette D.

Lynette D. designs web pages part-time for a small marketing firm. Her husband Al sells industrial products and travels three days a week. They have three daughters, one of whom is in her last year of high school and still living at home. Lynette's passion for horses had gotten a little out of control. Her stable of three horses had grown over the past decade to 40 horses and she stated that, "I used to be crazy about horses, but now I'm just crazy."

Lynette received regular gynecologic care with the same physician for 15 years. Even though she had gotten a tubal ligation 12 years ago, she had resumed taking cycle control pills because of their benefits of no PMS and no periods. Her only new complaint was a decreased sex drive.

Lynette's general health was perfect. She took no prescription medication apart from the cycle control hormone pills, and she had been taking the recommended supplements for years. Looking after the stables provided plenty of exercise as she "shoveled literally a ton of horse manure every day."

Lynette's exam and all of her routine tests were normal. She determined that she was in perimenopause wThursday by studying the wTimeLine (Figure 3-1). Her BMI was an excellent 23 (Figure 1-3). Lynette's wScore (Figure 1-2) was a very low 6 W, and the only items checked were lack of sexual desire and lack of orgasm. Her wSxScore (Figure 18-2) was a very high 29.

Lynette related, during their first twenty years of their marriage, she and her husband had gotten into a comfortable routine that revolved around Lynette being the one who always initiated sex. Their sexual frequency had been fairly regular, once or sometimes twice a week, but somewhere along the way, their frequency had tailed-off. Al eventually tried to initiate sex, but they both felt awkward with it. Within the past year, she said they had had sex only twice, both times on vacation. Lynette emphasized she and Al were married for life, and she felt 100 percent responsible for the "problem". Even though her love for Al was as strong as ever, she just never thinks about sex, unless Al makes some dark comment about it; and then, it smothers her with guilt. Lynette stressed this was now a critical issue in their marriage, and she needed urgent improvement.

Sexual function is a complex union of biological, psychological, and spiritual forces, and Lynette was reassured that long-term relationships often have periods of decline followed by rebirth and growth. Relationship dynamics are not static, and couples mature together or apart over time. Lynette was given the example about how a marriage is like a garden. The garden produces not only fresh whole foods that nourish you, but the act of creating a garden yields a satisfying sense of accomplishment even if you never eat a single tomato. When you step back and look at a garden in full bloom, there is a realization that the hard work of digging, planting, weeding, and nurturing is worth the struggle. Marriage provides a structure for love and continuity that are important to many people, but even a solid marriage can fall apart with neglect.

Lynette had a good handle on the psychological part of her relationship. Biological issues needed to be addressed.

Testosterone (T) produced in small quantities by the ovaries is important for sexual desire and arousal in women. There is a slight, gradual decline in testosterone production with age. By the time of menopause, 40 percent of women are relatively deficient in "free" active testosterone, and it may impact their sexual desire. Another confounding factor had to do with Lynette's cycle control pills (birth control pills, oral contraceptives). Through a complex series of metabolic changes, cycle control pills, in some women, may reduce the amount of available "free" active testosterone by binding up more of the total testosterone with sex hormone binding globulin. Reduced production coupled with reduced availability may spell reduced sexual desire and arousal.

Lynette had blood tests to check her testosterone level. Her "free" testosterone was calculated to be less than 0.5 (the lowest it could be measured), and her Sex Hormone Binding Globulin was elevated (SHBG soaks up "free" available testosterone). Lynette wanted to know if there was anything she could do to get back to normal.

Lynette was given the option of switching around her hormone therapy to one that was potentially a little more sex friendly. A good place to start would be stopping the oral cycle control pills. With time that may result in a decline in SHBG and subsequent rise in "free" testosterone, but it could take months for that to occur. Lynette decided to convert from cycle control pills to MHT consisting of Eva Mist, three sprays (transdermal estradiol) in the morning, coupled with oral Prometrium 100 mg at night. Because she had had a tubal ligation, her MHT did not need to cover birth control. Because of her urgency, she elected to simultaneously begin transdermal systemic testosterone (Testim) one drop applied to her wrist and rubbed in with the other wrist every morning. With no contact to the fingers, there is less chance of transferring it to someone else. Lynette and her doctor discussed all the potential benefits, risks, and side effects of each medication. She was instructed to increase the number of drops to 2 drops in 2 weeks if she had no unwanted side effects. Lynette was counseled about the five-night Sexercise assignment (Chapter 18), which she agreed to do on week four of her new regimen.

Four weeks later Lynnette returned. She and Al had crossed a new bridge in their relationship. For the first time they had had several discussions about their sex life, and both had expressed how important it was for them to please and satisfy the other. Lynette had experienced no problems, which she attributed to the menopausal hormone therapy. She was not completely sure whether it was the testosterone drops or the talk that helped her sex life; but in the end, she thought it was both. Six months later, she and Al felt their marriage was better than ever. Lynette tapered off the Testim and remained on the E+P. Her sexual desire and arousal remained excellent after that.

Part VI: Skinning and Winning

wBodyIdentical and CE/synthetic menopausal hormone therapy offer effective treatment for Hot Flash Fever, night sweats, Vaginal Sahara, and prevention of osteoporosis. There is growing recognition that transdermal wBodyIdentical estrogen has advantages over oral forms of estrogen (Figure 21-4). The difference between them derives primarily from liver metabolism of oral estrogen. The liver changes orally consumed estrogen as it passes through the liver (called first pass metabolism) before it has a chance to reach the rest of the body. Even if 17beta-estradiol wBodyIdentical hormone is swallowed, most of it is changed into a less active or different estrogen (E1) before it reaches the target tissue. If synthetic/conjugated non-human estrogens are taken by mouth the liver does not change them into wBodyIdentical estrogens either. The only way to get estradiol (E2) into the target tissues is to apply E2 to the skin. Absorption through the skin bypasses the liver and allows E2 direct access for action (Figure 21-3).

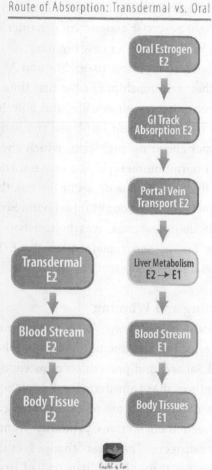

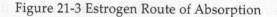

Figure 21-3 Estrogen Route of Absorption

Part VII:
I Never Promised You a Rose Garden

Imagine a vase of long stemmed roses on a sunny windowsill. It is a classic scene with a flower of unmatched beauty. However, if you grab those roses without looking them over carefully, you are likely to get pricked into the harsh reality of life. If you are not careful, even beautiful roses can cause grief.

Menopausal Hormone Therapy can provide unequivocal benefits. They must be examined carefully because each woman has important unique features that may factor into their suitability. The next chapter helps women choose a designer therapy that fits their specific needs.

All pharmaceutical-grade estrogens deliver effective relief of menopausal symptoms with proven safety. The differences between transdermal 17beta-estradiol wBodyIdentical estrogen, and all the others are subtle. Those slight differences may be more important to some women than to others. Lower than standard doses may be better tolerated and may have lower risks.

Delivering bona fide E2 to the body is not the only advantage of transdermal wBodyIdentical estradiol. As estrogen passes through the liver (as when taken as a pill), the liver changes its way of making other things. Four important changes have been proven, and there may be more known in the future.

1. Oral estrogen, but not transdermal estrogen, may change the way the liver works. Oral estrogen may make the liver produce substances that lead to increased risks of cardio-vascular disease. There is a rise in inflammatory substances (CRP) an associated marker and mediator of coronary heart disease and an elevation of triglycerides with oral but not transdermal estrogen. Women with hypertriglyceridemia should not take oral estrogen but may take transdermal estrogen because transdermal

TRANSDERMAL	ORAL
17b-estradiol wBodyidentical	other estrogen mixtures
stable serum levels	fluctuating serum levels
lower doses absorb through skin	larger doses to absorb through GI
>♀to♀ variation in dose	>uniformity in dose ♀to♀
decreasing triglycerides	increasing triglycerides
some improvement LDL & HDL	more improvement LDL & HDL
probably no effect on coagulation	more neg effect on coagulation
possible neg effect on liver disease	more neg effect on liver disease
fewer headaches	more headaches
may decrease BP	may increase BP
may improve diabetes	may worsen diabetes
treats hot flash fever	treats hot flash fever
treats vagina sahara	treats vagina sahara
may improve libido	may improve libido
treats mood matters	treats mood matters
improves the skinny on skin	improves the skinny on skin
may improve the insomnia queen	may improve the insomnia queen
reduces heart disease in wFriday	reduces heart disease in wFriday
prevents bone loss	prevents bone loss
reduces mortality in wFriday women	reduces mortality in wFriday women

Figure 21-4 Differences Between Transdermal and Oral
Estrogen Therapy

estrogen decreases triglycerides.

2. Oral estrogen changes the constituents of the coagulation
system, making the blood a little more likely to form a clot.
The hyper-coaguable state may lead to blood clots in the
legs that may dislodge and travel to the lungs causing a

life-threatening pulmonary embolus. It may also contribute to blockage of the coronary arteries and cerebral arteries resulting in a heart attack or stroke. Women with a history of oral hormone induced blood clots should avoid all oral forms of estrogen.

3. Oral estrogen may cause an increase in Sex Hormone Binding Globulin (SHBG) another liver-made protein that transports testosterone (and other hormones to a much lesser degree). Increases in SHBG seen in women on oral estrogen, both MHT and cycle control pills, may reduce the amount of "free" available testosterone with a resulting decrease in sexual desire and arousal (Chapter 18). Switching to transdermal estrogen may improve the amount of free testosterone.

4. Oral estrogen has a higher rate of causing breast tenderness than transdermal estrogen.

Part VII:
Summary: Preview

Deciding where to go on vacation can sometimes cause a lot of anxiety. Should we visit relatives? How about Florida? Could we do that trip to Paris? When should we go? Where should we stay? How much will this cost? The decisions go on and on. In truth, all the trips have some good points and bad. Staying home may indeed be the least expensive and safest, and if you are afraid of flying, France is definitely out of the picture. But you have to ask yourself, "Am I missing anything by staying home?" Many people choose not to travel for lots of reasons. For others, travel and vacations are one of the best parts of their lives.

Menopausal Hormone Therapy is a little like that. There are a lot of possibilities, and it's difficult sometimes to narrow down the choices. All MHTs have pluses and minuses, as do vacation destinations. Fortunately the FDA has visited all the hotels on the list, has slept in every bed, and has tasted every item on the buffet. All prescription hormones available in the U.S. are supported by a ton of scientific investigation, and all are FDA government approved.

The next chapter will build upon the information presented in this one and help women help themselves in the determination of whether or not MHT is right for her.

Taking hormones has known risks, and those will be detailed. Not taking hormones also has risks.

Part VIII:
The Womenopause Challenge: Pruning Roses

1. Look-up the word "bioidentical".
2. Look-up the word "wBodyIdentical".
3. Both words are made-up! One is used to sell/market hormones, and the other is used to explain hormones. Can you tell which is which?
4. Look-up the words "synthetic" and "bioengineered".
5. If you dare, research the word "natural". Does it have any relevance in the context of menopausal hormone therapy?

Chapter 22

Designer Therapy: Tailoring Hormones For Specific Needs

Part I:
A Dress and a Slip

Who doesn't love a great dress? When the right size, the right design, and the right fabric come together, a woman can handle just about anything. Dress power! Some dresses are a little too sheer or a little too clingy to wear without a slip, and a good slip can take a dress from good to great. However, no one would wear a slip under a dress unless they had to; and for sure, no one would go out on the town wearing only a slip. The same is true with menopausal estrogen and progesterone. Estrogen is the "dressy" female hormone that catches everyone's eye while progesterone is the slip of hormones that works behind the scenes. Just as no one would wear a slip underneath a dress that did not need one, women do not take progesterone unless they need to. The only reason to take menopausal progesterone is to protect the uterus; and in that case, the slip is absolutely required.

Menopausal Hormone Therapy (MHT) has a distinctive appearance because of the estrogen dress and almost all of the beauty and benefits are due to it. No one knows what a progesterone slip would look like alone because it is never worn that way. This chapter takes the wrap off estrogen and walks it up and down the runway so everyone can see it from all angles.

Part II:
"When You Get To a Fork In The Road, Take It"

The baseball sage, Yogi Berra, may have anticipated

271

menopausal women's decision dilemma about whether or not to take Menopausal Hormone Therapy (MHT). Almost everyone would probably like to walk down both paths to see what each one is like. Before we go any farther, it must be said, for the majority of healthy women there are no absolutes. Choosing to take or not take hormones is a personal decision. That determination is not then carved into stone either, and women may change their minds later. Anyone may initially start out going down the left path, change her mind, and go the other direction. For MHT it's left or right, *not* right or wrong. Every month, new information becomes available and ideas may change. Keeping informed by having regular medical care with a genuine expert healthcare provider is a good place to start.

The fork in the reproductive road does not usually appear suddenly out of the blue. Most women see it coming from a long way off. Perimenopause, for some women, may stretch-out for a decade with irregular periods. There is usually plenty of time to gather information and make an informed decision about what is best for you. However, keeping an open mind throughout the process is important. It is one thing to have an opinion about a certain topic, but it is another thing when it affects you personally; you might develop a different opinion. For instance, many pregnant couples plan on having a "natural" childbirth, without an epidural. *One of them* frequently feels a lot differently about it after a few hours of painful contractions. It almost goes without saying; everyone would prefer to not take any medication for any reason. On the other hand, there is nothing "natural" about antibiotics; the human body does not make amoxicillin, but where would we be without it?

Part III:
Going Naked: Estrogen Withdrawal and Deficiency

During perimenopause, estrogen production from the ovaries becomes erratic; and at menopause, it all but ceases. There are two distinct types of problems that low estrogen can cause in women: short-term estrogen *withdrawal worries* and long-term estrogen *deficiency drawbacks*.

There has always been clear appreciation of the short-term withdrawal worries, but many experts have never considered them serious health issues. They are. The long-term deficiency drawbacks have only recently been clarified. Although much more research will need to be done, it appears now that MHT has important long-term effects on women's health and well-being. For many women, going naked without an estrogen dress (and without the progesterone slip when needed) makes the following fashion statement.

- Short-term estrogen withdrawal worries:
  1. Hot Flash Fever and Cold Crashes
  2. Night sweats and drenched night gowns
  3. Insomnia Queen and daytime drowsiness
  4. Meno-Fog and impaired thinking
  5. Mood Matters and mood swings
  6. Crying spells
  7. Headaches
  8. Palpitations

- Long-term estrogen deficiency drawbacks:
  1. Vagina Sahara: vaginal discomfort and atrophy
  2. Impaired sexual response, low libido, and diminished arousal
  3. Osteoporosis with fractures of spine, hip, and wrist
  4. Cardiovascular disease, heart attacks and stroke
  5. Brain impairment with dementia, and fatigue
  6. Dry wrinkling skin
  7. Arthritis and joint pain
  8. Dry eye

You might be thinking, "Why wouldn't every healthy menopausal woman take hormones if it was that important?" Good question. The answer is complicated and has to do with the fine print.

Part IV:
Wardrobe Expense: MHT Risk

The Women's Health Initiative study (Chapter 19) published in 2002 determined hormone therapy to be risky and not worth it. Many women stopped taking hormones when that information was published; and even today, women often shy away from MHT because of what they thought they heard about the WHI report. Much has changed since 2002. Even though the WHI found some problems associated with hormones, re-analysis of the WHI data discovered some very positive aspects of hormone therapy.

It is often difficult to come to agreement on what is an "acceptable level of risk". The risks a doctor might be willing to let a patient take may be different than what the patient is actually willing to risk. Also, risk is stealthy and hidden everywhere. For instance, someone could eliminate their risk of dying in a plane crash by driving everywhere, but they turn around and increase their risk of dying in a car crash (which is more likely to begin with).

Risk assumption is often more emotional than practical. Risk is a gut reaction, and risk is hard to quantify. Say someone wants to hide in the closet to avoid getting mugged. Imagine the enormous risks she takes by staying in the closet: no exercise (bad for the heart), no social contact (bad for the soul), and so on. Avoiding one risk never means avoiding all risk; it just means risking something else.

Taking menopausal hormone therapy means taking on certain risks while avoiding others. Because hormones have been extensively studied, the magnitude of those risks is now well documented. Whenever risks of taking hormones are present, you can be sure there is a corresponding risk by not taking them. Some of the risks listed here are hotly debated even among experts. This is particularly common when the absolute risks are negligible, and it takes thousands and thousands of women studied over years and years to find the minute differences in order to compare the advantages and disadvantages. Many of the supposed risks of MHT derived from the WHI study have been subsequently refuted.

- Possible menopausal hormone therapy side effects and their solutions:

   1. **Fluid retention and swelling:** improves with exercise, water, and a change in hormone to transdermal estrogen or a change in the hormone dose.
   2. **Bloating:** improves by switching progesterone to wBodyIdentical Prometrium.
   3. **Breast tenderness:** improves with time or a change to a transdermal estrogen or a lower dose of estrogen. Decreasing caffeine, chocolate, decongestants, and taking vitamin E improves breast tenderness.
   4. **Headache:** improves with changing estrogen to trans-dermal formulation or reducing the dose.
   5. **Nausea:** improves by switching to a transdermal estrogen.
   6. **Vaginal bleeding:** is considered normal and fairly common during the first six months of MHT and improves with time and a change in dose or delivery method. If bleeding lasts longer than six months, a pipelle sample of the endometrium may be warranted.
   7. **Weight gain myth:** There has never been a study done proving MHT causes weight gain, but there are several studies demonstrating weight loss and decreased belly

fat.

8. **Patch irritation:** improves with topical OTC hydrocortisone and switching to transdermal gel, cream, spray, or vaginal ring.

9. **Patch dirt ring:** can be prevented with talcum powder and removed with mineral oil.

• Big-ticket items: menopausal hormone therapy risks and controversy:

1. **Breast Cancer:** The most hotly debated subject in women's health is the benefit/risk of MHT and breast cancer. The WHI said HRT (the term used before MHT) increased the risk of breast cancer, but the re-analysis said otherwise. With MHT consisting of estrogen only (no progesterone for women who have had a hysterectomy), there is a *reduction* of diagnosis of breast cancer by 33 percent (Figure 19-1). With MHT consisting of E+P (for women who have a uterus), there is an insignificant *increased* incidence of breast cancer diagnosis but a *reduced* risk of dying from breast cancer (go figure that one out). Oral conjugated estrogens (the only ones studied in the WHI) may have a different effect on breast disease than transdermal wBodyIdentical estrogen. (More on this topic in Chapter 27: Breast Cancer).

2. **Venous thromboembolism:** The WHI said the risks were elevated with HRT, but the re-analysis said otherwise. The risk of blood clots is elevated with oral forms of estrogen, but not with transdermal wBodyIdentical 17beta-estradiol (Figure 22-1).

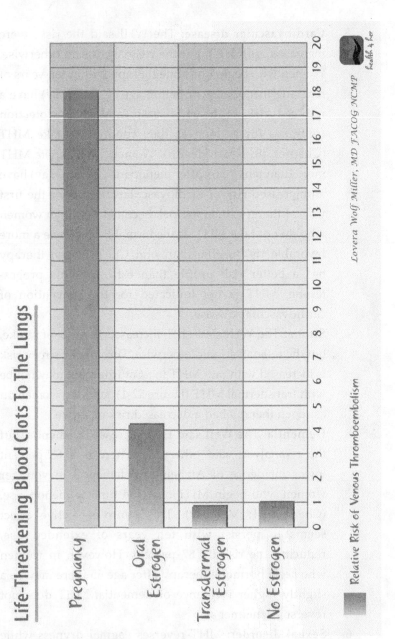

Figure 22-1 Relative Risk of Venous Thromboembolism

3. **Cardiovascular disease:** The WHI said the risks were increased with HRT, but the re-analysis said otherwise. Women who begin hormone therapy within ten years of reaching menopause or before age 60, (*w*Friday) have a reduced risk of heart disease, and that protection continues for as long as they continue to take MHT (Chapter 28: Heart Health). Women who *initiate* MHT more than tens years after menopause (*w*Saturday) have an increased risk of cardiovascular disease for the first year of therapy, then the risk becomes less than women who do not take MHT. Transdermal E may have a more favorable risk profile than oral CE. Estrogen therapy has a better risk profile than estrogen plus progesterone. MHT is not indicated for the prevention of cardiovascular disease.

4. **Stroke:** The WHI said HRT increased the risk of stroke, but the re-analysis said otherwise. Thrombotic stroke risk is increased with oral MHT in *w*Saturday, but may not be with transdermal MHT (Figure 22-1). *w*Friday women on estrogen therapy had a decreased risk of stroke.

5. **Dementia:** The WHI said HRT increased dementia, but the re-analysis said otherwise. There is a 65 percent lower incidence of Alzheimer's dementia in younger women who begin MHT near the time of menopause. (Chapter 31: Memory). This neuro-protective effect seems to persist with ten years of extended use, reducing the risk by 87 percent. However, in women who *begin* hormone therapy after age 65 there may be a slightly higher incidence of dementia. MHT does not reverse Alzheimer's.

6. **Sexual disorder:** MHT reverses vaginal dryness while restoring desire and arousal. Transdermal estrogen has advantages over oral CE by way of keeping SHBG lower (Chapter 18: Sexercise).

Part V:
Timing: When Not to Wear White Shoes

Unfortunately, most people (and most doctors) know about menopausal hormone therapy risks *only* through the WHI media reports. The WHI information is not relevant for the majority of menopausal women. The subjects in the WHI were *w*Saturday women who had been *w*UpSiders for almost 2 decades, and who were, at the beginning of the study, having no menopausal symptoms! WHI was not intended as a study about the treatments for menopausal symptoms, but it did provide some valuable information.

First, there is strong evidence now that there is a "window of opportunity" for starting MHT. Timing is extremely important. If MHT is started near menopause on *w*Friday, almost all of the bad things the WHI noted disappear. Second, if the type of MHT is examined, almost all of the bad things the WHI noted may have been due to the liver effects of oral estrogen. As detailed in the last chapter (Chapter 21), oral estrogen undergoes extensive first pass metabolism and results in increased clotting risk and increased inflammatory markers. Blood clots and inflammation may be behind all of the cardiovascular, brain, and venous thromboembolism problems seen in the WHI because the WHI *only* studied a fixed dose of oral non-human conjugated estrogen. Currently used *w*BodyIdentical 17beta-estradiol transdermal products do not have the adverse effects on clotting or inflammation and would, therefore, not be expected to increase the other risks like the conjugated estrogens of the WHI study.

There remain questions about what age is considered too advanced to start MHT. Just like there are loose fashion rules about not wearing white shoes after Labor Day, there are some developing conventions about when *not* to start MHT. We need a show of hands, who has ever worn white shoes after Labor Day? Well, probably just about everyone has broken that rule for one reason or another. There is little debate, the WHI data demonstrates excellent reward/risk value of MHT in women under age 60 or within ten years of menopause (wFriday). It is a grey area to begin MHT in women age 60 to 70 or more than ten years since menopause (wSaturday morning), and more risk to begin MHT after age 70 or more than 20 years since menopause (wSaturday afternoon). If a woman begins estrogen therapy younger than 60, her risk is rare and no greater than the risk associated with taking aspirin or lipid-lowering drugs. Women who begin MHT early may continue taking it as long as they desire the benefits, and there is no data to suggest there is danger of increasing cardio-vascular disease risk over time. This should be re-evaluated on an annual basis with your healthprovider to reassess your risk in light of ongoing research and changes in your personal health.

There is strong evidence about the benefits of Estrogen (E) alone, for MHT in wFriday early postmenopause women who have had a hysterectomy. Here are some of the confirmed benefits:

- Reduction of heart disease by 40 percent
- Reduction of stroke by 11 percent
- Reduction of new diabetes by 12 percent
- Reduction of fractures by 30 percent
- Reduction of breast cancer by 30 percent
- Reduction of colon cancer by 20 percent
- Reduction of dementia by 65 percent
- Reduction of Metabolic Syndrome
- Reduction of total mortality by any cause by 40 percent
- Reduction of skin wrinkles
- Reduction of depression
- Reduction of weak muscles
- Reduction of hair loss
- Reduction of vaginal dryness
- Reduction of sexual distress

Beneficial Effects of Estrogen Therapy

Improved Mood
Better Memory
Thicker Hair
Smoother, Softer Skin

Stronger Muscle
Lowered Cardiovascular Disease
Reduced Breast Cancer

Reduced Belly Fat

Improved Sex Response
Eliminates Vagina Sahara

Stronger Bone
Smoother Skin
Less Joint Pain

Stronger Nails

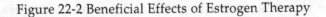

Figure 22-2 Beneficial Effects of Estrogen Therapy

There has never been a question about whether or not MHT reduces short term estrogen withdrawal worries like hot flashes, night sweats, and vaginal dryness, but there have been disputes about what MHT does for, or against, long term estrogen deficiency drawbacks and serious chronic diseases. That question now has some clarity. When MHT is initiated close to the time of menopause, there are health benefits that go far beyond the reduction of hot flashes. Because there are estrogen receptors scattered throughout many organs of the female body, it is no wonder estrogen therapy provides beneficial effects not only for short-term estrogen withdrawal worries but for long-term estrogen deficiency drawbacks, as well. Venus loves estrogen.

MHT for women over seventy requires a careful risk to benefit estimation. And it is absolutely true; some situations require white shoes to be worn out of season.

Conventional MHT is considered a higher risk for women with estrogen receptor positive breast cancer and is usually avoided. Alternate therapies are covered in Chapter 16. Breast cancer survivors with severe vaginal atrophy may be candidates for local vaginal estrogen and/or local vaginal testosterone, which restore the health of the vagina while not being significantly absorbed and distributed to the rest of the body.

MHT is also considered a risk for women who have had a hormone-induced blood clot or pulmonary embolus or a recent heart attack or stroke. With a history of liver disease, a woman should avoid oral hormone therapy but could consider the possibility of transdermal estrogen.

Part VI:
Progesterone Lingerie

A finely crafted slip with a nice lace edging is still just a slip. It is necessary to go under certain dresses; otherwise, you leave it in the closet. Because estrogen stimulates the endometrium to grow, it is necessary to pair estrogen with progesterone so that the growth is reigned in. Unopposed estrogen stimulation of the uterus may lead to an increased risk of uterine cancer and the addition of progesterone lowers that risk below non-hormone users.

During perimenopause the chosen progesterone style depends upon several variables (Figure 22-3: The Hormone Grid).

- If a perimenopausal woman, wWednesday or wThursday, develops irregular periods and hot flashes or other perimenopause symptoms, she may want to consider Yaz (cycle control pills); NuvaRing (vaginal birth control ring); or Ortho-Evra Patch (a birth control patch), particularly if fertility is still an issue. All cycle control therapies with the exception of two, contain both estrogen and progesterone; although none of them are wBodyIdentical. All may be cycled monthly to resemble regular periods or taken continuously to avoid having any bleeding at all. This style of dress is very sheer and always needs a slip.

- If a perimenopausal woman develops irregular periods and hot flashes and does not need birth control (she has had a tubal, or her partner has had a vasectomy, or she is not sexually active, or she would not mind becoming pregnant); she can control the symptoms with menopausal hormone therapy instead of cycle control pills or the NuvaRing. MHT has the advantage of containing less than one-fourth of the dose of hormone as cycle control pills, but has the disadvantage of taking a little longer to establish control of the periods. MHT is not strong enough to stop ovulation, so pregnancy remains a possibility while taking MHT. MHT consisting of a wBodyIdentical trans-dermal E plus an oral wBodyIdentical progesterone (P) would work. wBodyIdentical P (Prometrium) causes less bloating and depression than synthetic progestins. Prometrium is a kinder-gentler P and is a slip of a hormone that does not hang-down below the hem of the dress.

- If a perimenopausal woman, wWednesday or wThursday, develops hot flashes and has had a hysterectomy, then three important differences are present. First, with no uterus, irregular periods are not an issue. Second, with no uterus, pregnancy is not an issue. Third, with no uterus, progesterone would not be needed to protect the endometrium. MHT transdermal estrogen would be an appropriate start. This dress is made with the type of fabric that does not need a slip.

The Hormone Grid

	E	E+P	CCP BIRTH CONTROL PILLS
Perimenopause with a uterus		+	+
Perimenopause without a uterus	+		rarely
wUpSide with a uterus		+	
wUpSide without a uterus	+		

Figure 22-3: The Menopausal Hormone Therapy Grid

During postmenopause, wUpSide, the choices are simpler. MHT estrogen is paired with progesterone (E+P) for women with a uterus while women who have had a hysterectomy use MHT estrogen (E) alone. Transdermal wBodyIdentical estrogen has advantages over oral CE estrogen, and oral wBodyIdentical progesterone (Prometrium) has advantages over oral progestins.

Part VII:
A Hormone That Fits to a "T"

Although present in only small quantities in women, testosterone (T) serves an important role. Testosterone has an influence on sexual desire, and orgasm for women and facilitates bone and muscle growth. T also has a subtle effect on women's mood, sense of well-being, and energy levels. Unlike estrogen and progesterone that have a rather abrupt decline at menopause, testosterone slightly and gradually decreases over several decades and doesn't change dramatically at menopause.

Testosterone deficiency in postmenopausal women is a controversial subject; and to date, there has been no FDA approved indication for testosterone treatment in women. There is a growing body of evidence T therapy in some women improves the sexual response, and it warrants further investigation. Testosterone therapy remains off-label in the U.S. but not in Europe or Canada for women with Hypoactive Sexual Desire Disorder (HSDD).

Sex Hormone Binding Globulin (SHBG) transports testosterone in the bloodstream. Only a small percentage (1 to 2 percent) of the total testosterone is "free" and available to perform its function. This is important because all *oral* MHT appears to stimulate the liver to produce more SHBG. Higher amounts of SHBG soaks-up more testosterone leaving even less "free" T available to work. Therefore, the combined effects of *lower production* of testosterone in postmenopause with *reduced available* "free" T from oral MHT, result in a significant additional decrease in testosterone function in some *w*Friday and *w*Saturday women. Lowered bioavailable "free" T may manifest itself as diminished sexual desire and arousal.

Serum measurement of SHBG, free testosterone, and total testosterone may help guide therapy but remain somewhat controversial because laboratory measurements of such low levels of T in women may be inaccurate. Menopausal testosterone therapy in the U.S. consists of off-label male products (transdermal Testim, testosterone drops) or compounded vaginal testosterone cream 1-2 percent. Testosterone therapy is monitored by tracking the symptoms and/or side effects of the treatment. Dosage is adjusted to get just the right fit. If low sex drive is the reason for starting T therapy, then response may be measured by using the wSxScore (Figure 18-2).

Side effects of low dose testosterone for women with HSDD are mild and uncommon. The easiest way to monitor testosterone side effects is by monitoring its action on the skin. A very low dose of T therapy usually improves dry skin and restores softness to the surface. Slightly higher dose T therapy may begin to produce a noticeable skin-shine. Still higher doses may produce oily skin, and even higher doses may promote acne. In most circumstances, low doses required to restore sexual desire and arousal in women are associated with only positive skin changes. Unwanted hair growth may occur when the dose gets too high, but this should disappear with decreasing the dose.

The big question mark about testosterone therapy is what effect does it have in stimulating breast cancer? The FDA says there is not enough data to be sure, but the Canadian and European regulators believe there is sufficient data that Testosterone does not increase the risk of breast cancer.

Testosterone blood levels can also be increased by vigorous exercise and estrogen therapy (a small amount of E gets converted to T in the body). One of the best ways to improve internal testosterone production is by having more sex. Sexual activity induces the production of testosterone which increases sex drive; more sex leads to better sex. Raised testosterone levels have been correlated with improved feelings of confidence, decreased belly fat, improved muscle tone and bone strength, and improved vaginal health. In fact, testosterone may be applied directly to the vagina as a cream for the treatment of vaginal dryness for wUpSide women. Local topical testosterone therapy may be considered to treat vaginal dryness in some women with breast cancer.

Part VIII:
Creative Closets

The only women who should consider taking menopausal hormone therapy are those with short-term estrogen withdrawal worries such as Hot Flash Fever, night sweats, Cold Crashes, Mood Matters, Meno-Fog, Insomnia Queen, and Vagina Sahara or to prevent osteoporosis. Everyone else (if there actually is anyone else) can refrain and begin the effective lifestyle changes discussed earlier in the book to stop pausing and start living. Although MHT clearly improves long-term estrogen deficiency drawbacks such as cardiovascular disease, dementia, and sexual dysfunction when started near the time of menopause, it is not currently recommended as a specific therapy or prevention for any of these conditions. The long-term MHT effects are considered a side effect bonus by some experts and an essential objective by others.

Decisions about which hormone or combination of hormones is most suitable for you should take into account the following:

- *w*Score: Women with estrogen withdrawal identify symptoms on the *w*Score may warrant further discussions with a healthcare provider (Figure 1-2).
- **Uterus**: If you have a uterus then your MHT will consist of E+P. If you do not have a uterus you may take only E.
- **Fertility**: If you are perimenopausal and having periods (regular or irregular), then you may still become pregnant. Although fertility rapidly declines near menopause, cycle control pills (Yaz) or NuvaRing may be required to control menopausal symptoms and protect against unplanned pregnancy.
- **Risk**: Most women who have the following are not candi-

dates for MHT: pregnancy, undiagnosed vaginal bleeding, breast cancer, deep vein thrombosis or pulmonary embolus, recent (in the last year) stroke or heart attack, and severe liver disease.

- **Benefits**: The alleviation of menopausal symptoms may make a trial of MHT advantageous. It is appropriate to consider personal feelings and non-scientific qualities before beginning therapy.

- **Sexuality**: Sexuality, that is impaired as a consequence of estrogen withdrawal in perimenopause and beyond (Vagina Sahara), may improve with systemic transdermal E therapy (or E+P). Local vaginal estrogen therapy may also be required to fully restore the vaginal mucosa because systemic menopausal hormone therapy today uses very low doses of estrogen; and sometimes, it is not enough to reverse Vagina Sahara. Occasionally, testosterone therapy is needed to restore sexual desire and orgasm. Set goals and monitor results with the wSxScore (Figure 18-2).

- *w*Bodyidentical: MHT consisting of transdermal *w*Bodyidentical estrogen (17beta-estradiol) and oral *w*Bodyidentical progesterone (Prometrium) for women with a uterus is a preferred choice (Figure 21-2).

- **Route**: *w*Bodyidentical estrogen may be administered with equal safety and effectiveness via transdermal spray, gel, cream, patch, or vaginal ring. *w*Bodyidentical progesterone is available only as a capsule or as gel inserted into the vagina at the present time. Current progesterone skin cream is not absorbed well in a usable form and may not be protective of the uterus. Therefore, progesterone skin cream should not be used. Some women prefer oral estrogen therapy.

- **Dose**: The official recommendation for menopausal hormone therapy maintains that it should be given at the lowest effective dose to adequately control the menopausal symptoms. However, it must be admitted that the lowest effective dose to control hot flashes may not turn out to be the optimal dose for prevention of osteoporosis or heart disease. It's just not known. Younger women frequently require higher doses to manage estrogen withdrawal worries and to prevent estrogen deficiency drawbacks.

- **Duration**: The official recommendation for menopausal hormone therapy maintains that it should be used for the shortest duration of time to control the menopausal symptoms. Improvement of long-term estrogen deficiency problems may prove to be the greatest benefit of MHT, and continued therapy may turn out to be worthwhile. Since 5,000 estrogen research articles are published every month (another exaggeration, maybe only 4,000) the truth of the matter may evolve over time. It seems eminently prudent for women to reassess the safety of their hormone therapy every year with their healthcare provider. An experienced healthcare provider can guide you toward a balanced understanding of the current medical literature and minimize the temptation to chase the latest trend. Many women may choose to take menopause hormone therapy for the duration of their life.

The hormone closet is well-stocked with stylish choices. Every woman will feel relieved to know that there is no peer pressure to follow what is in vogue. Only you know what fits you best.

Jan D.

The first thing out of Jan's mouth was a clear warning, "Don't you dare try to take away my Prempro." Jan was 68 and had been happily taking Prempro, a combination conjugated estrogen plus progestin (CE+P) for 15 years. This past year her internist told her she had to stop because her blood pressure was going up, and she "didn't need hormones at *her* age." She could not decide which steamed her most, the hypertension, or that her doctor thought she was too advanced in years to need estrogen. Her internist sent her to the menopause specialist to "talk some sense into her."

Aside from controlled hypertension, Jan was perfectly healthy. She had been married to Jan (by a quirk in fate she married a guy with the same first name) for a million years and had raised two sons. "We tried to raise them, but they just won't grow up." Both boys were NASCAR pit crew workers and lived "racy lives." She had an uneventful menopause at age 53 and had started MHT within the first year. She attributes her health and vitality to "4-H" (not the farm kid club): **H**ormones, **H**ealthy foods, **H**eavy work, and **H**appiness.

She said she was not about to mix anything up. Earlier in the year her internist "scared me into stopping" the Prempro which she did for "two horrible weeks." She resumed taking them every other day as a compromise with her doctor's temporary approval. On her hormone "off" days, she had multiple hot flashes and moodiness. Jan wanted one thing: permission to take them everyday.

Jan's *w*Score during hormone "on" days was 11 W and during hormone "off" days was 33 W (Figure 1-2). Her blood pressure was 134/84, and her BMI was 26. Her mammogram and blood lipids were normal (total cholesterol was 165 and the good cholesterol, was extra good, at 80). Jan's only cardiovascular risk factor was her mild hypertension for which she was receiving Lisinopril. She had no family history of cardiac disease and had made excellent long-term lifestyle choices. She readily accepted additional information about the Womenopause Challenge and planned to step up her vitamin and mineral intake. She also made plans to schedule more time for regular exercise.

The benefits and risks of MHT, for extended time, were discussed. Jan realized taking MHT for decades has supporters and detractors even among hormone experts. The goal of hormone therapy, like the goal of any medical therapy, would be the lowest dose for the shortest period of time to take care of the problem. Jan asked, "When is my need for estrogen going to stop?" That is a great question. Jan was advised that there is no consensus on how long is too long, and it needed careful reconsideration every year. There has been accumulating evidence that many women prefer to continue MHT for as long as they think it serves a purpose in reducing symptoms while others continue to take MHT because they are doing great and see no reason to stop. Jan was advised that there is no evidence that the longer she takes MHT the higher her risk of cardiovascular disease. Extended use of E+P may increase her risk of being diagnosed with breast cancer, but at the same time E+P reduces her risk from dying from anything, breast cancer included. Jan was advised that there is some evidence oral conjugated estrogen may raise blood pressure, and transdermal estrogen lowers blood pressure. In the final analysis, Jan was advised she could take MHT as long as she wanted to continue receiving the benefits.

After about a millisecond of thought, she decided she wanted to continue MHT. Jan was given the following options. One, she could stay on Prempro. Two, she could change her MHT to wBodyIdentical, transdermal estradiol plus oral progesterone. During a discussion about risks, Jan revealed she had an allergy to peanuts. Aside from the sad situation of not being able to enjoy Reese's Peanut Butter Cups, Jan should not take Prometrium oral progesterone. Prometrium, the only wBodyIdentical progesterone in common use is suspended in peanut oil. There is another progesterone product, Prochieve, which is wBodyIdentical and is applied as a vaginal gel, but Jan was not interested in applying a vaginal medicine. As an alternative she could consider a transdermal patch, which delivers both estrogen and progestin.

Jan began her new MHT with Combipatch. The patch delivers estradiol and progestin continuously through a patch applied to her lower abdomen which she changed twice a week. After an exchange of information between her menopause specialist and her internist, her internist agreed to the plan. Four weeks later Jan reported she was back to normal, and everything seemed like it was when she took Prempro. She wanted to know again why she switched to the patch. Transdermal 17beta-estradiol has all the benefits of oral conjugated estrogen plus a few specific additional benefits. Among the several differences, a reduced risk of thromboembolism and blood pressure with transdermal estrogen are often reasons enough to consider switching to transdermal estrogen in a woman with hypertension. Jan said, "Thanks, but I'm not worried about blood clots, but I guess I'm glad my doctor is".

Part VIII:
The Womenopause Challenge: Sorting Through The Closet

1. Find yourself on the wTimeLine (Figure 3-1). Imagine your wTimeLine day is the first day of spring, so clear out all those dark heavy winter clothes!

2. Your spring clothes are all beautiful pastel colors, and they are all in season and just your size. They are all brand new brought to you by the clothes fairy. Clothing color key: pink=estrogen, white=progesterone, lime=cycle control pills.

3. If you are perimenopausal, why not try the pink jacquard dress with the small white pattern (E+P). As an alternate, you'd also look good in the sateen lime one (CCP).

4. If you are perimenopausal but have had a hysterectomy,

you might look best in the sheer silk solid pink dress (E), but if your ovaries are still acting up with PMS (rarely happens), you could try on the sateen lime dress for a while (CCP).

5. If you are *w*UpSide, you would definitely want to try on the pink jacquard with the white pattern (E+P).

6. If you are *w*UpSide but have had a hysterectomy, then hands down, the one for you would be the solid silk pink dress (E).

7. Now the *real* question: which shoes?

Chapter 23

Suzanne Somers Is Not Ageless

Part I:
No One Gets Out Alive

Nowhere in this book can the reader find the "O word" (you know, the one insinuating your age is advanced beyond caring). No one likes that word; and besides, it's just a number, right? Also in this book, the reader will not find a reference to any of the following: miracle, breakthrough, supernatural, age defying, or fountain-of-youth. Those things are part of an unreal fantasy world, not this world. *Womenopause* is about not pausing at menopause; it is about starting to live fully in the real world. It is possible for you to be healthier at age 60 than you were at age 40. It is possible for you to be stronger, leaner, keener, and happier. Those things are possible. It is not possible to stop aging, and it is not possible to become younger. Sorry, it's just not possible. It is also impossible to become ageless by taking hormones.

Suzanne Somers is the most notable celebrity identified with promoting the concept of high dose hormones as a miraculous fountain of youth. Interwoven with the high dose theory is the notion there are different hormone levels for different types of women, and women should check their saliva before menopause to find out what kind of woman she is. The theory of replacing women's hormones to so-called youthful levels is not new (and even precedes *ménage et tois* TV programs). Her book *Ageless* is an undeniably fun read and reflects Somers' public image as a feminine health revolutionary. Everyone loves the positive energy and lifestyle encouragement the book espouses. The writing style is as seductive as the book's cover. There are honest differences of opinion about the theory and practice of custom compounded bioidentical hormones.

Part II:
Double Trouble: Don't Compound Your Problems

Have you ever driven off the beaten path, gotten lost, but couldn't bring yourself to ask for directions? It's a classic case of compounding your problems. Usually only men pull that one. Women in midlife, faced with menopause, are pulled in many directions at once by competing opinions about how best to proceed. Be assured, no one has all the answers when it comes to what is best for you. Modern medical practitioners have powerful arguments of logic and science behind their recommendations; but in the end, each person decides with a little thought, a little intuition, a little advice, and a lot of guess. There is no doubt, menopausal symptoms may be a significant problem for many women. The treatment for those problems, hopefully, does not heap additional problems on top of it. That would be another example of compounding your problems. You can ask for directions at any time; and better yet, get this map.

Part III:
What Is a Compounded Hormone?

The universe of hormones can be divided into two planets: the sun and the moon. The sun represents commercially prepared hormones that are prescribed by a licensed healthcare provider and sold at conventional pharmacies. The pharmacy buys the hormone product from a pharmaceutical company who manufactures it. These hormone products undergo extensive testing before the Federal Drug Administration (FDA) approves them. The FDA is charged to oversee all drugs and to protect the public from unsafe products and unscrupulous health claims. The FDA tightly controls what a pharmaceutical company can say about a product and insists that they advise the public about *every possible* side effect and risk on the package insert accompanying the drug. The sun works in broad daylight.

By a quirk in the system, the moon of compounded hormones circumvents all of that and works in the dark. In this case, the moon eclipses the sun, and an eerie darkness ensues. Somehow compounded hormones get classified in the same category as a face wash and are not regulated by the FDA at all. Therefore, compounded hormones do not have to meet government standards and claims about their effectiveness, and safety may go unchecked. To a degree, this loophole has been exploited to the detriment of a potentially useful medical therapy.

Bioidentical hormone therapy (BHT) is based, in part, upon mixing customized amounts and types of hormones to suit the specific requirements of women with specialized needs. The practice of custom compounding of hormones is useful for certain unique situations such as intolerance to standard pharmaceutical grade conventional hormone therapy. There may be rare individuals who have allergies or sensitivities to dyes, fillers, and preservatives present in commercial products. For instance, Prometrium, a wBodyIdentical progesterone pill is made with peanut oil, and women with peanut sensitivity should avoid it. Before outspoken advocates like Suzanne Somers promoted compounded hormones, the use of them was limited to the few women with documented reasons not to take an FDA regulated product.

Compounded hormones are marketed by certain pharmacies as a safer alternative to conventional pharmaceutical-grade hormones. Many women have the mistaken belief that compounded hormones are not synthetic and are, thereby, more natural. Where do you think the pharmacies get the hormones they compound? Do you think they have a soy garden out back of the store and just harvest some estrogen when they need to restock? Of course not. Compounding pharmacies buy their hormones from a drug maker who synthesizes them ("bioengineers" them behind the scenes). Bioidentical compounded hormones are synthetic! Indeed ALL hormones are synthetic except those produced by an animal in its own body!

Part IV: Black Jack: 21 Questions About Compounded Hormone Therapy

The usage of unsupervised custom compounded hormones has expanded since the devastating news from the WHI in 2002 (Chapter 19). The WHI at first blush, seemed to report menopausal hormone therapy was risky, and women should avoid it. Although subsequent analysis appears to have successfully refuted most of the negative findings, in 2010 most women (and men) have still heard only the bad stuff from the original report and none of the good stuff from later work. Many menopausal women with symptoms of estrogen withdrawal and deficiency abandoned hormone therapy for fear of breast cancer and heart attacks as a result of the WHI news. Because of persistent severe estrogen deficiency symptoms such as Hot Dreads, Insomnia Queen, Vagina Sahara, and Mood Matters; many women subsequently searched for alternate therapies and in swooped bioidentical custom compounded hormone therapy to fill the void. Since compounded hormones are not FDA regulated, symptomatic women have been targets of exploitative marketing. Many women were led to believe that bioidentical compounded hormones are perfectly natural and safe: in short, a miracle. Bioidentical custom compounded hormone therapy continues to be promoted as a safer and more effective therapy than conventional pharmaceutical hormone therapy, even though, it has never been tested for safety or effectiveness.

All medical societies who are dedicated to looking out for the welfare of women's health are firmly against compounded bioidentical hormones as they are commonly used, including: North American Menopause Society, International Menopause Society, American Medical Association, American College of Obstetrics and Gynecology, and the Endocrine Society.

The following 21 questions about bioidentical custom compounded hormones (BHT) deserve answers:

1. **What is natural?** Only humans make human hormones, and there is no such thing as a human hormone donor. BHT does not provide hormones naturally made from a human being (Chapter 21). Bioidentical hormones are not more natural than conventional FDA approved hormones. They are both made from plant products.

2. **What is "bioidentical?"** The molecular structure of human estrogen hormones has been well-known for decades, and exact duplicates are available as either FDA approved or non-FDA approved (compounded BHT). Bioidentical is a marketing slogan not a scientific or medical term. The preferred term of *w*BodyIdentical describes hormone molecules that are the exact duplicates of the hormone molecules naturally made within the human female and are FDA approved.

3. **What is synthetic?** All hormones, FDA approved and compounded BHT, are synthesized in a lab *exactly the same way*. Compounded bioidentical hormones are synthetic like all of the pharmaceutical grade hormones.

4. **What are plant-based hormones?** Plant based hormones are the ones synthesized from plant ingredients. Most FDA approved pharmaceutical hormones are made from soy and yam raw materials *exactly* like most compounded BHT.

5. **Are bioidentical hormones safer?** No. Bioidentical hormones are real hormones and have at least the same risks as pharmaceutical grade hormones plus *additional risks* due to their unregulated nature. Bioidentical hormones are definitely not safer.

6. **Do bioidentical hormones have fewer side effects?** No. Compounded BHT are real hormones and have at

least the same side effects as pharmaceutical grade hormones *plus the added unknown side effects* inherent in the unknown. Bioidentical hormones are promoted without disclosure of their significant side effects.

7. **What are drugs?** Compounded BHT are drugs and meet all the criteria of the definition of the word drug: "products are drugs when they are intended for the treatment, mitigation, or prevention of a disease or intended to affect the structure or any function of the body of women". Pharmaceutical grade hormones are drugs, and compounded BHTs are drugs.

8. **Can BHT reverse aging?** No. Compounded BHTs are hormones like the ones present during the fertility year's *w*Monday through *w*Thursday. Every woman who had naturally produced estrogen in her youth on *w*Tuesday still aged to *w*Wednesday. Women who produce their own estrogen still advance in age and having hormones does not make you immune to time. Compounded BHT would not reverse aging any more than pharmaceutical grade hormones.

9. **Is BHT as safe as MHT?** No. Compounded BHT is a drug with all the pluses and minuses of pharmaceutical grade hormone. The safety of pharmaceutical grade hormones has been proven in peer reviewed scientific journals, but the safety of compounded BHT has not been proven. Bioidentical hormones are definitely not as safe as pharmaceutical-grade hormones.

10. **Are bioidentical hormones unique?** No. Some compounded BHTs have the identical chemical structure as naturally made human estrogen, which are *exactly* like many pharmaceutical grade available FDA approved products. There is nothing unique about BHTs, except they add pregnancy estrogen (E3) that is untested in postmenopausal women and progesterone

skin cream that woman's skin may not absorb.

11. **Do BHTs cause less breast cancer?** No. Compounded BHT are real hormones and have at least the same breast cancer risks as pharmaceutical grade hormones plus the uncertain risks due to their nature of being unregulated by the FDA. Bioidentical hormones are definitely not safer for the breast. In fact, the safety of bioidentical hormones and breast cancer has never been studied.

12. **Do BHTs provide a more natural mixture of hormones?** No. Women naturally make three estrogens: E1, E2, & E3 (Chapter 2). Estrogen affects the body by binding to estrogen receptors, and E2 performs the vast majority of the function during the reproductive years. There is no evidence that E1 or E3 have any additional properties except acting like weaker E2.

13. **Should hormones be measured in saliva?** No. The amount of estrogen in saliva depends upon the time of day, the state of hydration, the type of recently eaten food, the facility doing the test, and dozens of other variables. The hormone levels in saliva are not related to the amount of menopausal symptoms or blood levels, and saliva tests are not reliable.

14. **Are Triest and Biest safer?** No. The commonly compounded BHT containing large amounts of estriol 80 percent (E3) and small amounts of estradiol (E2) and estrone (E1) (trade named Triest and Biest) reduces menopausal symptoms, even though the compound is mostly composed of the untested weaker form of estrogen. Having E3 confers no known additional effectiveness or safety. In fact, the FDA has recently taken action against compounding pharmacies because estriol (E3) has NEVER been studied for safety in humans.

15. **Do Triest and Biest better resemble natural hormone**

mixture? No. Estriol (E3) is the major hormone component of Triest and Biest BHT. However, in healthy non-pregnant fertile women (*w*Sunday through *w*Thursday) estradiol (E2) concentrations are higher than estrone (E1), and estriol (E3) is present in significant amounts only during pregnancy. The human female tightly regulates the amount of E1, E2, & E3 by enzymes throughout the body.

16. **Are BHTs really customized?** No. Compounded BHT utilizes a "one size fits all" approach because of the unwarranted emphasis on saliva testing to determine the dose. Every reputable medical and scientific society recommends dosing according to the control of symptoms not according to blood levels and definitely not according to saliva levels.

17. **Are BHTs economical?** No. BHT is usually not covered by prescription insurance plans because they are considered experimental, since no one has yet, actually done the experiments on them. Saliva hormone testing may add thousands of dollars a year in unnecessary additional costs.

18. **Is progesterone cream effective?** No. Transdermal progesterone cream has poor and variable absorption. Progesterone serves no purpose except for uterine protection during estrogen therapy. Compounded BHT progesterone cream used with estrogen therapy may not be absorbed well enough to safely protect the uterus from cancer. Use of BHT progesterone cream paired with BHT estrogen may increase the risk of uterine cancer.

19. **Is progesterone safer than estrogen?** No. Compounded BHT progesterone cream is often promoted to take the place of estrogen for the symptomatic treatment of hot flashes and osteoporosis, but there is no evidence that

it is either effective or safe.

20. **Are BHTs pure?** No. Uncertainty of dose and purity pose additional potential dangers to women who use compounded BHT. The FDA, through independent testing, has found compounded BHT products failed tests for purity, potency, contamination, and uniformity 90 percent of the time.

21. **Is there a need for BHT?** Maybe. There are a great variety of menopausal hormone therapy products available that are molecularly identical to human made hormones and are produced by pharmaceutical companies with FDA approval. The proven effectiveness, safety, and purity of pharmaceutical grade MHT make compounded BHT unnecessary for the majority of symptomatic menopausal women. Compounded medications of any kind should be reserved for those circumstances when individuals, because of allergies or specific problems, need a medicine not made by pharmaceutical companies.

Jackie W.

Jackie was 48, a happily married mother of two who worked as the director of a large non-profit organization. At her annual gynecology appointment she disclosed a concern about her health. She was planning to see a specialist at a university center for a "sweating" disorder. When asked to describe her symptoms, she noted she had "sweating spells six to ten times a day," and she produced a notebook detailing the frequency and intensity of the episodes. She often had a feeling of "being trapped and anxious" with the spells, and they occurred day or night. Sometimes the night episodes were so intense her nightgown became drenched, and she woke up shivering. "It's driving me a little batty," she said.

Jackie was advised the episodes closely resembled vasomotor

symptoms of perimenopause. She said that is what she originally had thought, but she had already tried to treat it with a hormone prescription from her family doctor, and it did not work. Since hormones did not help at all, they were pursuing an evaluation by a sweating expert at the university. She was asked to describe how she and her family doctor had used hormones.

Jackie's family doctor had sent her to a pharmacy to get saliva tests to find out if there was any hormone abnormality and after reviewing the results, determined she was low only in progesterone. She was prescribed a compounded progesterone cream from the same pharmacy and applied it to the skin of her abdomen once a day for six months. Her saliva was retested four times, and dosage adjustments in her progesterone cream were made after each test, but her symptoms never improved. She was next referred to a psychiatrist to see if it was a psychological anxiety disorder. She tried taking Ativan, an anti-anxiety medication, but it made her feel worse; she stopped it in less than a week. After several more tests looking for a possible source of infection, she and her doctor decided it must be a primary sweating disorder. "After all, I'm still having my periods, so can it really have anything to do with menopausal symptoms?"

After a review of the wTimeLine (Figure 3-1), Jackie determined she was probably in wThursday; but quickly noted, she had none of the perimenopause symptoms. She denied having hot flashes, mood swings, memory loss or vaginal dryness. She felt strongly her poor sleep was due to her "sweating disorder". The wScore (Figure 1-2) painted a slightly different picture. Although she reported zero hot flashes, she reported 3 W for Hot Dread, 3 W for warm flush, 3 W for night sweats, 3 W for wet nightgown, and 3 W for Cold Crashes. Jackie also reported 3 W for not feeling myself, 3 W for Meno-Fog, and 3 W for anxiety. Her total wScore was 38 W.

Jackie's general health was excellent. She had had a tubal ligation ten years prior, and her menstrual periods were as regular as a British train. She took no medications. The exam and all of her gynecology tests (Pap, mammogram, and bone density) were normal. Jackie was advised it seemed more likely her "sweating disorder" was estrogen withdrawal frequently encountered by perimenopausal women, and MHT or cycle control pills or rings would probably stop them. Jackie said, "Yeah, but I've already tried all of that, and it didn't work." She was advised progesterone would not be the usual choice of treatment for the management of vasomotor symptoms. Progesterone cream is also not well absorbed through the skin in an active available form. Instead, conventional treatment would focus on stabilization of her estrogen level by delivering trans-dermal wBodyIdentical 17beta-estradiol coupled with oral progesterone. Jackie was wary and asked, "Are you talking about synthetic hormones? I've heard they cause breast cancer and are not as safe as bioidentical hormones."

Jackie was receptive to information refuting the claims she'd heard that compounded bioidentical hormones are safer than pharmaceutical grade hormones. The information she found to be most compelling was the hormone levels depicted on the Menstrual Cycle graph (Figure 2-1). She realized depending upon which day of her cycle a hormone might be real high or real low, and you could not tell what her absolute hormone status was without measuring it every minute of every hour, all month long. Coupled with the inaccuracies of saliva testing, hormone testing as a whole may not tell the whole truth about what is happening.

Jackie received printed information from the North American Menopause Society which outlined the principle that hormone therapy should be tailored to control the magnitude of the menopausal symptoms not to restore a blood level to some predetermined number (and saliva testing is considered unreliable, unnecessary and expensive).

There were four weeks between her gynecology appointment and her sweating expert consultation. Jackie was advised she had plenty of time to evaluate whether or not her sweating would go away with MHT. Because fertility was not a consideration, Jackie chose to begin treatment with Evamist topical spray (three sprays to the forearm each morning) and oral Prometrium (100mg at night). Four weeks later she returned.

"You should advertise as a sweating expert because after a year of trying, you got rid of mine in a couple of days," Jackie said. Her follow up *w*Score had changed from 38 W to 8 W. Her Hot Dreads (as she now referred to them) completely disappeared, as did the drenched nightgowns and her Insomnia Queen.

Jackie wanted to know, "How is it you are the only one who seems to think prescription hormones are safe?" Jackie was advised that the vast majority of Board Certified OBGyns who care for menopausal women have faith in the effectiveness and safety of conventional FDA approved medications and find very little purpose for compounded hormones and no use for saliva testing.

Chapter 24

Medicines 4 Menopause

Part I:
One Stop Shopping

The good thing about the Home Depot is that it has (almost) everything you need to work on your house, but don't expect to find a travel guide to the Canadian Rockies, and don't expect to find fresh pineapples. It has a lot of stuff, but it's pretty focused on home repair. This chapter will bring together, under one roof, (almost) all the non-hormonal medicines thought to be useful to treat menopausal symptoms. Most of the problems are so big they have their own chapters. Use this chapter as a guide to find a more expansive discussion elsewhere.

The most useful way to look at the medicines for menopause is by examining the problems they are supposed to help. The major menopausal symptoms are identified on the wScore (Figure 1-2). It is accurate to think of menopausal symptoms as directly related to estrogen withdrawal beginning in perimenopause and moving through postmenopause, the wUpSide. Some women don't need to take anything because their symptoms are mild and brief. Other women may have moderate or severe symptoms for months or years or for life. There is only one medicine that works well for the treatment of all moderate and severe menopausal symptoms: estrogen.

For a variety of reasons, some women can't or won't take menopausal hormone therapy (MHT). There are two well-known reasons for not taking hormones to relieve menopausal symptoms:

1. Estrogen positive breast cancer. Activation of the

estrogen receptor in certain breast cancers may stimulate the cancer to grow. For those women, systemic estrogen therapy is usually not recommended, but topical local vaginal cream may be considered. Most of these non-hormonal medicines in this chapter may be first-line therapies of great usefulness for women with estrogen positive cancers. There are evolving concepts about specific situations in which hormone therapy may be considered in breast cancer survivors (Chapter 27).

2. Just don't want to take hormones. It is perfectly acceptable to choose non-hormonal therapy (OR NO THERAPY OF ANY KIND!) for the treatment of menopausal symptoms. Some women have a fear of hormones because of something they read or something they heard, and they can't shake the uneasiness. Some are philosophically against one type of treatment or another. Treatments for menopause (and every other symptom) are supposed to make you better and happier not scared and stressed. If any treatment makes you scared and stressed, it is probably counterproductive, so don't take it. A reason that makes sense to you is reason enough.

As much as The Home Depot has, it does not have everything you want, and it stocks a ton of stuff you do not need, same as the medical treatments for menopause. One additional *cautionary* note: the predominant reason women choose not to take menopausal hormone therapy, is fear of breast cancer. Therefore, some women might be more inclined to use a non-hormonal medicine instead. It must be emphasized; however, none of the following medicines have ever been tested to see if they have an effect of causing breast cancer. They have simply never been tested. An *unknown risk* is not the same thing as *no risk*.

Part II: Hot Flash Fever Medicines

Hot Flash Fevers, Cold Crashes, night sweats, and drenched night gowns describe the vasomotor problems common among perimenopausal and *w*UpSide women. In addition to all the practical suggestions made in Chapter 9 many report improvement by trying some of the following:

- **Vitamin E** 400 IU a day. The mechanism resulting in the lessening of hot flashes with vitamin E is unknown. High dose vitamin E (over 800 IU a day) is associated with worse health outcomes and should be avoided.

- **Effexor.** The selective serotonin/norepinephrine reuptake inhibitor (SNRI) may reduce hot flashes by up to 60 percent. This medicine is primarily used to treat depression, but it helps vasomotor problems independently of helping mood. Women may notice an improvement of hot flashes in less than four weeks. Possible side effects are nausea, dry mouth, dizziness, and constipation. A newer formulation of the medicine, **Pristiq,** is thought to have some advantages over Effexor. Effexor and Pristiq do not cause weight gain and usually don't interfere with sexuality. Discontinuing Effexor or Pristiq may trigger dizziness and nausea.

- **Prozac.** The classic antidepressant of the selective serotonin reuptake inhibitor class (SSRI) may reduce hot flashes approximately the same magnitude as SNRI's, 60 percent. There are many medicines in this category that may be equally effective such as **Paxil, Zoloft, and Lexapro.** SSRI's may have minor side effects of nausea and dizziness. Prozac and other SSRI's may cause weight gain and interfere with sexuality. All SSRI's may interfere with liver enzymes making them incompatible with Tamoxifen, a medicine commonly used to treat breast cancer.

- **Gabapentin.** The brand name Neurontin (gabapentin) is a medicine for the treatment of seizures, and it has usefulness in calming vasomotor symptoms as well. It reduces hot flashes by up to 50 percent in some women. The side effects can be bothersome including: dizziness, double vision, fatigue, unsteadiness, and diarrhea. A newer derivative of gabapentin named **Lyrica** may also be useful for treating Hot Flash Fever.

- **Clonidine.** Clonidine is a medicine used to treat high blood pressure, and it may reduce hot flashes by 40 percent in some women. The side effects are tiredness, dizziness, and fatigue.

- **All the rest.** There are dozens of other medicines that might be tried for relief of menopausal hot flashes; but so far, none have been shown to work any better than a placebo, which decreases hot flashes by 30 percent. They all carry some risk, and some of those risks are known, and many are simply unknown. Responsible healthcare providers have a hard time recommending something that has little or no evidence for effectiveness and safety.

Part III: Mood Matters Medicines

The Mood Matters of perimenopause are like PMS on steroids, if you will. Estrogen fluctuations may trigger a distinctive mental change referred to here as *w*Worry. It is not major depression and includes symptoms such as "not feeling myself": mood swings, crying spells, Meno-Fog, anxiety, inability to complete tasks, and withdrawal from usual social activities. Chapter 12: Mood Matters covers all the usual approaches to improve the mood.

The medicines useful for menopausal mood matters are limited to **Effexor**, **Pristiq** (SNRI), and **Wellbutrin**. Those medications are preferred because of their effectiveness and low side effects. Two important aspects differentiate the Effexor group (SNRI) from the Prozac group (SSRI). First, the Effexor group does not stimulate weight gain, a particularly distressing feature of the Prozac group. Second, the Effexor group does not usually interfere with sexuality. Wellbutrin has unique features that tend to help reduce weight and improve sexuality. Incidentally, eating real whole food and exercising reliably improves mood, weight, and sex without causing any side effects.

When Effexor, Pristiq, and Wellbutrin are used for major depression, it frequently takes four months to see improvement. There are rare reports of young depressed patients (under the age of 24) having a worsening of their suicidal thoughts, during the first few weeks of therapy, but fortunately, it is not usually a problem for the typical menopausal woman (average 51 years young). wWorry is not major depression and menopausal women with wWorry are not suicidal. Effexor, Pristiq, and Wellbutrin are effective non-hormonal medicines for menopausal mood matters in four weeks.

Part III: Sexercise Medicines

Medical research for improved sexuality has been a little unbalanced in favor of searching for medicines for men. Treatments for male erectile dysfunction and low libido are a big business. Women's sexual health is about to come of age, and progress is seen on the near horizon. In the US, the FDA has stepped forward to acknowledge the link between vaginal health and the female sexual response (Chapter 18: Sexercise) and has approved a topical estrogen hormonal treatment. There are several other non-hormonal medicines currently under evaluation for a direct effect on women's sexual response, but none are at the stage of general recommendation at this time. **Flibanserin** is a new drug currently in trials.

Indirect effects on the female sexual response can be seen in any medicine that improves her general health, be it cardiac, pulmonary, or metabolic. This is especially true for the treatment of depression. Depressed women may have low sexuality, and it improves by treating the mood disorder. **Wellbutrin** is the most helpful non-hormonal medicine for improving sexuality.

Part IV: Vagina Sahara Medicines

There are a host of potential problems that may manifest as vaginal discomfort such as infections. The accurate diagnosis will lead to appropriate medical treatment (Chapter 10: Vagina Sahara). The vaginal dryness that results from estrogen withdrawal at perimenopause and beyond can be mitigated with over-the-counter moisturizers and lubricants. **Temovate cream**, a local topical steroid vulvovaginal cream, will help relieve some of the symptoms and treat some of the problems.

Part V: Skinny on Skin Medicines

Chapter 29 covers all the Womenopause recommendations for skin care. There are no non-hormonal medicines to cover menopausal skin related issues.

Part VI: Insomnia Queen Medicines

Sleep is a precious commodity, and during perimenopause, it is in short supply. Sleep is one of those things that can take a hit from all angles— night sweats: no sleep, Mood Matters: no sleep, unsexed: no sleep, and family general cluelessness: no sleep. Along the same vane, sleep cannot be improved independently from all those other problems. It takes the whole person (body and mind and spirit) working right to get good sleep (Chapter 11: Insomnia Queen).

Billions of dollars are spent each year in the search for a nirvana nap. Most of it is wasted. Taking care of the seventeen secrets for successful sleep will do more than a boatload of medications. That said, some women just cannot sleep without a sleep medication. Those individuals should consider seeing a sleep specialist to identify any other possible cause for their insomnia. Modern sleep medicines are superior to the past ones, and there is a reason why they are so expensive. It takes a lot of research money to prove a sleep medication works, is safe, and is not addictive for long-term use. Many women may benefit from properly selected medication for sleep:

- **Rozerem**: a distinctly different type of sleep medication that stimulates the melatonin receptors to generate a normal sleep pattern. There is a concern about Rozerem causing an increased secretion of prolactin, a pituitary hormone important in breastfeeding. High prolactin is associated with irregular menstrual periods, infertility, and depression.

- **Ambien**: the gold standard for modern sleeping medicines, and the first one approved for intermediate term use with low addiction potential. Low addiction potential is not: "no" addiction potential. Ambien is associated with a few quirky side effects such as Ambien-amnesia (forgetting everything that you say or do after taking an Ambien), and Ambien-activities (doing weird things at night you would not normally do, like driving to the zoo at 2 AM). No sleeping medicines should ever be taken with alcohol. **Ambien CR** is a sustained release version of Ambien and has a slightly longer duration of action.

- **Sonata**: a fast onset short duration sleep medicine. Sonata is useful for those who have trouble falling asleep or wake up early, 3 or 4 hours later. Because Sonata is cleared from the body so quickly that it can be used at 3 AM, if a woman still has another four hours to go before having to get up.

- **Lunesta**: the butterfly sleep medicine asked for by name. Lunesta has a slightly longer duration than regular Ambien and probably less daytime drowsiness side effect. About one third of women report a funny taste in their mouth after taking Lunesta but without the Ambien-type side effects.

- **A million others.** OK, that's an exaggeration too. There are a lot of sleeping medicines for two reasons: 1) there are a lot of people who can't sleep; 2) no single sleeping medicine works great for everyone. Let's face it, if one of the medicines worked well, there would not be a reason for the others to exist; there would just be one.

Part VII: Plumbing and Pain Medicines

The only women who do not experience pain are the ones who spend their entire life on the shelf. If you are living an active life, then there is bound to be some wear and tear. It's a good thing. The best way to minimize the effects is by managing your weight (Chapter 14 and 15) and strengthening your body (Chapter 16). Everyone experiences pain of one type or another. Pain is a useful signal urging you to pay attention to what hurts and to baby it for a while to let it heal. When pain interferes with your ability to enjoy life, then pain medicines may be in order.

Tylenol, acetaminophen, has a mild pain relieving effect and has been used for hundreds of years. It also reduces fever. It is safe at recommended dosages. The problem is, because it is so safe, many products contain some: cough medicine—throw in some Tylenol, flu medicine—throw in some Tylenol, sleep medicine—throw in some Tylenol. Before you know it, the safe dose of Tylenol is exceeded. Everyone should be aware that high doses of Tylenol might cause liver damage (one of those unappreciated organs you can't live without).

Aspirin, ASA, is another mild pain reliever that packs a little more punch than Tylenol. Aspirin inhibits an enzyme in the body's inflammation sequence and helps turn down the development of inflammation and pain. Aspirin also reduces fever. Aspirin may irritate the stomach and small intestines producing gastritis, ulcers, and GI bleeding. Aspirin interferes with platelets and prolongs bleeding. That may be a good thing for people with heart disease (low dose ASA reduces heart attacks, Chapter 28), but may be a bad thing if you get an ulcer of the stomach.

Anti-inflammatory medicines such as **ibuprofen** and **naproxen** (Advil and Aleve) are over-the-counter strong pain relievers and should be reserved for tough pain. The class of medicines is referred to as non-steroidal anti-inflammatory drugs (NSAIDS, pronounced 'en-sades'). Their mechanism of action and risks are similar to aspirin. High doses may also cause kidney injury (another one of those unappreciated organs you can't live without). Advil and Aleve have less effect on platelets than ASA.

Prescription pain relievers divide into two broad categories, narcotic and non-narcotic. **Non-narcotic NSAIDS** are the mainstay for the treatment of advanced arthritis. They work exactly like over the counter NSAIDS only they cost a lot more. Narcotic medications, bettered termed **opiates**, are strong analgesics, and are best managed by pain specialists.

Rose J.

Rose was having her first appointment with a gynecologist at age 47. Previously, she had seen only her male internist. She was really suffering. Unrelenting Hot Dreads were making her so anxious she was missing work half of the time. She wanted hormones, and she wanted them now. She'd been having irregular periods for two years, and had had no periods for six months. Rose had plenty of complicating health problems that would alter her treatment options.

Six months prior, Rose had suffered a heart attack and required two coronary stents. She had recovered reasonably well but continued with significant unaltered risk factors. She had been sent to cardiac rehab, "but it didn't take," she said, meaning she had not followed through with an exercise plan. She had been sent to the dietitian, "but it didn't take either." She had been given a prescription for Chantix for smoking cessation but did not fill it when she found out how expensive ($120) it was. (At $7 a pack and rising, one month's supply of cigarettes costs $210, and one year's worth of cigarettes costs a-pack-a-day-user over $2,500; double that for two-pack-a-day habits). She stated she was doing everything she could do by remembering to take her blood pressure medicine and her diabetes pill. "Just give me some hormone pills, and I promise to take them," she pleaded.

Smoking, hypertension, diabetes, BMI of 34, no exercise, poor food choices, and "stress" adds up to some serious cardiovascular disease risk. Incidentally, those are the usual suspects for hot flashes too.

Rose was told there was good news and was advised she could be healthier and happier at age 60 than she was at age 40. However, her health care providers could only point the way, and only she could decide to go, or not. As so often happens, when the urgent healthcare crisis abates, so does the motivation to stay on top of it. Rose was so desperate for relief of hot flashes (her present crisis and her least important health problem), she was now willing to reconsider her lifestyle choices. Rose was advised to fully consider the big commitment that would be required to become healthy because there are no short cuts. Prescribing medications into a vacuum of self-destructive lifestyle choices is futile, and Rose was so advised.

Rose's wScore was a remarkably high 75 W (Figure 1-2). Her Carroll Rating Scale (a test for depression) was also abnormally high with a score of 30. She determined she was probably a wThursday or wFriday woman (wTimeLine Figure 3-1) and suffering from vasomotor symptoms "and all the rest of that stuff," as the result of estrogen withdrawal. She was presented with information about how lifestyle choices can have direct effects on hot flashes (Chapter 9). She was advised that due to her recent heart attack she, unfortunately, could not use hormones to control her hot flashes. Rose's menopause makeover was about to begin.

Rose accepted the Womenopause Challenge. She decided to begin her transformation with three separate attacks.

1. She decided to start the Fast 4 Fit program: 15,000 steps a day, no sugar drinks, no potatoes, and no bread for four weeks (Chapter 15: Shape Your Waist).
2. She was going to start Pristiq 50 mg a day. This SNRI antidepressant has the ability to help her in two ways: reducing hot flashes, and improving her depressed mood.
3. She immediately took her cigarettes out of her purse and put two packs into the trash. Additionally, she agreed to take the Womenopause recommended supplements; a multi-vitamin, vitamin E 400 IU, vitamin D 4000 IU, calcium citrate 1500 mg, and fish oil 2 g daily.

Four weeks later, Rose returned. Rose returned "new and improved". After decades of decline, she recognized it did not have to be that way. Her hot flashes were more than half gone. She weighed-in, with two full points off of her BMI. She showed her logbook of how many steps she had taken every day since her last appointment. It showed a steady improvement throughout the month, and she was now taking 10,000-15,000 steps a day. Her mood was "better" but still not up to par, and she had missed only two days of work. She had stopped smoking for good.

Three months later Rose reported continued enthusiasm for real food and vitamin-X exercise. Her Carroll Rating Scale was 6 indicating significant improvement in her mood, and her hot flashes remained well controlled. Her BMI was now 30 (down from the original 34). Rose was congratulated on her impressive efforts and reminded that the work she had done to reduce her hot flashes would pay even better dividends for reducing the risk for heart disease, diabetes, hypertension, insomnia, and depression.

Part VIII: The Womenopause Challenge: Medicines & You

1. Make a list of all of your prescription medicines along with the reason you are taking them, and put the list in your purse. If you are like *some* people, you might need to make 20 copies to put one in each of your purses! Show the complete list to your healthcare providers at every visit (even if they don't ask to see it).

2. Do the same thing with your non-prescription vitamins and supplements.

3. Make sure you keep your medicines in a safe place where children and other snoopy people will not stumble upon them.

4. Check your medicines for drug interactions at: www.drugs.com/ drug_interaction (or similar).

Chapter 25

*Man*opause: The Next Big Thing

Part I:
It's Not a Typo

Men are people too. The subject wouldn't even come up; except for the fact, many women have to deal with a man on a regular basis. Peoples' hormones change with time. This entire book examines some of the many facets of how changing hormones may affect a woman's health and well-being in midlife and beyond. Guess what, a similar process goes on in men, too. Maybe they are human after all.

*Man*opause, low testosterone production in adult males, is common. It is distinctly different from *Women*opause, low estrogen production in women, in a variety of ways.

- *Women*opause is universal; every woman who lives long enough (average age 51) will reach menopause and stop having menstrual periods (Chapter 3: *w*TimeLine). Not all men will reach *Man*opause, but many will.

- Men do not have a uterus; and therefore, there is no easy way to understand their hormone status. Women have a uterus that broadcasts their hormone status on a regular basis (Chapter 4: Uterus News).

- When women reach menopause there is a decisive line in the sand, no more menstrual periods (Chapter 6: Menopause). When a man reaches *Man*opause no one seems to notice, not even him.

- When women have fluctuating estrogen levels in perimenopause dramatic symptoms frequently occur: Hot Flash Fever, Cold Crashes, night sweats, Mood Matters, fatigue, Meno-Fog, and Insomnia Queen (Chapter 5: Perimenopause). Men get all of those symptoms, but at a much slower pace and milder.

- Both men and women may experience declines in sexual desire and receptivity, but the patterns for each are quite different (Chapter 18: Sexercise).
- Diagnosis and treatment for Womenopause is well studied, but most men do not know about *Man*opause. They soon will because it's going to be the **next big thing.**

Part II:
Testosterone and Tomatoes

Testosterone in men may begin a natural decline any time after age 30 – which is well before they reach their peak in life. Among men at age 50, one-in-three have documented low testosterone levels, and over half at age 80 are low in testosterone. However, those numbers may be deceiving. The actual number may be higher. Look at it this way. If you were growing ten tomato plants, and six of them were five feet tall, two of them were four feet tall, and two of them did not get enough water and never got more than two inches tall, you might say the "average" tomato plant was only three feet four inches tall (the numerical average). Wouldn't it be more accurate to say the average healthy tomato plant is a little less than five feet tall not a little over three feet tall? The dwindled plants skewed the average height much lower, but if you exclude the obviously stunted plants, you get a height estimate that is closer to what an average healthy tomato plant is supposed to look like. "Average" testosterone levels for adult men are just like the average tomato plant height. Because there are so many adult men with very low testosterone naturally, the lab averages are skewed toward the low end of the scale. No one knows exactly what an optimal "normal" testosterone level should be for a healthy adult man, but it should probably be more like an average healthy man in his thirties

(500-750 ng/dL) rather than an average man in his eighties. Laboratory reference values put "normal" testosterone for adult men somewhere between 300 and 1100 ng/dL. If a man's blood test shows 301 then he might be considered normal just like a 3 feet tomato plant, but he shouldn't. Some lab reference values go as low as 200 ng/dL as the lowest end of the "normal" range.

Part III:
*Man*opausing Is Not Refreshing

It's not all about sex. Men with low testosterone (T) gradually develop a constellation of symptoms that may be related to decreased testosterone. None of them taken out of context seems very important at first, but as *Man*opause is more fully explained later in the chapter, the symptoms of low testosterone may be strong predictors of impaired health and well-being.

1. Lower sex drive: Okay, maybe it is a lot about sex. Reduced sexual fantasies, absent or reduced spontaneous morning erections, reduced desire for sex, and impaired sexual performance (erections and orgasms) may all indicate low testosterone production.

2. Lower energy: Age is not the only reason for feeling tired and run-down.

3. Lower strength and endurance: Muscle development and maintenance requires testosterone.

4. Lower happiness: Decreased enjoyment and disinterest in life along with a grumpy mood may be due to low testosterone.

5. Lower mental sharpness: Impaired attention span, lack of humor, loss of memory, and low vitality may reflect low levels of testosterone.

6. Enlarged breasts: Man breasts – not considered attractive.

7. Infertility: Low testosterone = low sperm count.

On the positive side, men with low testosterone do not have to shave their beards as often, and they do not go bald as fast; but other than that, there is no great advantage. Men may feel refreshed after taking a quick nap during a time-out of a TV ball game, but they do not get refreshed when their testosterone takes a pause. Low testosterone in adult men is beginning to generate research interest because testosterone has been found to play an important role in many chronic diseases.

Part IV:
Seriously, It's Not All About Sex

Serious health problems may accompany low testosterone production, and much like menopausal hormone therapy for women, restoring testosterone in men can provide remarkable health advantages. Co-morbidities are diseases that go in virtual lock-step together. The list is eerily familiar (they are exactly the ones that are in lock-step with women with long-term estrogen deficiency).

- Diabetes: The intermesh of glucose/insulin/testosterone /estrogen/fat is real, and it is really complicated. For simplicity's sake, it can be stated that normal testosterone levels in men significantly reduce the occurrence of diabetes (as does estrogen in women).
- Cardiovascular disease: Normal testosterone levels have favorable affects on blood lipids and other risk factors (ditto estrogen levels for women).
- Osteoporosis: Normal testosterone levels are essential for bone metabolism (ditto estrogen for women).
- Metabolic syndrome: Normal testosterone reduces the incidence of metabolic syndrome and reduces belly fat (ditto estrogen for women).
- Depression: Normal testosterone is associated with reduced rates of depression (ditto estrogen for women).

- Sleep: Normal testosterone improves sleep (ditto...).
- Dementia: The male brain loves testosterone (and the female brain loves estrogen).

Part V:
Hey Testosterone, What's Up?

When it comes to male sexuality, testosterone is *numero uno*. A good blood supply to the penis is second; the autonomic nerves are fundamental; strong pelvic floor muscles are also a factor. A romantic mood probably figures in somewhere, but they are still looking for that one.

The penis is like a circus-clown balloon that engorges with blood if the blood valve gets turned to the "on" position, and there are no leaks. The nerves, arteries, veins, and muscles must all pull together to create a properly inflated flirtation devise. Seriously, just like women (Chapter 18: Sexercise), men have desire, arousal, satisfaction, and intimacy components to their sexual response. Unfortunately, the male sex response is often reduced to one of two performance factors: the man gets a proper erection, or he does not get a proper erection. However, it is way more complicated than that. Focusing exclusively on medication for erectile dysfunction is shortsighted.

Every woman who reads this book now understands the rich interaction between lifestyles and menopausal sexual health. The exact same process underlies male sexual health as well. The following conditions lead to impaired erections in men:

- Chronic obstructive pulmonary disease (COPD): It is one more reason to stop smoking.
- Over-weight, high BMI: Improper nutrition and lack of exercise impact every aspect of health and well-being. Fat cells convert testosterone into estrogen through the enzyme aromatase. Estrogen feminizes men.
- Diabetes: Adult-onset-diabetes is often related to improper

nutrition, being over weight, and lack of exercise. Diabetes and hypertension wreck havoc on the arterial blood supply to the penis (and everywhere else for that matter).

- Excessive alcohol: "A few too many" will convert what testosterone there is, into estrogen, which is a real deflator of arousal.
- Cardiovascular disease: Plaque in the arteries of the heart foretells plaque in the artery of the penis. It's like someone playing a prank on the circus clown by turning off his gas supply, so he cannot inflate the funny balloons.

Men may have sexual dysfunctions that parallel the ones seen in women (Chapter 18: Sexercise). Certain men may have low testosterone with a resultant erectile dysfunction (ED) or normal testosterone with an erectile dysfunction because the ED/testosterone relationship is not one-to-one. In a similar arrangement, sexual desire has an unpredictable relationship to male testosterone level. It's complicated further by the relationship, health, mood matters, self-image, stress, and so on (just as it is in women). Some men's "sexual neutrality" state takes a lot more external input to move it into the aroused state (Figure 18-1). Therefore, male sexual behavior, like female sexual behavior, is modified by their hormones but not exactly driven by them.

The long-term solution for these problems would be the "man version" of the Womenopause Challenge and nothing less. Lifestyle, lifestyle, lifestyle. In spite of good lifestyle habits, many men will develop low testosterone. There are two recognized mechanisms underlying low testosterone: 1) The Leydig cells within the testes simply reduce their production of testosterone. Even though the brain is calling for more testosterone, they cannot meet the demand: they poop-out. This is termed primary hypogonadism. 2) A less common cause of low testosterone is when the brain (hypothalamus or pituitary) slows down or stops sending the "I need more testosterone" signal to the testes. In this case the testes are willing, but no one asks them to; therefore, they do not put out. This is termed secondary hypogonadism. There is a long list of other uncommon causes of low testosterone such as certain medications, injury to the testis, infection, and a bunch of rare inherited syndromes. For the majority of men with hypogonadism (primary or secondary), there is no known cause.

Part VI:
Prostate: The Male Breast

Just about everything that is said about the female breast (Chapter 27: Breast) can be said about the male prostate, except few men have a strong emotional attachment to their prostate. Men are more emotionally attached to their penis. The prostate is a small gland hidden away just above the genitals below the urinary bladder. It serves two functions: 1) the prostate adds pleasurable volume to ejaculations. 2) It causes trouble. The trouble it causes is also of two types: 1) Gradual benign enlargement of the prostate (benign prostatic hypertrophy, BPH) can obstruct the outflow from the urinary bladder. 2) The prostate can develop cancer. Cancer of the prostate kills about 40,000 men each year in the U.S., almost exactly the number of women who die from breast cancer.

Both the prostate and the breast share another very weird property. Both develop cancers that may be stimulated by their respective hormones, estrogen for the female breast, and testosterone for the male prostate; and inexplicably, both of the types of cancers become more apparent when those hormones are at the lowest levels later in life. It is well-documented that women who have taken menopausal hormone therapy (MHT) have better survival from their breast cancer than do women who have never taken MHT. The same is seen for men with prostate cancer. It sort of goes against the grain, but normal amounts of reproductive hormones appears to be protective in some way against the worst kinds of breast and prostate cancer.

There is a very high tech way to examine the prostate. It is so high tech; it is actually "digital". The technique involves having the healthcare provider put one of his fingers (a digit, if you will), up into the rectum to feel the size and consistency of the prostate. Yearly digital rectal exams combined with a blood test for prostrate specific antigen (PSA) are crucial for the early detection of prostate cancer, beginning at age 50.

Part VII:

The *Manopause* Solution

Adult men who have the symptoms listed in Part III above: low sex drive, erectile dysfunction, low energy, low strength and endurance, low concentration and memory, increased belly fat, hot flashes, and Mood Matters (tell the truth, do you know *any* man who does not fit at least one of these criteria!) should seek a medical evaluation by a competent healthcare provider. After a normal medical exam, a man should have a morning total testosterone blood level determined. If it is under 300 ng/dL, a more thorough discussion about risk factors should be done including medical diseases like cardiovascular disease, medications, and nutrition. A second confirmatory morning total and "free" testosterone level should be checked along with a measurement of LH and FSH (the brain signals that tell the testis to make more testosterone), prolactin, sex hormone binding globulin (SHBG), prostate specific antigen (PSA), hemoglobin, and thyroid function. If the only abnormality identified were the confirmed low testosterone, a discussion about testosterone therapy would be appropriate.

*Manopause is low testosterone. It can be corrected with testosterone therapy. However, just as seen in menopausal symptoms for women, lifestyle changes alone may be all that is needed to boost the return of testosterone. The following are the sex friendly lifestyle recommendations:

- Smoke Free (another reason to quit)
- Real Food (Chapter 14: Real Food)
- Weight Loss (Chapter 15: Shape Your Waist)
- Vitamin-X Exercise (Chapter 16: Vitamin-X Exercise)
- Kegel pelvic floor muscle exercises (Chapter 18: Sexercise)
- Relaxation Practice (Chapter 12: Mood Matters)
- Vitamin D 4,000 IU daily (decreases prostate cancer Chapter 17))
- Zinc 50 mg daily
- Soy protein supplement
- Vitamin C 1,000 mg daily
- Vitamin E 400 IU daily
- Vitamin B6
- Multivitamin daily
- Modification of all the cardiovascular risks (Chapter 28: Heart Health)
- Avoid grapefruit
- Avoid excessive alcohol

Testosterone production and sexual performance will benefit from these lifestyle changes. As a bonus to an improved sex life, every other aspect of a man's health will follow along too!

Testosterone can be administered by giving an FDA sanctioned product via one of several different routes:

- Injection: This is the original. It may need to be given every week or two (75-100 mg weekly or 150-200 mg every two weeks). Injections result in more erratic blood levels, and therefore, are not recommended. This route of administration is the least expensive.
- Patch: Testosterone in a patch gets changed every day (2.5-7.5 mg applied nightly). This provides stable blood levels.
- Gel: Transdermal gel applied to the abdomen or shoulders every day provides fairly consistent blood levels. This is

the most popular route of administration and comes in the brand names: AndroGel and Testim.

- Oral tablets: Testosterone lozenges are effective when taken twice a day (30 mg). The levels may not be as stable as other routes.

- Pellets: Testosterone pellets are implanted under the skin every three to six months (150-450 mg). This route may prove to be the most reliable way to provide the most stable dose of testosterone for the long run.

Carl M.

At age 52, Carl was a commuter airline pilot with a great (second) wife, Carla, and three boys all under the age of ten, Danny, Darrel, and Doug. He reported a flagging sex life for the past two years and was very concerned. He noticed a "sinister and progressive" inability to perform sexually. He and his wife had become much less frequent with sex, and when they did have sex, his erections were unreliable. He had been trying to chalk it up to being overworked, but now his exhaustion seemed out of proportion to his workload. His schedule had not really changed that much in the past five years, but his energy level sure had. He dreaded disappointing the boys by not playing soccer with them. He admitted feeling blue and drinking too much on his off days.

Carl's health was excellent. He took no medications and had regular medical care. He was trim, athletic, and possessed a world-class, dry sense of humor. He found almost nothing funny to say about his "grounded" sex drive.

His physical exam was completely normal, and his prostate was small and soft. His mSxScore (Figure 18-3) was 24. Carl's total testosterone was checked the next morning and was abnormally low at 290 ng/dL (below the cutoff of 300 ng/dL). Carl was given information about Manopause and encouraged to begin supplements and to cut way down on the alcohol. A repeat testosterone blood test, along with other tests, was ordered.

He returned the next week for the results. Carl's total testosterone was confirmed low at 282 ng/d; his LH and FSH were normal (the brain signals telling the testes to make testosterone); his thyroid function was normal; his prolactin was normal (one of the other pituitary hormones); his PSA (the prostate specific antigen) was normal; and his hemoglobin was low normal at 13.2 g. Carl was advised the sex symptoms and fatigue may be the result of low testosterone, and the labs confirmed the potential problem as hormonal.

After a review of lifestyle optimizations, Carl was offered a trial of testosterone therapy. He reviewed the benefits and risks of therapy and began by taking AndroGel 5g a day applied to his abdomen. Three months later he returned.

After 90 days of therapy, Carl had not noticed anything dramatically different other than a little more energy. His total testosterone measured 410 ng/d; his PSA was normal; and his hemoglobin improved to 13.9g. He was offered an escalation of his testosterone dose with the objective of getting it into the mid-normal range for healthy young men. For the next three months, Carl was instructed to apply 10g of AndroGel daily.

"Home run," said Carl, "I'm all the way back". Carl's total testosterone was now 607 ng/dL; but more importantly, his sex drive and erections had returned. His *mSxScore* had recovered to a 5. He felt as energetic as ever and said, "The boys think I'm playin' soccer like *Beckham*, and I think Carla is lookin' like *Posh Spice*."

Part VIII: The Manopause Challenge: Salute the Flag

1. Men have feelings, and their relationship dynamics affects their sexual response. He may initially resist, but have a sex talk today.

2. All tired, run-down, and bored men should have their

testosterone level checked.

3. All men who have lowered sex drive or erectile dysfunction should have their testosterone level checked.

4. All men with cardiovascular disease, hypertension, pulmonary disease, or diabetes should have their testosterone level checked.

5. All men who have gained weight or have a waistline problem should have their testosterone level checked.

6. All men who have any concerns identified on the mSxScore should have their testosterone level checked.

7. All men...

Chapter 26

Boning Up 4 Osteoporosis

Part I:
How Not to Build a Hospital

Everyone has had the experience of trying to find her way around a hospital. It can be pretty frustrating. There are usually plenty of zigzags, turns, ramps, and dead ends. The reason it's that way is because the typical hospital has undergone a couple dozen remodels, revisions, and additions. It is hard or impossible for hospital administrators to anticipate the services and technologies the future will bring, so they add-on, tear-down, and make-do. Our bones are like that.

Imagine a hospital that is always in a state of adding-on. After it expands all the way to the curb, it has to start tearing down the existing stuff to make room for the new. The hospital employs two teams to get the work done: a *construction* crew that is always building, and a *demolition* crew that is constantly tearing down the unneeded outdated parts. Ideally, there is one boss overseeing the whole process in order to make sure the construction does not get too far ahead of demolition or vice versa. If the construction crew chief goes on vacation, you might expect a little slack in the amount of bricks that get laid that week. If she goes to Europe for the rest of the season, there will be a serious imbalance between what the construction crew gets done compared to what the demolition crew does. The demolition crew chief continues to spur on the crowbars and jackhammers to take down the original parts of the hospital because that's what her orders are. At some terrible point, the amount of demolition exceeds the construction. Can you imagine the two crews working side-by-side along the same scaffold? On one end are the bricklayers, and on the other end are the brick breakers—and the brick breaking demolition crew is gaining ground on the construction crew! That's when the hospital begins to shrink. The construction crew is still showing up every day for work, but they just get less work done than the demolition crew. Bones are exactly like that.

Part II:
Bones Alive

If you have ever held a bone in your hands, you recognize it is like a cross between a stick and a rock; it's lightweight and yet hard. Bones can survive thousands of years after the person who made them has ceased living. It's tempting to think of bones as lifeless little poles that hold us up. Not true. Bones are a living, breathing tissue, as are all of our organs. Like the hospital, we constantly add-on and tear-down our bones in a dynamic equilibrium that suits our needs. If we are active, we build stronger bones; and if we are inactive, we don't need such strength; we let the bones shrink down. The construction crew bone cells are called osteoblasts, and the demolition crew cells are called osteoclasts. The construction osteoblasts need orders to build. The build order comes in the form of genetics, activity stress (the good stress), metabolic signals, and hormones; and once it gets the blue prints, it needs a lot of bricks and mortar to carry out the plans. Bone bricks and mortar are like the bone essentials, calcium and vitamin D. All the while the construction osteoblasts are building, there are demolition osteoclasts knocking down the brick walls that had been constructed years ago. When the osteoclasts work harder than the osteoblasts, bone becomes weaker. Weak porous bone is called osteoporosis.

Part III:
Osteoporosis: So What

Women make great bone. Given adequate amounts of activity,

sunshine, and real food, women continue to build bone strength for over three decades. Then they "reach the curb" and do not physically get any bigger bones. At that point they can maintain their bone strength by urging on the construction crew, or they can take a long holiday and allow the demolition crew to get the upper hand. All the factors for preventing bone loss can be avoided, but what does it matter?

Death, for most women, is such an abstract concept, it holds little power to motivate. Even so, many women find it astounding that osteoporosis factors into women's death more than breast cancer does. For some reason, no one seems to fear a fracture like they fear breast cancer, but they should. Over 50,000 women die in the U.S. each year from complications following a fracture as compared to 40,000 who die from breast cancer (Chapter 30: Death Prevention).

Disability, to most women, sounds like a young worker who gets laid up for a back injury. Osteoporosis causes women more real pain than any other single thing ever imagined. In the U.S. there are over 1.5 million osteoporotic fractures a year. Cardiac angina pains are brief, but osteoporotic back fractures may hurt forever. Being unable to do simple life-fulfilling activities (disability) causes even more misery than pain. Osteoporosis causes suffering through two mechanisms: pain and misery, and *they do not* take vacations.

The number of osteoporotic fractures doubles every seven years after menopause. The average age of a hip fracture is 82, and the average age of the first vertebral fracture is 70. Yikes. Since the average life expectancy is something north of 87, every woman should take a good hard look at how to keep her bones strong.

Remember seeing that elegant 5ft 8in woman at age 80 glide across a room with perfect posture? No, probably not. By age 80, the average woman has lost three to four inches of height and is bent over as the result of multiple vertebral compression fractures. It is all totally preventable.

Part IV:
Osteoporosis and Estrogen

Estrogen deficiency causes osteoporosis. The (lucky) women who have a late natural menopause (after age 55) have a delayed onset of osteoporosis. The (unlucky) women who have an early menopause or an induced menopause (Chapter 8) may have a premature onset of osteoporosis if measures are not taken to prevent it. It does not take a genius to figure out the role estrogen plays in the development of osteoporosis. The construction crew osteoblasts respond to the presence of estrogen, and when she is gone (the extended vacation we call postmenopause *w*UpSide), they will not lay as many bricks in a day. It may be more complicated than that too. The number of bricks is not the only thing that gives a wall its strength. The number of supporting braces and side walls are just as important and don't forget the quality of the mortar; it's holding everything together! Estrogen covers all of that.

There is a period of time when bone loss is accelerated. Maximal bone loss begins two years before the final menstrual period (FMP) and continues on for another four years after the FMP. During this critical time, a woman may lose 12 percent of her bone strength. What took 50 years to build can be torn down pretty quickly. As they say, a sledgehammer works a lot faster than a regular construction hammer. After the quick loss of bone strength surrounding menopause, there is a continuous drain of bone strength of about 1 percent a year throughout the *w*UpSide. Osteoporosis is more of a menopause problem than an age problem.

Part V:
Osteoporotic Fractures: Rounding Up the Suspects

Bones are a living breathing tissue, and there are a number of known risk factors that directly affect their health and well-being. The following is a list of the **primary causes of osteo-**

porotic fractures:

- Menopause: estrogen deficiency
- Genetics: blame your parents for one more thing
- Inadequate calcium intake
- Inadequate vitamin D intake
- Smoking: one more reason to quit
- Low body weight: weight less than 127 pounds or a BMI less than 21 (so it *is* possible to be too thin!)
- Previous fracture: if you already had a fracture after menopause
- Parent had a hip fracture: see second point above
- Low bone mineral density: more on that later
- More than three alcoholic drinks a day
- Steroids for more than three months
- Poor vision
- Poor balance
- Hazardous environment: pets, rugs, and steps
- Poor general health
- Dementia

Part VI:
Osteoporosis: It's Not Just a Number

The strength of a hospital wall depends not just on the number of bricks but also depends upon the quality of the mortar and the number of supporting braces. Bone strength is partially dependant upon the amount of calcium but also depends upon the quality of the bone matrix glue and the number of the trabeculae supports. The amount of bone calcium can be measured by a test called a DEXA. A DEXA is like a special kind of x-ray that can measure the bone density. Bone density is an approximation of bone strength but, as you can see, does not tell the whole story. Just like counting the number of bricks in a wall does not predict if it will hold up in an earthquake. Unfortunately there are only two ways to measure bone strength: 1) the easy way: lay down on an x-ray table and get a DEXA scan (painless), or 2) the hard way: fall down and get a fracture—then we know for sure your bones are weak (painful). As a rule, getting a DEXA is the preferred way to estimate bone strength.

Determination of bone density is frequently used to figure out who should receive osteoporosis treatment or not. Beware. Broad public health guidelines, such as who should be getting a DEXA scan or who should be prescribed treatment for osteoporosis, are devised to *save money* not necessarily to save individuals. Your healthcare provider may take many things into account in counseling you about when you should get a scan and about the risks and benefits of treatment.

DEXA screening should be performed on the following women:

- All women with any known medical cause of bone loss regardless of age (menopause and any of the previously mentioned risk factors)
- All *w*UpSide women who sustain any type of fracture
- All *w*UpSide women with a BMI less than 21 (too thin?!)
- All *w*UpSide women whose parent sustained a hip fracture or has been diagnosed with osteoporosis
- All *w*UpSide women who currently smoke (say what?)
- All *w*Saturday women
- All women who, in consultation with their healthcare provider, believe it is prudent to know their bone density or risk of osteoporotic fracture

Part VII:
How Bad Is Bad Enough?

There is some disagreement among professional organizations when it comes to recommendations for osteoporosis treatment. The North American Menopause Society (NAMS) guidelines are promoted here. The following are criteria used to determine **who should receive prescription osteoporosis treatment**:

- All *w*UpSide women who sustain a vertebral fracture
- All women with a bone mineral density "T" score less than -2.5 (minus two point five)
- All women with a bone mineral density "T" score between -2.5 and -2.0 plus a risk factor: low BMI less than 21, personal history of a fracture that happened after menopause, or hip fracture in a parent

An advanced bone strength estimation tool is the FRAX. Your healthcare provider may input data about your bone density and personal risk factors (such as your mother's hip fracture) into an online formula to determine your FRAX number. This number will soon be available on your DEXA results, along with your T score. That value may also help determine whether or not you need treatment for osteoporosis.

Part VIII:
So Many Choices, So Little Bone

Osteoporosis is better prevented than treated. Like a 401k retirement program, bones deserve an automatic deposit plan to ensure adequate strength after the ovaries retire. Bone density nosedives after menopause, and the more strength that is stored up before hand, the better the bones can withstand the loss.

All women should supplement their diet with **calcium citrate** (1500 mg a day) and **vitamin D** (4000 IU a day) beginning at puberty and ending a day or so after their funeral. Although bricks are not the only things holding up a hospital wall, they are pretty darn indispensible. A **real food diet** (Chapter 14) and **regular exercise** (Chapter 16) are of upmost importance.

If a woman has no contraindication (Chapter 20), **menopausal**

hormone therapy (MHT) should be considered as first-line treatment for the prevention of osteoporosis. In addition to elimination of Hot Flash Fever, Insomnia Queen, Meno-Fog, and Mood Matters, MHT stimulates the construction crew osteoblasts to make more bone. MHT at low doses restores bone formation to a similar level as it was during the reproductive years. MHT is known to increase bone density over 5 percent in just two years of therapy and reduces the risk of fracture by 30 percent. For women who are not candidates for MHT, fortunately there are other effective alternatives. A class of medicines called **bisphosphonates**, have become very popular in the treatment of osteoporosis. Keep in mind, the only reason women need bisphosphonate today is because of extended life expectancy and many years spent living in the wUpSide without estrogen.

Osteoporosis is a problem of long term estrogen deficiency coupled with poor diet and sedentary lifestyle. The following are currently available osteoporosis medicines:

- Fosamax: the original
- Actonel: the contender
- Boniva: who doesn't like Sally Field?
- Reclast: restricted use, must be given IV and very expensive

As far as anyone knows, all bisphosphonates work the same way, and they all have the same high level of effectiveness. As you might guess, they have the same risks and side effects as well. These medicines are approved for the prevention and treatment of osteoporosis. The side effects include GI irritation, and users are advised to take the pill on an empty stomach with a full glass of water and remain upright for at least 30 to 60 minutes. Rarely, women on chemotherapy for cancer who take a bisphosphonate, may develop osteonecrosis of the jawbone

(ONJ). There are some reports of bones becoming brittle with long-term use, but there are no specific guidelines to know just how long a woman needs to stay on the medicines.

Another class of osteoporosis medicines is **Selective Estrogen Receptor Modulators (SERMs)**. This type of medicine may have huge implications in the future for the treatment of menopause. Right now they are very limited in their usage. The ideal SERM would do all the beneficial things estrogen does, (vasomotor, vagina, sex response, heart health, sleep, mood, bone, skin, and on and on...) without doing any of the supposed bad things (risk of breast cancer and endometrium cancer). There may come a day when a woman can take a designer collection of SERMs specifically tailored to manage her unique physiology. Right now there is only one available in the US for the osteoporosis indication, Evista. Evista is a weak estrogen receptor activator in some tissues (like the bone) and an estrogen receptor blocker in other tissues. Because of that, Evista can cause bone growth but trigger hot flashes. There does not seem to be a good reason to trade bone strength for hot flashes unless the side effects of the bisphosphonates are intolerable. Rarely, Evista, like oral estrogens (but *not* like transdermal *w*BodyIdentical), can increase the risks of blood clots and pulmonary embolism. Evista also may cause flu-like symptoms, leg edema, cramps, and joint pains. On the positive side, Evista may be safely used in breast cancer survivors, and it actually reduces the risk of invasive breast cancer like its cousin, tamoxifen (more on this in Chapter 27: Breast Cancer). Unlike tamoxifen, Evista does not cause an increased risk of endometrial cancer.

Tattyanna

An exotic beauty originally from Malta, Tattyanna age 57, worked as a freelance writer. She has been happily married for 35 years to Lorenzo, and together, they owned an Italian restaurant. They had two married daughters. Tattyanna reached menopause at age 52. She had experienced severe hot flashes, night sweats, insomnia, and mood swings until she started hormone therapy. She obtained excellent relief of her vasomotor symptoms on Vivelle dot 0.05 mg, (wBodyIdentical 17beta-estradiol) coupled with Prometrium 100 mg to protect her uterus. At age 53 her bone mineral density T score of +1.1 put her in the twenty something range. She knew about vitamin D and calcium supplementation but always had excuses for not taking them right now; she would "get to it later". Her BMI was a trim 21, and she exercised, but irregularly. Her favorite foods were pizza, pizza, pizza, and popcorn.

After her hysterectomy for fibroids at age 54, she tried switching her estrogen to Estrasorb but did not like getting the medicine on her hands. She switched back to the low dose Vivelle Dot without the Prometrium. At about this time, she was diagnosed with hypertension and began treatment with Benicar. She skipped one year of follow up with her gynecologist, and when her MHT prescription ran out, she tried for two weeks to go without it. She gave up and made an appointment. Everything was good again; except now, at age 55 her bone density T score had gone down to -2.2 (minus two point two). Tattyanna and her gynecologist were both concerned. After a thorough review of osteoporosis risk factors, it became readily apparent that Tattyanna had not done her best in taking the recommended supplements, nor did she exercise as frequently as she could. In addition, she reported she had sustained a toe fracture, stubbing it on the stairs at home six months earlier.

Tattyanna was given the opportunity of going on a bisphosphonate or going up on her dose of estrogen because of her continued night sweats. Either way, she was going to have to take vitamin D 4000 IU a day with calcium citrate 1500 mg a day. Everyday. Tattyanna opted for the increased estrogen dose and went up to Vivelle Dot 0.075. She also accepted lifestyle advice about real foods and Vitamin-X, exercise.

One year later, Tattyanna's bone density T score had improved from minus 2.2 up to minus 0.8. Her blood pressure was slightly lower, and her cholesterol had improved. She noticed improved skin quality and no night sweats with the Vivelle Dot 0.05 to 0.075 dosage change. She had faithfully taken the vitamin D and calcium almost every day. She had somehow gotten Lorenzo interested in yoga, and they exercised with a DVD instructor four days a week, and on the off days, she and Lorenzo walked three miles (she knew that three miles were exactly 5486 steps because she wore a pedometer every day). She reported she had limited her pizza consumption to twice a week (not counting lunches).

The lowest effective dose to control vasomotor symptoms and other short-term estrogen withdrawal symptoms may not be the optimal dose to prevent osteoporosis and other long-term estrogen deficiency health problems.

Part IX:
The Womenopause Challenge: Rock Your Bones (It's Not Hard)

1. Take the following "Bone Pledge".
2. I swear to make my bones stronger today than they were yesterday.
3. I swear to take 4000 IU of vitamin D today.
4. I swear to take 1500 mg of calcium citrate today.
5. I swear to walk at least 10,000 steps today.
6. I swear to eat only real food today.
7. I swear to dance at every opportunity today: rock, pop, or country.
8. I swear to forgive my parents for the genes they gave me.

Chapter 27

Breast Cancer Prevention

Part I:
The Breast Cancer Pyramid

If someone pulls you aside and whispers, "I have the most terrible news to tell you about our friend Marie," probably the first terrible thing that comes to mind is breast cancer. The fear of breast cancer transcends the usual concerns for disease and death because of its potential to threaten physical disfigurement of an important part of a woman's feminine sexual identity, her breasts. Breast cancer ranks highest among women's health concerns. Treatments for breast cancer steadily improve, but 120 American women continue to die from it each day.

It might be helpful to think of breast cancer disease as a pyramid (Figure 27-1). The very top stone is the one everyone seems to be pointing toward: **The Cure**. Finding the cure for breast cancer disease has garnered tremendous public and scientific attention. A great deal of research money continues to be raised and invested for this important purpose. Significant advances have been accomplished, and women diagnosed with breast cancer today have effective treatment options including:

- Pioneering chemotherapy
- Progress in hormonal approaches
- Advances in radiation treatment
- Novel surgical care.

All of this adds up to improvements in survival rates for women diagnosed with breast cancer today compared to women diagnosed ten years ago.

An important fact came out of the breast cancer disease treatment research; women diagnosed with early stage breast cancer have significantly better outcomes than women with a more advanced cancer. For example, women diagnosed with stage I breast cancer survive more than five years, 96 percent of the time; whereas, for women with stage IV breast cancer, the five year survival drops off to 65 percent. This leads us to discuss the next component of the breast cancer pyramid: **Early Detection**.

Since we know the earlier the breast cancer is detected the better the outcome, doesn't it make sense to put at least as much effort into improving early detection technology as we put into breast cancer treatment? The central section of the breast cancer pyramid emphasizes the vital importance of finding breast cancer disease before it reaches an advanced stage and becomes hard to treat. By now, everyone should know the **Big Six Tests for Breasts,** but let's review them to be sure.

1. **Breast Exam:** Each woman is encouraged to examine her own breasts monthly, in order to tell if anything changes. If anything about the breast is different, then a breast exam by an experienced healthcare provider should be performed. All women should have a clinical breast exam as part of their regular annual medical care; 80 percent of the time, a breast lump does not mean cancer, but it should always be checked-out.

2. **Mammogram:** The gold standard for the early detection of breast cancer is the annual mammogram beginning at age 35. Literally thousands of women are alive today because their breast cancer was detected at an early stage by a screening mammogram before they or their healthcare provider noticed any symptoms or lumps.

3. **MRI:** The role of MRI screening for breast cancer disease is expanding but is still somewhat uncertain. MRIs have proven to be helpful in examining dense breasts where

standard mammograms are inconclusive, but they have the drawback of "finding" a suspicious lesion when, in fact, there is nothing there. It remains difficult to get insurance coverage for breast MRIs, and they are very expensive.

4. **Ultrasound**: Ultrasound is frequently used to further the diagnosis of a lump or an abnormality seen on a mammogram. It is not sufficient by itself for screening breasts for cancer.

5. **Biopsy**: If there is a lump or a suspicious finding on the mammogram or the MRI, then a tissue biopsy is important to categorize which type of cells are present in the lump. Knowing exactly what type of cell is present determines the treatment options available. Frequently this can be done through a fine needle, sometimes by a local surgical excisional biopsy, and occasionally by a non-invasive ductal lavage.

6. **Chromosome**: Two separate genes, BRCA 1 and BRCA 2, have been linked to breast and ovarian cancer. The vast majority of women who develop breast cancer do not have these cancer genes, and it remains uncertain whom to test. This is also a very expensive test.

As important as early detection is, wouldn't it be better to protect the breast from ever having something *to* detect? Breast cancer **prevention** is a relatively new concept and forms the foundation of the breast cancer pyramid. Very little research used to go into breast cancer disease prevention, but that is changing.

Several large-scale studies have identified certain lifestyle characteristics that reduce the risk of developing breast cancer disease. That is certainly great news. Women can adopt healthy choices and are no longer relegated to passively waiting for their mammogram results. Maintaining a low Body Mass Index, regular exercise, eating whole foods with plenty of vegetables, not smoking (and yet another reason...), not drinking alcohol in excess, and taking extra vitamin D, all predict lower breast cancer disease rates. If you notice, all the Womenopause lifestyle recommendations for the treatment of menopausal symptoms reduce your risk of breast cancer as a special bonus.

The Gail Model is a risk assessment tool used to determine a

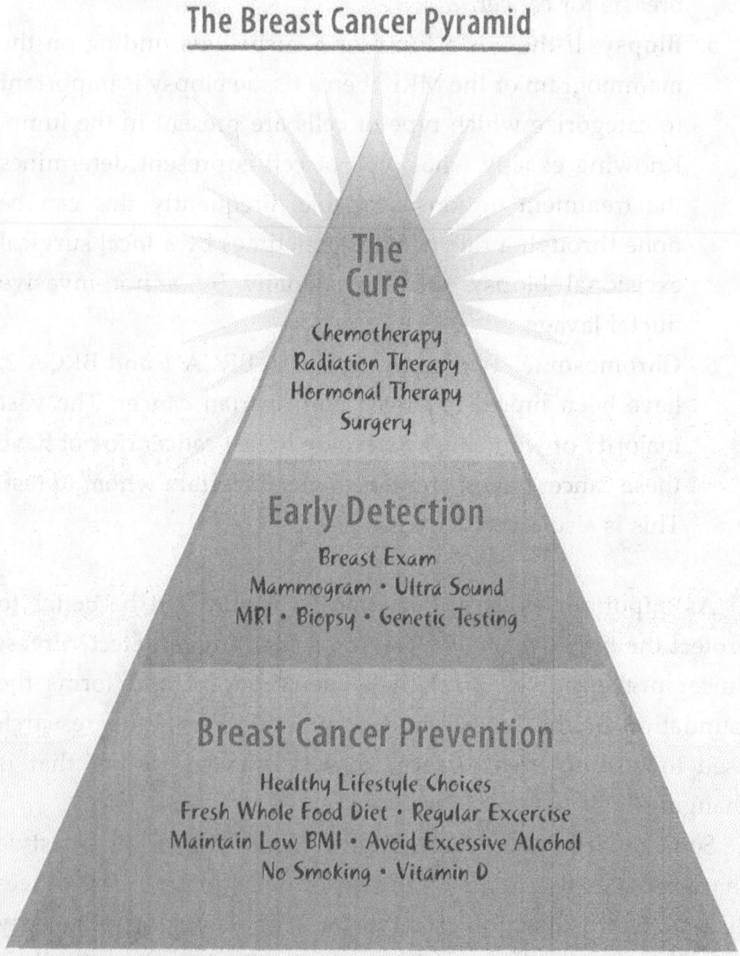

The Breast Cancer Pyramid

The Cure
Chemotherapy
Radiation Therapy
Hormonal Therapy
Surgery

Early Detection
Breast Exam
Mammogram • Ultra Sound
MRI • Biopsy • Genetic Testing

Breast Cancer Prevention
Healthy Lifestyle Choices
Fresh Whole Food Diet • Regular Excercise
Maintain Low BMI • Avoid Excessive Alcohol
No Smoking • Vitamin D

Figure 27-1 Breast Cancer Pyramid

woman's risk for breast cancer. It combines 7 different risks into a single Gail score, which helps guide women to consider pre-treatment to prevent breast cancer. Some very high-risk women may choose to take tamoxifen, a complicated estrogen-like compound, for chemoprophylaxis depending upon their Gail score.

Part II:
Breast Cancer Logic

Women have a distinct feminine physiology that is determined at conception. From the very beginning the die is cast for estrogen and progesterone to dominate over testosterone. To say breast cancer is the result of estrogen and progesterone is like saying the game of baseball is caused by the ball. Of course it is. You cannot have one without the other. If a woman does not have estrogen and progesterone, she will not develop female characteristics; she will not have female breasts; and it is unlikely she would get breast cancer. Blaming estrogen is howling at the moon. Women are susceptible to breast cancer because they are made like a woman. "Why is there breast cancer?" is a great question for philosophers and theologians.

There are so many contradictions when it comes to breast cancer and menopausal hormone therapy (MHT); it's hard to know whom to believe. The best advice is, "do not take the advice of someone who is totally dogmatic about MHT and breast cancer, one way or the other." There is no doubt that breast tissue is rich in estrogen and progesterone receptors, and stimulation helps breasts grow and maintain function. It is not so clear how menopausal hormone therapy affects the breast.

By the way, men are dominated by testosterone and subsequently develop a prostate gland. Without testosterone, men do not get prostate cancer, and just as many men die each year from prostate cancer as women die each year from breast cancer. Very few men, willingly, get castrated as a preventative treatment for prostate cancer. Men expect their testosterone to carry on without interruption until the end. If men get prostate cancer, then they consider the option of life without testosterone; but until that time, no way are they giving up their T. On the other hand, women are generally encouraged to let their estrogen go after menopause. Hmmmm…

Part III:
Breast Cancer by the Numbers

One woman in eight will contract breast cancer sometime in her lifetime. Although there are numerous TV shows and movies that seem to demonstrate otherwise, breast cancer is usually a disease of wSaturday late postmenopause women. The incidence climbs gradually with age. Some think breast cancer is more tragic for a young woman, but it's not a good deal no matter what the age. Less than 2 percent of women under the age of 50 have the diagnosis of breast cancer. That figure climbs slowly to 5 percent of women in their sixties, 7 percent in their seventies, and finally to 10 percent in their eighties. Interestingly, women have peak levels of estrogen and progesterone during their reproductive years in their thirties and forties, but rarely, get breast cancer then. Decades after they stop making large amounts estrogen or progesterone, they develop breast cancer. Breast cancer is not considered to be triggered by menopause.

Early detection, more than anything else, has resulted in significant improvement in survival rates for women diagnosed with breast cancer. When a cancer is found early and has not spread to the lymph nodes, over 96 percent of women are alive and well after five years. Because of that, breast cancer has taken on a transition to being more of a "breast disease" than a terminal condition. There are many breast cancer survivors who require special consideration for their long-term health problems.

Part IV:
Breast Cancer Prevention

The following is a list of risk factors for contracting breast cancer:

- Being born a woman. No kidding.
- Age. Breast cancer incidence rises with age. Whatever age you are today, thank God, and pray you will be around next year to celebrate another birthday.
- Breast cancer. If you already had a breast cancer, you are at a higher risk of developing another.
- Family history of breast cancer. If a first degree relative, mother, sister, or daughter contracted breast cancer *before* menopause age, you are at an increased of getting breast cancer too. However, most women with breast cancer (80 percent) have no family history.
- Early or late menstrual cycles. If you started having menstrual periods before age twelve and or stopped having menstrual periods later than age 55, there is an increased risk of breast cancer. It is true that the greater the total number of menstrual cycles a woman has in her lifetime, the greater the relative risk of developing breast cancer.
- No children or late-in-life children. If you have had no children or your first child was born after you turned 30 (probably due to more menstrual cycles, as above), there is a slight increased risk of breast cancer.
- Weight gain. Gaining more than 20 pounds after menopause increases your risk of breast cancer.
- Excessive alcohol. More than three alcoholic drinks a day are correlated with increasing your risk of breast cancer.
- Smoking. Smoking increases your risk for breast cancer. This is another good reason to quit.
- Inactivity. Exercising less than four hours a week increases

your risk of breast cancer. So, what do you think no exercise does to breast cancer risk?

- Low vitamin D. Low blood levels of vitamin D may significantly increase your risk of breast cancer.
- Fake food diet. Diets low in real food, like vegetables and fruit, are associated with increasing your risk of breast cancer.
- Radiation therapy. If you had to receive radiation therapy to treat a previous cancer, like a lymphoma, that will increase your risk of breast cancer if the breast was exposed to the radiation beam.
- MHT. There have been dozens of studies examining this important issue, and there are conflicting reports. Currently, the evidence favors a small *reduced* risk of breast cancer with estrogen alone (E), but a small increased risk of breast cancer diagnosis with long-term use (more than 5 years) of conjugated estrogen plus progestin (CE+P); and yet, a decreased chance of dying from breast cancer by taking either. More on this later.

All women are encouraged to examine this list and identify the risks they can personally modify. If you smoke and drink too much, you know where to start to reduce your risk of breast cancer. It seems like a broken record, but all the lifestyle recommendations for the Womenopause Challenge have universal benefits. The lifestyle habits that reduce Hot Flash Fever also improve Insomnia Queen. The lifestyle habits that improve Insomnia Queen also improve Mood Matters. The lifestyle habits that improve Mood Matters also improve cardiovascular system (and weight, and diabetes, and metabolic syndrome, and osteoporosis, and sex) and as a super bonus: ta-daa, reduce the risk of developing breast cancer!

Performing a self-breast exam monthly, just after your menstrual period is over, is the best time. The normal confusing tender lumps felt during PMS will have disappeared. A yearly clinical breast exam should be performed as part an annual gynecology evaluation. Annual mammograms beginning at age 35, or sooner if there are abnormal lumps or other risk factors, are recommended.

Part V:
Menopausal Hormone Therapy and Breast Cancer

There are conflicting reports about the effects menopausal hormone therapy has on breast cancer. The WHI, published in 2002, reported an increased risk of diagnosis of breast cancer for women who took oral conjugated estrogen with oral progestin (CE+P). wBodyIdentical 17beta-estradiol and progesterone were not studied in the WHI, and some believe they may have different effects, not showing an increase in breast cancer. However, even though the incidence of diagnosis was increased, the number of women who died from breast cancer decreased with oral conjugated estrogen plus progestin. It is a strange arrangement that future research must sort out. The WHI reported an overall decrease in the incidence of breast cancer for women who took only oral conjugated estrogen (women who had received a hysterectomy do not need progestins). These women who took the oral estrogen only, also had a decrease in breast cancer deaths.

Some experts point out that breast cancer is believed to arise very slowly in the breast tissue. There has been a tremendous amount of research studying how breast cancer develops. Breast cancer arises from a mistake in replication of a single breast cell, and it takes seven to ten years for a breast cancer to become large enough to be seen on a mammogram. When clinical studies report an increase in the number of breast cancers within a couple years of CE+P, MHT (as in the WHI study and others), there may be something else going on. It would be unlikely any breast cancer can start and become apparent on a mammogram in just a couple of years. It may be that MHT causes *a breast cancer that is already present before therapy* to become diagnosed sooner rather than later. If that is true, then MHT, even though there may be a higher incidence of diagnosis of breast cancer, may be to the woman's advantage because those tumors are a lower grade, easier to treat, and result in lower mortality. If the MHT did not bring the cancer to view early, then that cancer may develop slowly into a higher-grade tumor and be more difficult to treat when it is eventually discovered, resulting in a higher death rate.

Breast cancer associated with MHT consisting of oral conjugated estrogen and progestin (CE+P), tends to be estrogen receptor positive, lower grade, lower stage disease, and have better survival rates than breast cancer in women who do not take MHT. When women stop taking MHT, there is a reduced diagnosis of breast cancer, not necessarily a reduced risk.

Women with estrogen receptor positive breast cancer are traditionally not offered menopausal hormone therapy. Many of them are managed with a cancer-suppressing drug Tamoxifen. Tamoxifen is the original SERM that has positive and negative effects on the estrogen receptor. Tamoxifen blocks estrogen in

General Population	1.0
Vitamin D 2000 IU Daily	0.32
Oral Estrogen (CE)	0.76
Oral Estrogen Plus Progestin (CE+P)	1.26
College Graduate	1.28
1ˢᵗ Pregnancy After Age 30	1.37
Excessive Alcohol	1.52
Obesity	1.8
One Relative With Breast Cancer	2.2
Two Relatives With Breast Cancer	14.0

Figure 27-2 Breast Cancer Relative Risk

breast tissue and effectively reduces cancer recurrence. That blocking comes with a big price tag. By blocking estrogen, Tamoxifen induces menopausal symptoms like Hot Flash Fever, Mood Matters, Meno-Fog, Vagina Sahara, and all the rest. It also stimulates the endometrium like estrogen and increases the risk of uterine cancer and causes an increased risk of blood clots. Tamoxifen also increases the risk of osteoporosis. Recent data reveals that for women who have had a hysterectomy, MHT consisting of estrogen alone (E) have a 33 percent reduction in breast cancer, which is approximately the same reduction seen with Tamoxifen but without all the hot flashes, and osteoporosis.

Breast cancer survivors may experience menopausal symptoms and usually obtain relief with standard lifestyle changes (Womenopause Challenge). When lifestyle interventions are inadequate, there are now many effective non-hormonal agents for most of the specific estrogen deficiency problems such as Hot Flash Fever, Insomnia Queen, osteoporosis, and Mood Matters (Chapter 24).

For breast cancer survivors, a decision to initiate hormone therapy may be based on quality of life issues. The decision to take menopausal hormone therapy after breast cancer diagnosis should be done only after consultation with an oncologist. There are now several studies supporting the safety of MHT in selected breast cancer survivors. Because MHT reduces the risk of many other serious diseases, breast cancer survivors who began MHT had better overall quality of life and a lower death rate from all causes than did breast cancer survivors who did not use MHT. Local vaginal wBodyIdentical 17beta-estradiol may be considered a safe option for some breast cancer women who suffer from severe vaginal atrophy. Local vaginal testosterone may also be considered. There have been some women who have successfully initiated low dose systemic hormone therapy ten years after breast cancer treatment. MHT may be used in all pre-malignant breast disease without known deleterious effect.

Part VI:
Hormone Quibbling

Since 1990 there have been more than 20 large scientific studies looking at the risk menopausal hormone therapy has on breast cancer. There are conflicting conclusions and honest differences of opinion about the relative risks. For example, of the 22 studies looking at conjugated estrogen alone, there are nine studies that report a decreased risk of breast cancer, nine studies that found an increased risk of breast cancer, and four studies that found no change. The largest study in this group, WHI, found the largest reduced risk of breast cancer with MHT conjugated estrogen (CE) used alone. These studies involved thousands and thousands of women over combined hundreds of thousands of years. It seems the only results that ever make it into newspapers, magazines, and TV shows are the negative ones that pronounce unequivocally that hormones are dangerous. It's no wonder why many women have concerns about the safety of MHT. In truth, *if* there is a risk of breast cancer with MHT, then the risk is obviously quite low; otherwise, all of the studies would agree. Oral conjugated estrogen coupled with oral progestin (CE+P) probably results in a small *increased* incidence of finding a breast cancer on a mammogram, but it probably did not *cause* the cancer; and furthermore, the E+P *improves* the chance of surviving the cancer compared to women who did not take E+P.

At this juncture it is imperative to step back and look at the big picture. Breast cancer is one part of women's overall health. It is frightening to be diagnosed, and the treatments are difficult to go through. However, few women die from breast cancer. Women die from heart attacks, vascular disease, stroke, dementia, fractures, lung cancer, and a lot of other stuff. The frequency of dying from breast cancer is way down the list (Chapter 30). It is likely that MHT, when started in perimenopause or early postmenopause (wThursday and wFriday), reduces the risk of developing all of these high-mortality problems (Figure 30-2).

The complete understanding of how MHT affects risks for each individual should be carefully considered. A healthcare provider needs to be well-informed about both your personal health risks and how the specific risks of MHT might affect your health. In the end, only you can choose what is best for you.

Too many women dismiss hormone therapy because of a misunderstanding about the small debatable breast cancer disease risk. At the same time, they completely underestimate the huge affects lifestyle choices have on breast cancer. The affects of our daily life activities are dramatically more important in determining whether or not we get breast cancer.

- Vitamin D: Reduction in breast cancer by taking Vitamin D 4000 IU
- Alcohol: 50 percent reduction in breast cancer by reducing alcohol consumption
- Weight: 50-60 percent reduction in breast cancer by maintaining low BMI
- Exercise: Walking 3 hours per week reduces breast cancer by a whopping 50 percent
- Diet: 20 percent reduction in breast cancer by eating real food, green is good

Another way to think about breast cancer is to compare "relative risk" numbers. In relative risk statistics, the normal average chance for getting diagnosed with breast cancer is set to be 1.00 (one point zero zero). If the *relative risk increases*, the number *raises above 1.00* to a more positive number, like 1.80. If the *relative risk decreases* below the average risk the number *drops below 1.00* to a decimal number like 0.80 (zero point eight zero). Figure 27-2 charts some of the calculated relative risks for breast cancer. As can readily be seen, MHT, consisting of oral estrogen alone (CE), causes a reduction in the relative risk of contracting breast cancer (0.78 relative risk). Oral conjugated estrogen plus progestin (CE+P) causes a slight increase in the relative risk of contracting breast cancer to 1.26. This slight increase was so minimal that the researchers determined it was not statistically significant. Therefore, the risk of contracting breast cancer when taking CE+P was similar to the risk of breast cancer in women who did not take hormones.

Alice B.

At age 66 Alice had a BMI of 21 (slim figured), she exercised six days a week and was very well read on whole food diet. She had worked in the radiology department of the hospital as an x-ray tech for over 30 years. Her husband Allen owned a music store, and her three boys were all career military. Alice's health was excellent except for one thing; she had breast cancer.

At age 51 Alice underwent wide excision of a low grade stage I ductal cell breast carcinoma that was ER+ (estrogen receptor positive). She underwent chemotherapy and had several years of tamoxifen. By all measures Alice was cured of her breast cancer disease. She was highly motivated to control all her risk factors by carefully regimenting her lifestyle. In spite of all of that, she had persistent hot flashes and vaginal dryness. Over the years, she had tried Effexor, Neurontin, Clonidine, Elavil, and Valium to control hot flashes but to no avail (Chapter 9). She had doused her vagina with every moisturizer and lubricant available (Chapter 10). She continued to use plain mineral oil into which she put a drop of vanilla extract from her kitchen, twice a day and just before intercourse. This procedure helped some, but her vaginal opening and labia had experienced a long gradual atrophy. It had gotten to the point that no matter how much mineral oil she used, sex hurt.

No sex for the past six months had put Alice and Allen's relationship on edge. Sexual intercourse was an important part of their life, and they could find no mutually acceptable alternatives. Her wScore demonstrated a "perfect score" on the Vagina

Sahara and Sexercise sections with all "W" circled (Figure 1-2). Her wSxScore was a dismal 39. She wanted advice about anything new to try.

Alice had been asking to go on hormones, off and on, for more than a decade. Her oncologist had forbid her from doing so. Alice was delighted to learn several recent publications reported good relief of vaginal atrophy with local vaginal estrogen. Estrogen applied locally to the vagina had been found to have little appreciable systemic effects; and therefore, it could be safe for breast cancer survivors. After an exchange of information with her oncologist, Alice was cleared to give it a try.

Estrace wBodyIdentical 17beta-estradiol local vaginal cream was prescribed to Alice. She applied it once a day. For the first two weeks, she applied 2 gm vaginally by using the applicator and the following two weeks, only 1 gm of Estrace a day. She agreed to try the new SNRI drug, Pristiq, for her hot flashes, and she began by taking 50 mg daily in the morning.

Four weeks later Alice reported improvement in the condition of her vagina. She no longer had the continuous burning sensation, and it had become much easier to insert the applicator for dosing. She did not especially care for the mess that the Estrace cream made, but she was encouraged enough about the progress she definitely wanted to continue with it. When she was informed about the Estring, the local vaginal ring; changed every three months, no mess no fuss; she decided to give it a try. She reported moderate improvement in the frequency and intensity of her hot flashes. She and Allen had not had a romantic encounter the past month, and she was apprehensive about how to restart sex. She thought her vagina had recovered enough to try intercourse. She said, "If Allen was just a little guy, maybe we wouldn't have this problem, but he's definitely not little." She was receptive to detailed instruction in the use of vaginal dilators and decided it was worth a try. Alice accepted information about the Womenopause Five Night Sex Assignment (Chapter 18) and thought it could be a fun way to get reacquainted in the bedroom. She continued taking Pristiq 50 mg daily.

Four weeks later Alice claimed victory over breast cancer and brought flowers for the entire office staff. Her hot flashes were 70 percent better, and at a level she could easily live with. Her pelvic exam revealed her vagina and labia had become dramatically restored with the local vaginal estrogen. She and Allen had rediscovered how much they liked touching each other, and they had spent more time in bed together than ever, "And I don't mean asleep."

Breast Cancer: HOPE

Hope is the dew on an April morning
When a hungry farmer borrows money
To buy corn but instead of eating
He plants it

Hope is the clack clack clacking
That squeezes entrails
For the slow first hill ascent
Of the rollercoaster

Hope is the crispness of the astronauts' sheets
Folded with routine precision
In quiet aloneness
On launch morning

Hope is the juice flowing in the sprout
Of an Easter Lilly
Willing it's way up
Through three inches of snow

Hope is the edema of a mother-to-be's ankles

Lying on her left side eating celery
When every fiber of her soul
Begs for pizza

Hope is a glint of gold
Reflected with startling brilliance
On the hands of a couple of sixty-year-olds
Renewing their vows

Hope is red lipstick
Skillfully applied
Just before the knock on the door
By the summoned paramedics

Hope is the glimpse of light
That the heart almost abandons
Because everyone you trust
Turns the switch off

Hope is the abyss
Between this minute and the next
A great distance to travel alone
And damn near impossible
Without God

Part VII:
The Womenopause Challenge: Breast Cancer Survivor's Guide

1. Continue to take all medications prescribed by your healthcare providers.
2. Report all new problems to your doctor:
   • Unusual headaches
   • Bone pains upon awakening

- Shortness of breath
- Change in appetite

3. Consume real food.
4. Exercise like you mean it.
5. Take all of the recommended vitamins and supplements.
6. Make regular appointments with your healthcare providers.
7. Write a poem.

Chapter 28

Heart Health: Get Pumped

Part I:
Heart Disease: It's Not a Men's Club

Women don't give heart disease enough respect. Again, this year, more women than men will die in North America from heart disease. If the mortality due to heart disease, stroke, and peripheral vascular disease were all combined (termed cardiovascular disease, CVD), the total, over 500,000 deaths, is greater than the next 14 causes of women's death combined! About 1,400 women die every day from CVD. Cardiovascular disease is *thirteen times* more fatal than breast cancer. How did this sneak so far under the radar with hardly anyone noticing? Well, actually, the entire medical establishment has been on high alert about this problem for decades. Apparently the only thing missing from heart disease getting noticed is a good celebrity endorsement or a brilliant marketing plan. It's well past time for a Womenopause Heart Health Makeover.

Part II:
Risky Business

Arteries, supplying necessary oxygen and nutrients to the heart (and the brain, and the kidneys, and the legs, and the so on), can get clogged with atherosclerotic plaque. Plaque is a nice term for globs of inflamed fat. If the plaque exceeds a critical size, there is disruption of blood flow to the heart muscle, and the heart yells out with angina (chest pain) signaling a heart attack. Sometimes the heart is silent and gives almost no warning its arteries are blocked.

A lot is known about how plaque forms. (Another name for

plaque is atherosclerosis). First, lipids (fat) from the blood stream infiltrate the lining of the vessels and accumulate within the wall of the artery. If the growing plaque ruptures within the arterial wall, then an inflammatory reaction occurs drawing in white cells that eventually develops into a calcified plaque. Calcified plaques are bad because they can grow scars that rupture through the arterial wall and induce an immediate blood clot. Platelets and thrombin form a clot that is usually the "final clogging straw that breaks the blood flow's back". If the blood flow is blocked, then everything down stream suffers from lack of oxygen. How long can you hold your breath? That's about how long the heart muscle can go without oxygen.

How, you might ask, does plaque get into the blood vessel wall in the first place? Lipids are *invited* into the walls of heart arteries by special engraved invitations, of course. They do not generally crash the vessel party. Invitations come in the following forms:

- **Smoking**. Another reason to quit, convinced yet?
- **Hypertension**. High blood pressure is a major cause of cardiovascular disease.
- **Sedentary lifestyle**. Seems like that has come up somewhere before.
- **Diabetes**. Glucose intolerance and insulin deficiency spell trouble for the entire body.
- **Poor blood lipids**. High total cholesterol and especially high LDL-C (low density lipoprotein that carries choles-terol, so-called "bad" cholesterol) coupled with low HDL-C (high density lipoprotein that carries cholesterol, so called "good" cholesterol) and high triglycerides.
- **High BMI**. Seems like that one has come up before, too.
- **Fake food diet**. This is becoming very familiar by now.
- **Metabolic syndrome**. No kidding, that one, too.
- **Family history**. If your father had a heart attack before age

55 and/or your mother had one before age 65, you are born (but not bound) to be at a higher risk of heart disease.

- **Menopause.** Before menopause, women have a low rate of heart attacks (much lower than men's). After menopause, heart attack rates for women accelerate and pass the men's rate of heart attack.
- **Depression.** Our mood is connected to our body in both positive and negative ways. This is a big negative one. Depression is not just a problem with our mood. Depression is a whole body disorder.

There is really great news here! Look carefully at the preceding list. There is only one thing on the list that you cannot do anything about. You cannot change who your parents are. Besides, you would not be you without them. By the way, have you heard having children is genetically acquired? If your parents did not have any children, chances are really good that you won't have any either! (Give your parents a hug today).

Aside from your parents, everything else on the list is somewhat under your control. Being smoke free reduces your risk of heart disease by three-fourths. Reducing your cholesterol from 250 down to 200 cuts your heart disease risk by 50 percent. Exercising regularly cuts your cardiovascular disease risk by over 30 percent. Adult-onset-diabetes and the Metabolic Syndrome are often caused, amplified, and maintained by poor food choices and inactivity. Nutritious real food and regular Vitamin-X exercise improves mood better than any pill. Maintaining, or better yet, improving the BMI effects blood pressure, diabetes, metabolic syndrome, mood, and lipids all in one fell swoop. It's fantastic news. Everything that improves midlife women's menopause transition improves their risk of dying from cardiovascular disease. Ironic in a way, but getting a handle on Hot Flash Fever through lifestyle improvements, has tremendous long-term health benefits.

Part III:
Hormones and Heart Health

The effects of estrogen on the development of atherosclerosis plaque, has been hotly debated for decades. Although initial information from the WHI seemed to signal heart problems related to MHT, re-analysis has clarified important parts of the dilemma. The best evidence today, points toward a "window of opportunity" when menopausal hormone therapy has heart benefits. Before the WHI study, this was not fully understood. For the majority of women at menopause, the coronary vessels do not have significant atherosclerotic plaque (yet). Hormone therapy instituted at or near the time of menopause allows the estrogen to interact with the cells lining the heart arteries (and the brain arteries, and the kidney, and the legs, and so on) and help preserve them. If there is a delay, and atherosclerosis has become advanced, estrogen cannot interact with the lining of the vessels because it is blocked by a slathering of plaque.

Confusing information came out initially from the WHI because they lumped all ages of women together. Since the WHI mainly studied women over age 65 who had been without estrogen for about twenty years (and who had no symptoms of menopause), the results were skewed toward harm rather than help from MHT. After several years of re-crunching the data, it became apparent *w*Wednesday, *w*Thursday, and *w*Friday women on estrogen or estrogen plus progesterone had quite different effects than *w*Saturday late post menopausal women who began combination, E+P. Hence the belief there is a period of time, the "window of opportunity" lasting about a decade, in which starting (and continuing) menopausal hormone therapy proves to be very beneficial to women's hearts.

When the researchers separated women out according to specific decades, those starting hormones (E and E+P) in their fifties significantly decreased their risk of heart disease; those starting hormones in their sixties also significantly decreased their risk of heart disease; but those starting hormones for the first time in their seventies had a small increased risk of heart disease, although, only for one year. There were so many in their seventies that the premature analysis led to the wrong conclusion: hormone therapy was bad for the heart. In the original WHI report, all age groups were lumped together; the women on estrogen only, had an overall decrease in heart risks even in the original report.

Another important point about the results from the WHI involves the type of hormones studied. Only oral conjugated estrogen (CE) was studied and a relatively high dose at that. As was demonstrated previously (Chapter 21), oral estrogen may stimulate the clotting system and may increase blood clots. See the problem? Heart attacks are often preceded with a clot on top of a plaque, and anything that would induce more clots might raise the chance of a heart attack. One might conclude; therefore, transdermal wBodyIdentical 17beta-estradiol would have less affect on acute coronary blockage because they do not effect clotting (Figure 22-1).

Although the WHI has been the largest hormone therapy study, it is certainly not the only and will not be the last. Since 1990, there have been 23 scientific studies looking at different aspects of hormones and heart health. The cumulative data indicates estrogen therapy for menopause significantly reduces heart disease. If women begin estrogen only (E) under age 60, or within ten years of menopause, their risk of heart disease drops by 40 percent compared to women who do not take MHT (Chapter 30: Death Prevention). This is very important since, as already referenced, heart disease is the number one killer of English speaking women. Estrogen therapy, for women who have had a hysterectomy, is as effective as lipid lowering medicines (like Lipitor) in reducing heart disease plus has innumerable other quality of life benefits that lipid medicines do not have. Hormones and Lipitor-like drugs can be used safely together and complement each other.

Speaking of mortality, the WHI data and other studies make clear the dramatic point that for women who begin menopausal hormone therapy before age 60, oral estrogen (E) or estrogen plus progestin (E+P) reduces overall mortality by an astounding 40 percent. There is not any other medical intervention that comes close to the magnitude of death prevention as is seen for women who take menopausal hormone therapy. This data emphasizes the importance of timing of the initiation of MHT. If MHT is begun early and continued, there is a substantial affect on the prevention of heart disease. Even though estrogen is only "approved" for the treatment of menopausal symptoms like hot flashes etc, a case could be argued for starting estrogen at menopause solely for the purpose of heart disease prevention.

For women over age 70, who have been without estrogen for two decades, there is a temporary risk of increased heart events with E+P during the first year of therapy. After the first year, the risks reverse to below that seen in women who do not take hormones. The presumed reason for the difference between 70 something's and 50 something's is the amount of plaque already present on the coronary arteries at the time the hormones are started. When arteries of women in their seventies are examined, they invariably have substantially more plaque than arteries of women in their fifties. The plaque blocks the estrogen from having access to the cells lining the arteries, and the estrogen temporarily appears to cause the plaques to loosen. After one year, the coronary arteries adjust to the presence of estrogen; the plaques stabilize; and the risks of heart events diminish. After that vulnerable year, the risks are actually lower than the heart event risk of women who have never taken hormones, and that reduced risk appears to persist as long as they continue to take the MHT. The reasons are still hypothetical, but there appears to be a negative aspect of progestins on the wSaturday women's coronary arteries for one year. Still, that should be taken in the context of specific individual factors. The overall health benefits of taking E+P or E alone in wWednesday, wThursday and wFriday women, the heart not withstanding, were remarkably positive, with a reduction of total mortality by 40 percent.

The preponderance of the positive data about heart disease and hormones was obtained in studies looking only at oral conjugated estrogen (CE). Because of the well-documented problems CE has with the clotting system (Chapter 21), there is intense interest in looking at transdermal estrogen formulations to see if there would be even greater cardiovascular disease prevention by taking those. Several positive attributes of transdermal 17beta-estradiol have been found that would be expected to further reduce heart disease risk.

Transdermal Estrogen therapy has the following favorable cardiovascular affects:

- Reduces coronary artery calcium
- Reduces coronary artery atherosclerotic plaque
- Reduces hypertension
- Reduces diabetes
- Reduces metabolic syndrome
- Reduces weight gain
- Reduces total cholesterol
- Reduces bad cholesterol, LDL-C
- Increases good cholesterol, HDL-C
- Reduces triglycerides
- (Does not affect who your parents are)

Symptomatic menopausal women under age 60 with Hot Flash Fever, night sweats, Mood Matters, Vagina Sahara, and Meno-Fog, may seek relief by deciding to take menopausal hormone therapy. It is reassuring to know that estrogen therapy substantially improves heart health as well, and improved cardiovascular risks may be evident in as little as four weeks.

Pearl C.

"A purveyor of the world's last best legal socially acceptable drug" was how Pearl described her work; by that, she meant she sold coffee. She and her husband Mike owned three hugely successful upscale "caffeinated experience boutiques". Success had not come easily, and the long hours of private entrepreneurship had taken a toll on Pearl's health. She was 52; both her daughters were married with two kids of their own. Her husband Mike, somehow, still found the time to be a scratch golfer. Pearl could not find the time to turn around. She opened all three shops, managed the crews all day long and personally closed them just in time to get six hours of sleep in preparation for doing it again the next day. Her diet: coffee and pastries (they were free).

She made a big deal about taking time out of work to come to her gynecology appointment and was appreciative of her appointment being on time. To streamline the process, Pearl had gotten her annual labs drawn the week before. Her complaint was, "hot coffee showers ten times a day and less sleep than ever." Her blood pressure was 135/80; her BMI was 32; her waist measurement was 38 inches; her HDL-C was only 38 (good cholesterol); her triglycerides were 197; and her fasting blood sugar was 112.

Pearl anxiously paced around the exam room asking, "Can I have a prescription and get back to work?" Pearl needed a little more in-depth discussion (and maybe a lot less caffeine).

Pearl received information about the risk factors for cardiovascular disease. She was advised her Hot Flash Fever was probably the most obvious problem, but something more sinister could be brewing underneath. Pearl's father had died of a heart attack at age 57, and her mother had died in a car crash the following year. She had recently quit smoking "for the ninth time."

In short, Pearl was a poster child advertizing the risks of

cardiovascular disease. Her lifestyle allowed no time for exercise or relaxation; she had constant access to fake food-like substances; and she continued to smoke. All of which takes the hot flashes up a couple notches. All of her labs indicated she had met criteria for the Metabolic Syndrome (MBS): low HDL, high triglycerides, boarder-line high blood pressure, and an abdominal fat expanding waistline. That spelled t-r-o-u-b-l-e. On top of all that, she attempted to cover her daytime drowsiness with gallons of espresso coffee and tried to "unwind" with two (usually five) quick glasses of wine before bed. Her wScore was 39 W (Figure 1-2).

Pearl was advised that today was the day to begin her menopause makeover. She said she was willing to do whatever she needed to get rid of the hot flashes.

Pearl reviewed the real food nutrition suggestions (Chapter 14: Real Food) and Vitamin-X exercise (Chapter 16: Vitamin-X). It was time for Pearl to make decisions about work. Did she want business success at the expense of personal illness and possible premature death, or did she want healthful happiness for decades to come? Did she want to know her grandchildren and be there to know her great-grandchildren? Pearl was reassured, she could be healthier at 60 than she had been at 40, but it would not happen without thought and effort. Pearl accepted the Womenopause Challenge.

Her first order of business was to recruit Mike to help her scale back some of her 70-hour work weeks by hiring an assistant manager, or two. She would exchange opening the coffee shops with working out at the health club one block away. She was encouraged to seek a fun activity that had nothing to do with work. (She had previously said that cleaning the coffee grinders was her most fun thing to do!) Pearl was particularly impressed with the advantages of real food and converted the coffee shop offerings to mostly whole foods.

For her Hot Flash Fever, she chose Evamist (three sprays in

the morning) transdermal *w*BodyIdentical 17beta-estradiol coupled with Prometrium (100 mg orally at night). She obtained a pedometer and began the Fast 4 Fit program the same day (15,000 steps a day to lose weight, no pop, no potatoes, and no bread). She would try cutting out caffeine to see how it goes for one month.

Four weeks later Pearl sat relaxed in the exam room chair. Her *w*Score had dropped from 39 W to 8 W; her BMI had dropped from 32 to 30; and her waistline had contracted two inches. Her blood pressure had improved, and she reported seven solid hours of sleep at night. Her hot flashes were "G-O-N-E". Pearl produced her workout journal demonstrating excellent consistent exercise and 15,000 steps everyday for four weeks. "It works, you know, eating right and exercising does really work." Really.

For fun she had decided to teach her granddaughters how to paint. She had always held a romantic notion, about how relaxing it would be to sit outside with an easel, painting landscapes.

"The girls loved it, for about ten minutes, then we were off riding bikes, then swimming in the pool. Sooo-ooo much more fun than painting."

Six months later, a recheck of her blood lipids demonstrated significant improvements. Her HDL-C had increased to 45, her triglycerides were down to 125, and her blood sugar was normal at 98. Pearl asked if it was the estrogen or the lifestyle changes that were making the difference? The answer, of course, is yes.

Part IV:
The Womenopause Challenge: Have a Heart

1. Because heart disease is not just a plumbing problem, your relaxation exercises from Chapter 12 (Mood Matters) can serve double duty: improve your mood and help your heart.

2. Check your pulse rate while relaxed sitting in a chair. If your resting pulse is less than 65 beats per minute, great. If your resting pulse is greater than 75, not so great.

3. Make an appointment with your healthcare provider to have blood pressure, cholesterol, triglycerides, blood sugar, weight and belly circumference measured.

4. If you are still a smoke slave, it's time to become free at last.

5. Remember, there is no cholesterol of any kind in vegetables. Eat 'em up.

6. Substitute Benecol Light Spread for butter or margarine.

Chapter 29

The Skinny on Skin

Part I:
Skin Enemies

Skin is the body's largest organ. As it defends the body from invasion by outside forces, it sometimes takes a beating. Two basic problems are encountered with skin: first, skin can age poorly, and second, there can be just too much of it! The five horseman of the skin-apocalypse are:

1. Sun
2. Soap
3. Smoking
4. Spans of time
5. "S"trogen deficiency

Sun causes "photoaging" which is ironic, because the more sun the skin gets, the worse the photos look over the years. Sun destroys the connective tissue within the skin, producing wrinkles, frown lines, roughness, dryness, brown spots, spider veins, and even skin cancer. Who needs it? Great tans are definitely not so great for the skin; they come at a high price. Add smoking and excessive drinking to the life long beach party, and you've got a cosmetic cataclysm.

Part II:
Only Skin Deep

Skin is like a computer keyboard; it's the interface between the internal hard drive guts and the outside world. Skin is the contact point for both visual and touch interactions with other people.

Skin is important, and much like the internal organs, it can be assisted and protected or used and abused. Understanding the anatomy of skin helps explain the problems that might occur.

The outermost layer of skin, the epidermis, consists of layers of dead cells. These cells have squeezed out all of their water and loaded up with keratin to form a protective barrier. Below the epidermis lies the dermis, which provides the nutrient blood supply for the skin and produces the hair follicles and sweat glands. The dermis also produces the rich dense network of lacy connective tissue that gives the skin its softness. Deeper still is a variable layer of adipose tissue called the sub dermis, which supports the skin smoothness. The epidermis is "dead and shed", the dermis is "copious collagen" (98 percent) and "adequate elastin" (2 percent), and the subcutis is "satisfactory fat".

Near menopause women begin to appreciate their skin in ways they did not in their youth, and judging from the number of skin products available, almost every one is willing to invest some effort into keeping their skin healthy. The following vignette, unlike all of the others, is totally fictional. It is representative of many types of skin care problems menopausal women frequently encounter.

Scarlett's Skin

At 59, Scarlett left nothing to chance when it came to her skin. She was a natural beauty and had every intention of working hard to keep it that way. Let's follow her through a day and see what wisdom she has accumulated.

Scarlett's husband's alarm goes off at 6:15 am, giving him enough time to go downstairs to prepare her non-fat skim milk latte, so she can sip on their way to the gym. Scarlett is absolutely sure the health of her skin depends upon her taking care of her entire body, which means vigorous exercise six days a week. She loves it. She remembers to drink plenty of water during workouts. Afterwards, she and her husband Max, eat an egg white omelet with spinach and dry wheat toast with V8 juice to drink. She believes her skin deserves only the best nutrients.

Scarlett prefers tub baths to the shower, and she closes all the doors and windows to get the bathroom warm and steamy. She likes to listen to music rather than watch the bad news newscast because she believes a positive attitude is important to well-being. Into her warm (but not scalding hot) bath, she pours a cap full of Neutrogena body oil (fragrance free of course). She soaks and relaxes for ten minutes and washes her face, neck, and chest with MD Forte soap-free, oil-free facial cleanser with glycolic acid, which helps erase fine lines. As an alternative, she may wash her face with Cetaphil cleanser, a more soothing and affordable choice. Scarlett never washes her face with strong soaps or scented products. She washes her armpits and any dirty areas with a very small amount of Softsoap Nutra-oil moisturizing body wash with almond oil and shea butter. Scarlett uses Cetaphil Cleanser for the vulvovaginal area because it has the same pH, reducing the risk of infections or drying out the vagina. She proceeds to wash her hair, not with any soap, but with conditioner only. She likes Redken Fresh Curls Conditioner as a hair cleaner. Then, after rinsing with fresh water, she applies a small amount of Redken Smooth Down for conditioning and leaves it in her wet hair. After rinsing her entire body with fresh warm water, Scarlett steps out of the tub and gently pats, never rubs, her skin with a towel. Quickly, before the moisture leaves her skin, she applies Vaseline Total Moisture Conditioning with vitamins E & A. She knows moisturizers work by trapping water into the skin not by applying moisture to the skin. She then applies a coating of pure mineral oil to her labia and vagina (sometimes with a drop of vanilla extract added to the bottle). To her face and neck, she applies Trish McEvoy Protective Shield SPF 15 Moisturizer and spreads the leftover sunscreen onto the back of her hands. On her lower eyelids, she places a small amount of N. V. Perricone Eye Area Therapy containing Alpha

Lipoic Acid, NTP Complex, and, DAME to diminish and treat the fine lines and crows feet. Next, around the entire eye she gently rubs in a little Trish McEvoy Intensive Eye Therapy and finishes up with Trish McEvoy Line Minimizer around her mouth. After her makeup (various Trish McEvoy products), she applies additional moisturizer to her hands. She uses a firm toothbrush with Crest Vivid White toothpaste, three sprays of Evamist to her foreman, and off she goes to work.

During the day, aside from applying hand lotion and lip-gloss a dozen times (Trish McEvoy), she may touch up her powder just before dinner, but that's about it, all day long. She wears a hat if she ever goes out into the sun between 10am and 2pm. She keeps a humidifier going in the office to keep her skin moist. At night a different set of skin problems are addressed.

Before bed, Scarlett often applies Ureacin-20 Crème containing 20 percent urea in mineral oil to rough dry areas on the heels and soles of her feet. It's a prescription product she gets from her gynecologist. Occasionally Scarlett may get dry, itchy fine bumps on her legs or arms. Lac-Hydrin 12 percent cream containing ammonium lactate, also a prescription product, or just plain Crisco softens them and makes them disappear. On the back of her hands Scarlett applies hydroquinone 4 percent to a couple of pesky brown-pigmented spots. . Usually, before bed, Scarlett applies a small amount of Trish McEvoy Vitamin C cream all over her face and neck alternating with MD Forte Facial Cream with glycolic acid, super concentrated for the wrinkles. On nights when her face feels particularly dry or irritated she puts on MD Forte Replenish Hydrating Cream before always flossing and brushing her teeth.

Scarlett estimates her time commitment to keeping her skin healthy to be less than a half of a TV episode of American Idol; therefore, she skips the TV, has great skin, and has an extra 30 minutes to spend on beauty sleep. Scarlett takes a daily dose of estrogen to control her otherwise bothersome hot flashes, but she considers the beneficial effects the estrogen has on maintaining her skin more important than Hot Flash Fever.

Part III
More Skin Secrets

Midlife women frequently notice annoying skin problems, and they think that they are the only ones who have ever had them. The "dirty dozen" common skin problems and their solutions are next.

1. Pimples on the buttocks—try Ban Roll-On Deodorant.
2. Pimples on the buttocks that do not go away with two weeks of Ban—try prescription Cleocin cream.
3. Scaly skin patch on the cheek or forehead—try selenium sulfide Nisoral shampoo one percent
4. Facial pimples—try washing the face with Cetaphil cleanser.
5. Facial pimples during perimenopause—try the prescription cycle control pill, Yaz.
6. Facial pimples during perimenopause that do not go away with Yaz—try adding doxycycline oral antibiotic.
7. Facial pimples during perimenopause that just won't quit—try consulting a dermatologist and consider accutane or spironolactone.
8. Facial wrinkles that seriously bother you—try prescription Retin-A, Avage, Tazorac, Zorac, or MHT.
9. Deep facial creases—try consulting a plastic surgeon or cosmetic dermatologist and consider collagen injections and Botox.
10. Rash under the breasts—try washing with luke warm water, and blow-dry completely with a cool blow-dryer, then rub in some anti-fungal cream like Lamisil. Tucks pads under the breasts provide some relief.

11. Uneven skin tone—try Clinique even better skin tone corrector with Clinique even better skin tone correcting moisturizer SPF 20.

12. Thinning hair—try Rogaine, green tea, and vitamin B6 for 6 months.

Part III:
Hormones and Skin

Estrogen supports several important skin functions, and all levels of the skin are loaded with estrogen receptors. Estrogen has an important role in the dermis where collagen and elastin are produced. Collagen and elastin are the critically important structural components giving skin its soft fullness. Estrogen is known to limit collagen loss, maintain skin thickness, and improve skin elasticity and firmness. Estrogen also improves skin moisture. The dermis is the site of oil glands that release protective oils onto the surface and helps prevent skin drying. Estrogen reduces skin pore size. Estrogen also promotes the sub-dermal fat layer that smoothes-out the skin's contour. Estrogen has been found to reduce the small fine wrinkles by stimulating regrowth of the epidermis. Estrogen has also been found to lessen deep wrinkles by stimulating the production of collagen and elastin in the dermis. And finally, estrogen has been found to improve skin smoothness by restoring the thin layer of subdermal adipose tissue. There is advancing evidence that estrogen, when directly applied to damaged skin, may exert a direct local affect to stimulate skin recovery to reduce wrinkles. One can only imagine the marketing potential if it becomes proven that estrogen face creams decrease crow's feet and smile lines. Many menopausal women who begin hormone therapy for the control of hot flashes and night sweats remark about how much better their skin looks and feels since starting hormones. Improvements can be seen (and felt!) in as little as 4 weeks. Some women go so far as to say menopausal hormone therapy literally saved their skin.

Part IV:
Where's My Hair?

It comes as a shock that hair loss at menopause effects almost 50 percent of women. Hair loss for women looks different than men's hair loss although the underlying biological cause for both is similar. Men have a distinctive top of head and frontal hairline loss while women experience predominantly a more uniform top thinning. Everyone seems comfortable with male pattern baldness on men, but hardly anyone accepts female hair thinning and balding.

Androgenic alopecia is the primary cause of female hair thinning. It is usually inherited, begins slowly (with an onset as early as puberty), increases with age, and affects half of all women by the age of 50. In some women, the small amount of testosterone that the ovaries make, may affect the hair follicles on the scalp and cause them to cease making that beautiful mane. Rarely, other causes for female hair thinning are present: malnutrition (extreme dieting), stress (self-induced?), thyroid disease, diabetes, chemotherapy, burns, infections, rheumatoid diseases, and a few others. If the problem is significant, a couple of lab tests should be considered, TSH, liver and kidney function, total and free testosterone, SHBG, DHEAS, estrogen, and FSH.

Prevention and treatment of hair loss has little to be lost and much to be gained. After excluding the rare causes, it can be assumed the problem is benign, and the following are believed to be reasonably safe and effective treatments for female thinning hair.

- Creative hairstyles: Never underestimate the value of a good salon and good hair products.
- Rogaine (minoxidil 2 percent or 5 percent solution): Rogaine should be applied once (or preferable twice) a day for at least four months to see if your scalp will be responsive. Rogaine works better as a hair thinning preventer than a restorer and must be continued to remain

effective.

- Menopausal hormone therapy: Some menopausal women will stabilize their scalp by initiating MHT.
- Cycle control pills or vaginal rings: Some perimenopausal women will obtain improvement with birth control pills.
- Treatment for anorexia: Severe dieting may result in hair loss.
- Low dose steroids: Under the direction of an experienced dermatologist, some women will respond to oral steroids.
- Metformin or spironolactone: Daily medication for thin hair occasionally helps.
- Green tea and vitamin B: No risk options.
- Weight loss: You will look and feel better while you work and wait for your hair to respond.
- Hyaluronic acid shampoo: It has been successful in European trials.
- Local topical estrogen: It has been tried with some success in Europe.
- Hairpiece: It becomes a personal decision.
- You will notice a difference in your skin and hair in just four weeks.

Part V:
The Womenopause Challenge: Skin Savers

1. Become smoke-free.
2. Avoid all harsh soaps.
3. Apply moisturizer to your damp-ish skin immediately after bathing.
4. Invest at least as much in your skin care products as you do for hair products.
5. Apply SPF 15 or higher UV protection to your face everyday.
6. Tanning is for wrinkly women only.

Chapter 30

Death Prevention

Part I:
Paris in the Spring

Everyone traveling to Paris for the first time anticipates seeing the Eiffel Tower, but that's not all France has to offer. Imagine champagne and cheese in a little café on the Left Bank of the Seine River. There is no view of the Eiffel tower, but the experience is exceptional. Similarly, good health is more than postponing death; but as end points go, death is the final destination. Knowing where it's located is important. On the trip to avoiding death, there are wonderful excursions of health and well-being that are just as graceful as that terrific steel tower. The best travel advice begins with something like, "Forget the destination, enjoy the journey."

A recent Gallup survey asked women what they thought caused most women's deaths. Forty percent guessed breast cancer, and 4 percent guessed heart disease. In actuality, those death rates are exactly the opposite. Apparently, there is much confusion about the real risks to women's lives. This chapter lays out the big picture, so there will be no more guessing. If a woman seeks any health information (for instance, someone who might read a book about menopause), it can safely be assumed that she desires to live life optimally and as long as possible. Knowing precisely what usually causes death is the important first step to preventing it.

The top 20 causes of death for American women paint a stark reality. Women die after suffering unnecessarily. Women die prematurely. Detection and treatment of diseases are important but not enough. Death prevention requires knowledge of lifestyle choices that result in absolute reduction of acquiring diseases.

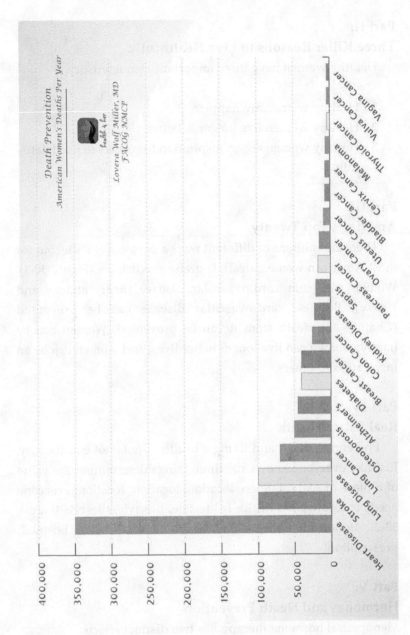

Death Prevention
American Women's Deaths Per Year

Lovera Wolf Miller, MD
FACOG NMCP

Figure 30-1 Death Prevention

Part II:
Three Killer Reasons to Live Healthfully
Healthy women have three important characteristics.

1. Healthy women are happier.
2. Healthy women live longer & better.
3. Healthy women are an inspiration for others to live healthfully.

Part III:
America's Top Twenty
There are millions of different ways a person *might* die, but for most American women, death is pretty predictable (Figure 30-1). Women die from cardiovascular disease (heart attacks and stroke). Because cardiovascular disease can be prevented (Chapter 28), death from it can be prevented. Women can be happy; women can live longer better lives; and women can be an inspiration to others.

Part IV:
Real Estate Health
Preventing death and living a healthy life is not exactly easy. Just like everyone knows the three things determining the value of a piece of real estate are location, location, location; everyone needs to know good health is lifestyle, lifestyle, lifestyle (Figure 30-2). Important notice: good health is *not*: doctor, hospital, prescription!

Part V:
Hormones and Death Prevention
Menopausal hormone therapy has two distinct effects.

1. Menopausal hormone therapy reduces the short-term symptoms of **estrogen withdrawal** in perimenopause and

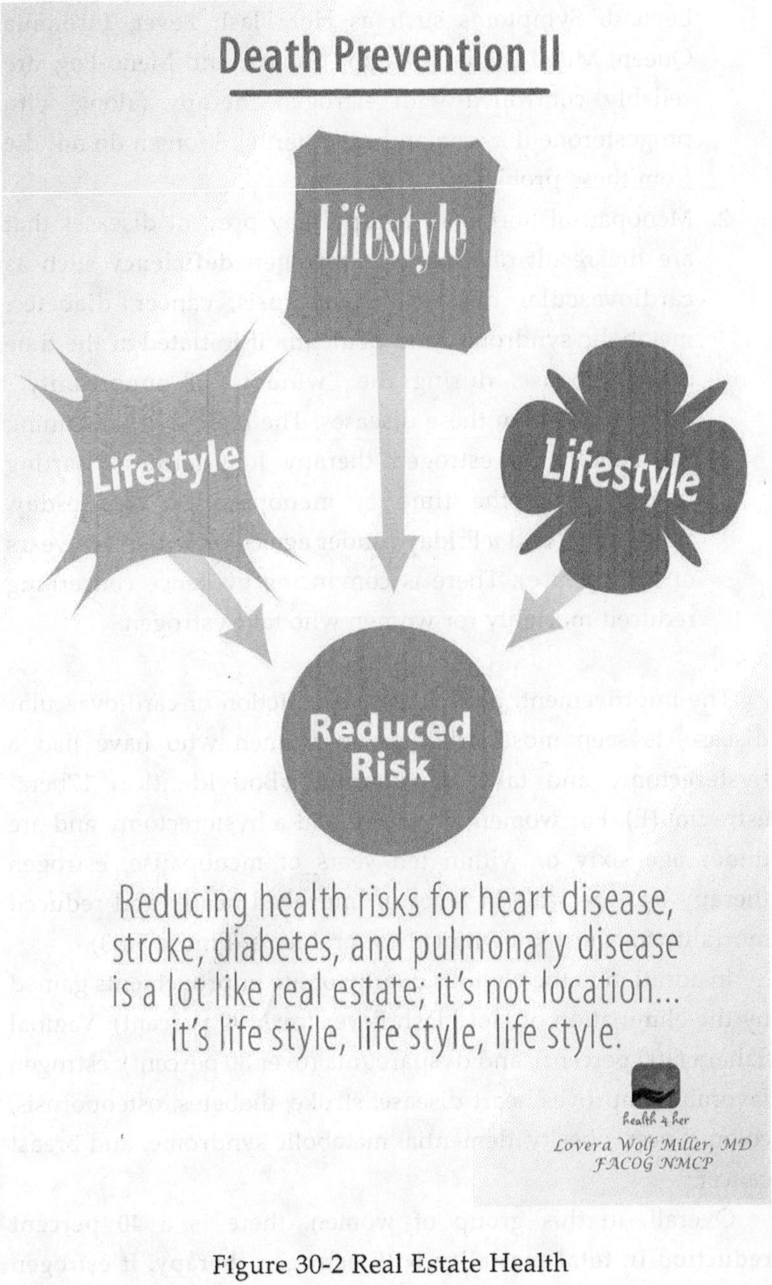
Death Prevention II
Lifestyle
Lifestyle
Lifestyle
Reduced Risk
Reducing health risks for heart disease, stroke, diabetes, and pulmonary disease is a lot like real estate; it's not location... it's life style, life style, life style.
health 4 her
Lovera Wolf Miller, MD
FACOG NMCP

Figure 30-2 Real Estate Health

beyond. Symptoms such as Hot Flash Fever, Insomnia Queen, Mood Matters, Vagina Sahara, and Meno-Fog, are reliably controlled with estrogen therapy (along with progesterone if a woman has a uterus). Women do not die from these problems.

2. Menopausal hormone therapy may prevent diseases that are the result of long-term **estrogen deficiency** such as cardiovascular disease, osteoporosis, cancer, diabetes, metabolic syndrome, and dementia if initiated at the time of menopause, during the "window of opportunity". Women die from these diseases. The real key to obtaining the benefits of estrogen therapy long-term is starting therapy near the time of menopause, wWednesday, wThursday, and wFriday (under age 60 or within ten years of menopause). There is convincing evidence concerning reduced mortality for women who take estrogen.

The improvement, particularly a reduction of cardiovascular disease, is seen most strikingly in women who have had a hysterectomy and take transdermal wBodyIdentical 17beta-estradiol (E). For women who have had a hysterectomy and are under age sixty or within ten years of menopause, estrogen therapy tips the scale in favor of improved health and reduced mortality for most known medical problems (Figure 30-3).

In addition to the obvious quality of life improvements gained by the elimination of Hot Flash Fever (over 90 percent), Vaginal Sahara (100 percent), and dyspareunia (over 80 percent); estrogen favorably improves heart disease, stroke, diabetes, osteoporosis, colon cancer, obesity, dementia, metabolic syndrome, and breast cancer.

Overall, in this group of women, there is a **40 percent reduction in total mortality with estrogen therapy**. If estrogen therapy were combined with the Womenopause Challenge lifestyle changes, there would certainly be additional death delay.

Weigh the Death Prevention Benefits
ORAL ESTROGEN (E) FOR wFRIDAY WOMEN

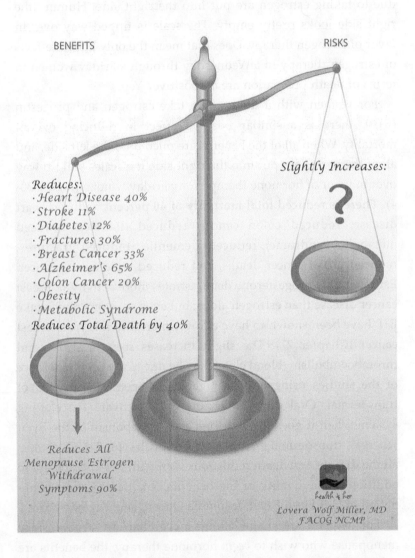

BENEFITS

RISKS

Slightly Increases:

?

Reduces:
· Heart Disease 40%
· Stroke 11%
· Diabetes 12%
· Fractures 30%
· Breast Cancer 33%
· Alzheimer's 65%
· Colon Cancer 20%
· Obesity
· Metabolic Syndrome
Reduces Total Death by 40%

Reduces All
Menopause Estrogen
Withdrawal
Symptoms 90%

health & her

Lovera Wolf Miller, MD
FACOG NCMP

Figure 30-3 Weigh the Death Prevention Benefits of Estrogen for wFriday Women

In Figure 30-3, all of the known benefits of estrogen therapy that reduce mortality for wFriday women are piled into the left side of the scale; while, all of the risks that would hasten death due to taking estrogen are put into the right side. Humm...the right side looks pretty empty. The scale is tipped way over in favor of estrogen therapy. Does that mean the only known effects of estrogen therapy in wWednesday through wFriday women in terms of death prevention are all positive? Yep.

For women with a uterus who take estrogen and progestin (E+P), there is a similar positive effect in reducing overall mortality. When all of the benefits are piled onto the left side, and all of the harms are put into the right side the scales still tip way over in favor of hormone therapy for wFriday women (Figure 30-4). **There is reduced total mortality of 40 percent,** reduced heart disease, reduced colon cancer, reduced diabetes, reduced metabolic syndrome, reduced dementia, reduced fractures, reduced breast cancer deaths, and reduced endometrial cancer. Estrogen plus progesterone demonstrates more activity in breast cancer disease than estrogen alone; but even so, women who take E+P have been shown to have a lower mortality rate from breast cancer (Chapter 27). The slight increases seen in stroke and thromboembolism (blood clots) may be due to the preponderance of the studies using oral conjugated estrogen (CE) instead of transdermal. Oral estrogen is known to activate the clotting system when it goes through first pass metabolism in the liver; whereas, transdermal estrogen does not (Chapter 21). Of course, all the disease and death reductions seen with E+P therapy are in addition to the quality of life benefits obtained by their elimination of Hot Flash Fever, Insomnia Queen, and Vagina Sahara.

For women over age 60 or more than ten years since menopause who wish to *begin* hormone therapy, the benefits are still substantial. It is known that therapy with estrogen (E) or estrogen plus progesterone (E+P), results in a **reduction of total mortality by 40 percent** for all ages of women compared to

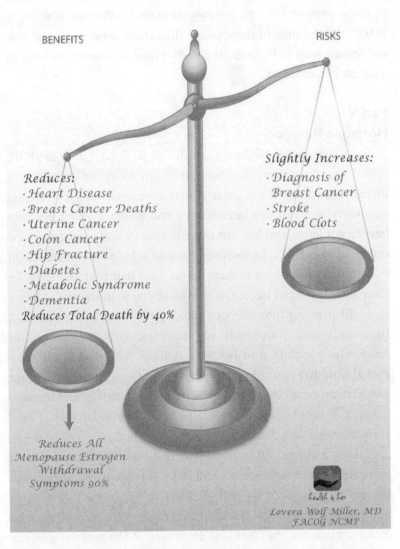

Weigh the Death Prevention Benefits
ORAL ESTROGEN PLUS PROGESTERONE (E+P) FOR wFRIDAY WOMEN

BENEFITS

RISKS

Reduces:
- *Heart Disease*
- *Breast Cancer Deaths*
- *Uterine Cancer*
- *Colon Cancer*
- *Hip Fracture*
- *Diabetes*
- *Metabolic Syndrome*
- *Dementia*
Reduces Total Death by 40%

Slightly Increases:
- *Diagnosis of Breast Cancer*
- *Stroke*
- *Blood Clots*

Reduces All Menopause Estrogen Withdrawal Symptoms 90%

health 4 her
Lovera Wolf Miller, MD
FACOG NCMP

Figure 30-4 Weigh the Death Prevention Benefits of Estrogen
Plus Progesterone for wFriday Women

women who do not take menopausal hormone therapy. Women, over age seventy (twenty years after menopause) who *begin* MHT at that time, are vulnerable to heart events for the first year of therapy; but after that, their cardiovascular risks are lower than in those women who do not take hormones. Women who *begin* MHT near the time of menopause (like most women do) the risk reductions seen in Figures 30-3 & 30-4 may remain for as long as therapy is continued.

Part VI:
Hormone Reunion

School reunions can be a blast. It can be great fun to catch up with friends you have not seen or heard from for decades. It's interesting to see if the class clown ever grew up, if the class egghead ever overcame her shyness; and whether or not the class beauty got any wrinkles. But there is always that someone you'd rather not see, too. Remember the one who always seemed to make some off-handed remark about your hair that would make your little teenaged heart crack. Would you skip the entire party to avoid running into that one mean girl? What if the class had thousands and thousands of students, and the chance of randomly bumping into her was remote; would you still stay away? Couldn't you think of ways to avoid or ignore her? Would you give up on all the friends, the food, the dancing, and the new dress and shoes—just to avoid the slim chance of seeing her? Well, it would be your choice.

Taking menopausal hormones is like that. There are loads of potential benefits and some small risks. If you never bumped into the bratty girl, you'd be real glad if you had gone to the party because it was sooo great seeing everyone, and you'd already be making plans for the next one. However, if she was assigned to your table, and you were trapped all night with her, you might think otherwise, but what are the odds of that happening? The odds of MHT benefits are significantly higher than their risk of causing harm in some women, but everyone has to consider her personal preferences in making her own decision.

Begin right now to prevent your own death so stop pausing and start living.

Malika C

Malika C. was a one-woman-culture-crashing-odds-defying-gender-defining paragon. Born and raised in urban Los Angeles, she met her "soul-mate" on a faith-based Internet dating service. The love of her life, Lester, was a funeral director of a family-owned business in a small mid-western town. Incredibly, Malika with two masters degrees in hand, moved three thousand miles to live and work in a place her family considered to be, "the far side of the moon". She made it work and the entire community loved her and benefited from her presence. She helped out at the funeral home, worked part-time with a local accountant (she was a CPA), taught watercolor painting, volunteered two days a week at the soup kitchen, copy-edited magazine articles from home, and still managed to help with her brother's warehouse business located in California. And then in the afternoons she...

At her third annual visit with her not-so-new gynecologist, she posed an interesting question. Could she please have a prescription for hormones? At age 51, Malika had reached menopause two years prior at age 49. She had a BMI of 18 (a notch below slim figured) and zero health problems. Her question sprang from concerns about her mother's health. Malika's mother was recently transferred here from a nursing home in California. She was 71 years old and in very poor health. Suffering from progressive Alzheimer's dementia, she had fallen last year, fracturing a hip from which she never recovered. Now bedridden, calling-out in constant pain, Malika's mother neither recognized her daughter nor cared. Recently, the attending internist told Malika that her mother's grave condition was made worse by end-stage congestive heart failure which was the result of her cardiovascular disease. In short, Malika recognized that her mother was not ever going to recover and make it home.

Most of us prefer not to consider death, not our loved one's and, definitely, not our own. Occasionally, we are forced to confront our mortality, and our response will determine how our life plays out. Malika was staring at her mother's death, choosing to make her personal health optimal to avoid her own premature death. No one gets out alive, but the duration and manner of our time in this world can be improved. Malika was motivated to improve.

Up to now, Malika had never considered lifestyle choices as important. She accepted the Womenopause Challenge and vowed to begin an exercise program and a real food diet. Her wScore totaled 3 (only three!) W. She indicated 1 W for hot flashes, 1 W for insomnia, and 1 W for dry skin. Obviously, the wUpSide had been kind to her so far. All of her annual tests were normal including a bone density T score of -1.6. She had had a hysterectomy ten years ago.

Malika had recently edited an article for an online health news service that covered the effects of hormones for postmenopausal women. She asked if it was true that hormones reduced the risks of osteoporosis, dementia, and heart disease; the very problems that were presently ravaging her mother?

Malika was advised that the answers to these questions were never simply, yes or no. The majority of menopausal hormone therapy is initiated for the control of moderate or severe vasomotor symptoms (Hot Flash Fever, Cold Crashes, and drenched nightgowns). Sometimes, menopausal hormone therapy is prescribed for vaginal dryness (Vagina Sahara). Occasionally, menopausal hormone therapy is prescribed for the sole purpose of prevention of osteoporosis. She said, "I can't lie to you; I don't really have any menopause symptoms. I just want hormones because that's what my body use to make, and it seems to me that I need them to stay healthy. Isn't it true that women who take hormones are healthier? That's what the article said."

Although there has been a lot of accumulating evidence, the FDA has not approved hormone therapy for the prevention of any chronic illness other than osteoporosis: not dementia, not depression, not cardiovascular disease, and not cancer. There remain some experts who feel the long-term risks of hormones outweigh their benefits particularly in terms of breast cancer, blood clots, and stroke. There are other experts who believe the opposite: hormone therapy (especially transdermal hormone therapy), when started at or near menopause, provides health benefits of reduced heart disease, reduced stroke, reduced dementia, reduced mood disorders, reduced cancer, and an overall reduced mortality from all causes. She was advised that her present gynecologist favored the later opinion, but new evidence was published every month, and opinions may change with time. Malika asked, "Well, shouldn't we do the best we can right now, while I'm still a wFriday woman?" Yes, of course, we should always do the best we can right now because now is the only time we have to stop pausing and start living.

Divigel 0.5mg was prescribed, specifically, for the accepted purpose of osteoporosis prevention; although, as far as Malika was concerned, the hormone was for the prevention of heart disease and dementia. She accepted that there are risks and side effects to estrogen therapy, and as she pointed out, "It seems that for me there are a lot more risks by not taking estrogen."

One month later, Malika returned for a follow up appointment. Her mother had passed away soon after the last appointment, and she and Lester had mixed feelings about it. On the one hand, they knew her mother's quality of life was non-existent, and it was beyond their control, but on the other hand, they missed her terribly. As far as her own health was concerned, she had successfully completed her "first month of the rest of my life." She had committed whole-heartedly to eating a real food diet and exercising everyday. She felt it honored her mother to become as healthy as possible. Her follow-up wScore was 0 (zero) W. She was advised that a zero score had never been reported before. She said, "That must mean I improved more than anyone else."c

Two years later Malika remained healthy and happy. She was enthusiastic about a couple of new projects she had begun. She had maintained her Womenopause Challenge activities, and now, could not imagine a life without healthy lifestyle commitments. Her bone density remained normal with a T score of -0.4. She reviewed the current information about the pros and cons of continuing menopausal hormone therapy, and decided for her, the benefits definitely outweighed the risks. She elected to continue it for another year and reassess then.

Part VII:
The Womenopause Challenge: Choose Life

1. Choose *not* to die prematurely from cardiovascular disease: become smoke free today.
2. Choose *not* to die prematurely from cardiovascular disease: eat real food (and not too much of it) today.
3. Choose *not* to die prematurely from cardiovascular disease: exercise like your life depends upon it.
4. Choose *not* to die prematurely from cardiovascular disease: get your blood pressure checked and treated today.
5. Choose *not* to die prematurely: make an appointment to see a NAMS Certified Menopause Practitioner (NCMP) today. www.menopause.org

Chapter 31

Almost Forgot the Chapter About Memory

Part I:
Grey Mush

The human brain is about two handfuls of soft grey mush. Unfortunately, that is how many people treat their brain, like mush. Womenopause Challenge intends to rehabilitate the brain's reputation. The menopause brain makeover starts right now.

The human brain is the single most impressive part of this created world, and it gets taken for granted. If a person put half as much energy into improving her brain as she spent following who would win *Dancing With the Stars*, or half as much energy as she spent raising her bowling average, or half as much energy as she spent picking out shoes...well, you get the picture. Everyone assumes the brain just does what the brain will do, and there is nothing that can be done to change it.

Brain Makeover point #1: The brain is like a puppy craving attention, and if we throw it a bone from time to time the brain will be forever devoted. Everyone should discard the grey image of the brain. Instead, think of it as a clear light blue breezy sky with fluffy white clouds and a bright blazing sun with a corner of inky black containing twinkling stars. The brain is as expansive and beautiful as all of that and more. Everyone assumes the brain is endowed at birth with certain capabilities, and that's the end of the story. Not true.

Brain Makeover point #2: The brain is a life-long child capable of learning new stuff—good and bad. Since the brain is encased within a nice thick skull, everyone also assumes if they do not allow the skull to be smashed (very often); they have done their part in protecting it.

Brain Makeover point #3: The brain is a living breathing organic psyche, and it thrives on health and dives on disease.

Part II:
How to Keep Your Brain Young

Remember the childhood song, "The ham bone's connected to the, thigh bone, and the thigh bone's connected to the, knee bone...?" It's true, every word of it. It's all connected. Knowing how to keep your brain young is *exactly* like knowing how to keep your heart young, and your skin, and your liver, and your muscles, and so on. Knowing how to keep your brain young is like knowing how to manage the problems of menopause. By this point you hardly need the list, but here it is anyway (besides, repetition is one of the best ways to remember things):

- Mood Matters: Being happy is not always easy, but it is always the better choice. Seeking happiness and fulfillment in constructive ways is an *action* not a thought. Peace comes to those who seek it (Chapter 12: Mood Matters). The brain loves peace and rails against animosity. Treating depression, when present, gives a thirsty brain a drink.
- Real food: The brain is a real biological entity and requires real fuel, the kind of fuel God put on the planet for us to eat: not fast food, junk food, snack food—real food, and not too much of it (Chapter 14: Real Food). Think green.
- Vitamin-X exercise: The brain is part of a physical dynamo that performs best when everything is in shape (Chapter 16: Vitamin-X: Exercise).
- Mental activity: Mentally challenging work; and get this, even mentally challenging leisure activities strengthen the

brain and helps preserve its function. Learn a new language, play a musical instrument, take a class in photography, play chess, or do crossword puzzles. They all stimulate the brain and eliminate Meno-Fog.

- Waistline: Trimming the waistline improves more than your self-image. It also improves how well your brain can take, process, and remember the images! (Chapter 15: Shape Your Waist)

- Cardiovascular disease: The brain doesn't *like* blood; no, it's way more than *like*, it's *desperate* for blood. Atherosclerosis that clogs cerebral arteries spells death to the neurons that make up the brain. Managing all of the cardiovascular risk factors helps protect the brain: hypertension, diabetes, smoking (another reason to quit), metabolic syndrome, weight, mood, did we miss anything? (Chapter 28: Heart Health)

- Diabetes: The brain prefers normal blood sugar. Do everything you can to make it so.

- Alcohol: The brain likes balance. A little alcohol (three drinks) appears to have favorable effects on memory, but more tends to have the opposite effect. Moderation is the key.

- Juice: One glass of juice (fruit or vegetable) a day has positive affects on memory.

- Supplements. A good multivitamin, extra calcium, vitamin D, folic acid, and fish oil every day seems prudent (Chapter 17: Vitamins).

- Socializing: Intimate relationships with friends and family have profound affects on brain function. Investing time and energy into friendships comes back to you in love and memories!

- Menopausal Hormone Therapy: No surprise. Since MHT for *w*Wednesday, *w*Thursday, and *w*Friday women, reduces the risks for cardiovascular disease, reduces the risk of diabetes, reduces the incidence of metabolic syndrome, reduces the risks of high BMI, and improves Mood Matters, it is no wonder hormones have beneficial effects on the brain. In addition to preserving blood flow, neurons all over the brain have estrogen receptors and, no doubt, there is a reason for that. Estrogen helps protect *w*Wednesday, *w*Thursday, and *w*Friday women from Alzheimer's (Chapters 21 & 22) and Meno-Fog. Given during the "window of opportunity", estrogen may reduce Alzheimer's disease by as much as 67 percent. If continued for 10 years, the risk may actually be decreased by 87 percent, but if wSaturday women with no symptoms, begin menopause hormone therapy after age 65, they may increase their risk of Alzheimer's.

- Sleep. While you are sleeping, the brain does some of its most important "thinking": making and storing memory. The brain formulates memories better with eight hours of adequate sleep (Chapter 11: Insomnia Queen).

Part III:
Brain Spa

While you were dreaming of a perfect spa day: cut, color, and style; manicure and pedicure; and a foot massage, your brain was dreaming of a perfect brain spa day.

This is what your brain might have been thinking. Get up whenever you wake up after eight hours of uninterrupted cool dark refreshing sleep. Ride your bike into the gym for a yoga class with friends. The last 5 minutes are devoted to child's pose with focused breathing and wind chime music playing softly in the background with the scent of sandalwood wafting through the breeze. Then head home for an oatmeal breakfast with a couple of egg whites and a glass of V8 juice (ready and waiting made by that wonderful husband of yours). After a leisurely shower, you apply your estrogen spray, take all your vitamins, minerals, and fish oil, dress; and then, off you go to work (but you feel guilty calling it work because it's so much fun). You make a break-through and solve a problem that had everyone stumped for a week, before having a spinach salad with grilled chicken for lunch with your mother. Back at work, you tie up some loose ends and have a cottage cheese snack before heading home. Before changing into your comfort clothes, you and your husband make plans for a hike and picnic with friends this coming weekend. Then, the two of you play 30 minutes of tennis before you hop on the mower, and he cleans the shed. Next, you both wash up for a dinner of your special 15-bean Tuscan soup and a salmon fillet. After dinner, you go for a walk and discuss the interesting and unintentionally hilarious things the kids told you both today. After returning home, you practice the harp and read some more of that book about the history of Renaissance painting. You are so engrossed in the reading you did not notice your husband had poured you a glass of wine, lighted some candles, and turned on your favorite music in the bedroom. Ahhh, your brain is so happy.

Part IV:
Don't Tease Your Brain

Brainteasers are cruel: you give your brain a taste of something interesting then snatch it away. The brain craves a steady diet of challenging activity—both mental and physical. It is better to think of the brain more like a mental muscle than mental mush. The brain wants to workout not to checkout. Relaxing has its place, but the brain prefers having thought-sweat running down its grey (or should we say sky-blue?) folds. Like any muscle, the memory muscle is a lot stronger the harder it is worked. TV is mental abuse, which could result in vacuous incarceration.

Brain health is exactly like menopausal health; you get what you work for. Get the best.

Part V:
Meno-fog and Menopause

Memory complaints are common in midlife women. Meno-fog appears to track along with Mood Matters but may have a distinctly different neural cause. For instance, Mood Matters of menopausal women respond well to anti-depressants such as the SNRIs, which modulate the neurotransmitters serotonin and norepinephrine in the brain, but that kind of treatment does not have a benefit for Meno-fog and memory. Memory disorders may have an alteration of acetycholine neurotransmitter, and antidepressants do not improve it. Estradiol (E2), however, has important effects on all three neurotransmitters, and that explains why it is so effective for both Mood Matters and Meno-fog.

Clinical memory tests have documented that women have a decline in verbal memory as they transition through perimenopause, and that estrogen reverses the effect for women who start therapy younger than age 65. In fact, there is a relationship between the severity and duration of hot flashes and the magnitude of the Meno-fog. The frightening thing about all of this research is the strong association between verbal memory deficits in midlife and the later development of Alzheimer's Dementia. Women with induced menopause have an even greater risk of verbal memory problems. Despite the favorable evidence, estrogen is not recommended as a prevention or a treatment for cognitive dysfunction. Fortunately, Meno-fog usually lifts during the postmenopausal time.

Fay C.

Fay was 64 years young, a married mother of nine (9!). She played the organ for a large church and taught piano out of her home. She and her husband Al were very active in the ski patrol and had just returned from the ski patrol convention. She was shocked and saddened to learn some of the younger members wanted to put a mandatory retirement age of 65 on high mountain active patrol members.

Fay was in excellent health, and there was a reason for that; she worked at it. She was not compulsive, neurotic, or extreme in any of her health habits. She was careful and disciplined because there was a lot of stuff she wanted to do, and sitting around at home in a recliner was not one of them. She took Divigel 0.5 g daily (wBodyIdentical 17beta-estradiol) and had been taking some form of estrogen since menopause 12 years ago. She had a hysterectomy 20 years ago and did not require progesterone. Other than that, her medical history was a blank. Her BMI was 22, her blood pressure was 110/74, and her waist measured a trim 29 inches.

She and Al learned to speak French two years ago because they had become active in a humanitarian group with work in Haiti. She believed her memory and reasoning powers were still improving. She excitedly discussed a renewed love for Bach organ music and thought she had finally matured enough to express the music properly. Fay was healthy and happy. She was not going to give up mountain ski patrol because of someone else's misguided notion about age.

From a medical standpoint, Fay did not need to change anything. In fact, maybe she could teach the medical staff a few things. She asked if there was a test for Alzheimer's she could take to prove she was mentally okay. She knew she could out-ski everyone; that would not be questioned. Fay received information about Alzheimer's dementia.

Alzheimer's Dementia (AD) is a brain disorder affecting 8 percent at age 65 and 30 percent at age 85. AD is an impairment of the brain's cerebral cortex, resulting in problems, especially with verbal memory, problem solving, attention, and language. A specialist in neurology or psychiatry usually makes the diagnosis.

The following tests may help confirm the suspicion of mental impairment:

1. Modified Mini-Mental State Exam: administered by the health care provider, taking about fifteen minutes to complete.
2. Blood tests: to *exclude* other causes like vitamin deficiencies, toxins, and metabolic problems.
3. Brain imaging: a CT scan or MRI to view the structures of the brain.

Fay was advised there would be no need to spend two thousand dollars for an MRI that would show her brain to be perfectly normal. There is always a temptation to trust an "objective" measurement over a clinical judgment; but in her case, there was no doubt. Fay was advised about the risk factors for AD and given information about how to improve and maintain the brain's ability to think. "I already do all of that," was the only reasonable comment she could make. Yes, of course. She was offered a letter attesting to her physical and mental medical clearance, but she changed her mind. "If they want me to step aside, they will have to think smarter and ski faster than I can. I'm not going to argue with them; I'm going to show them. I intend to ski until I'm 80, and then I'll decide about 90." She's living not pausing.

Part V:
The Womenopause Challenge: Memory Lane

1. Mind games: challenge your brain to a game of chess, or bridge, or black jack, or The Times crossword puzzle, or better yet, do 'em all.
2. Spring brain cleaning: remove, throw away, eliminate, and delete all unnecessary junk thoughts that cause such a messy clutter.

3. Brain business: give your brain a break and let it hike a new trail, sing a new song, and imagine a better world.

4. Head case: choose to think good thoughts; no seriously, believe in something or someone great and let your mind expand into loving it.

5. Brain food: eat real food; thoughts become memories only when everything stays connected and improves with feeding yourself real food.

6. Thought process: exercise your body's muscles to improve your brain strength.

7. Total recall: reduce your risk of heart disease; the brain absolutely requires a satisfactory blood supply and *anything* that reduces cardiovascular disease boosts memory power.

8. Brain pleaser: tell a joke; a sour or blue mood slows down thought process; whereas, a joke, or even a lame pun, brightens-up the brain's day every time.

EPILOGUE

Health and well-being are the sublime ash of a bright-burning life.

RESOURCES

Website one stop shopping:

#1) North American Menopause Society: menopause.org

#2) WebMD.com

#3) Mayoclinic.com

Other useful websites:

#1) The Women's Health Initiative: nhlbi.nih.gov/whi

#2) American College of Obstetricians and Gynecologists: acog.org

#3) Medline Plus: nlm.nih.gov/medlineplus

#4) National Cancer Institute: cancer.gov

#5) The American Heart Association: americanheart.org

#6) American Academy of Family Physicians: familydoctor.org

#7) National Institute of Mental Health: nimh.nih.gov

#8) U.S. Food and Drug Administration: fda.gov

#9) National Osteoporosis Foundation: nof.org

#10) American Urological Association: urologyhealth.org

#11) National Sleep Foundation: sleepfoundation.org

#12) American Academy of Dermatology: skincarephysicians.com

#13) International Society for the Study of Women's Sexual Health: isswsh.org

#14) National Center for Complementary and Alternative Medicine: nccam.nih.gov

#15) American Diabetes Association: diabetes.org

#16) Womenopause Book: womenopausebook.com

Recommended Books on Menopause:

#1) *The Cleveland Clinic Guide to Menopause*
   Holly Thacker, M.D.
   Kaplan Publishing: 2009

#2) *Hot Flashes, Hormones, and Your Health*

JoAnn E. Manson, M.D.

McGraw-Hill: 2006

#3) *The Hormone Decision*

Tara Parker-Pope

Rodale Books: 2007

#4) *Is it hot in here? Or is it me? The Complete Guide to Menopause*

Barbara Kantrowitz and Pat Wingert Kelly

Workman Publishing: 2006

#5) *A Woman's Guide to Menopause & Perimenopause*

Mary Jane Minkin, M.D., and Carol V. Wright, PhD.

Yale University Press: 2005

#6) *Could it be...Perimenopause?*

Steven R. Goldstein, M.D., and Laurie Ashner

Random House: 2007

Other Recommended Books:

#1) *Complete Guide to Women's Health*

Nieca Goldberg, M.D., with Alice Greenwood, PhD.

Ballantine Books: 2008

#2) *In Defense of Food*

Michael Pollan

Penguin, 2009

#3) *The Female Brain*

LuAnn Brizendine, M.D.

Broadway Books: 2006

#4) *You: Staying Young*

Michael F. Roisen, M.D. and Mehmet C. Oz, M.D.

Free Press: 2007

#5) *Sex and the Brain*

Gillian Einstein PhD editor

The MIT Press: 2007

#6) *Younger Next Year for Women*

Chris Crowley and Henry S. Lodge, M.D.

Workman Publishing: 2005

#7) *This is Your Brain on Music*
   Daniel J. Levitin, PhD.
   Penguin Group: 2006
#8) *Prayer is Good Medicine*
   Larry Dossey, M.D.
   Harper Collins: 1997
#9) *Why People Believe Weird Things*
   Michael Shermer, PhD.
   Henry Holt: 2002
#10) *The Road Less Traveled*
   M. Scott Peck, M.D.
   Touchstone Books: 1998
#11) *The Purpose Driven Life*
   Rick Warren
   Zondervan: 2002
#12) *The Brain That Changes Itself*
   Norman Doidge, M.D.
   Penguin Books: 2007
#13) *Timeless Healing*
   Herbert Benson, M.D., with Marg Stark
   Fireside: 1997
#14) *Body for Life*
   Bill Phillips
   Collins Living: 1999
#15) *Dr. Dean Ornish's Program for Reversing Heart Disease*
   Dean Ornish, M.D.
   Ivy Books: 1995
#16) *The Testosterone Syndrome*
   Eugene Shipper, M.D., and William Fryer
   M. Evans: 2007
#17) *A Woman's Guide to Sleep Disorders*
   Meir H. Kryger, M.D.
   McGraw-Hill: 2004
#18) *Getting the Sex you Want*

Sandra Labium, PhD. and Judith Sachs
Crown: 2002
#19) *Reclaiming Desire*
Andrew Goldstein, M.D., and Marrianne Brandon PhD.
Rodale: 2002
#20) *Fit to Live*
Pamela Peeke, M.D.
Rodale: 2007

Selected Reference Material

Menopause Practice a Clinician's Guide 3rd Edition, Wolf H. Utian, M.D., PhD.

Vitamin D Deficiency in Pre- and Postmenopausal Women, Munir MD and Barge MD, *Menopause Management,* 17, Number 5, 2008.

Pharmacologic Treatment Options for Menopausal Symptoms, Hess MD et al, *The Female Patient,* May, 2009

Identifying Patients at Risk for Osteoporotic Fracture, Silverman MD, *Menopause Management, vole* 18, Number 3, 2009.

Bioidentical Hormone Therapy: A Review of the Evidence, Cirigliano MD, *Journal of Women's Health,* Vol 16, Number 5, 2007.

Women, Hormones, and Therapy: A Practitioner's Guide to Balancing Benefits and Safety, Simon MD, Saia MD, and Minchin MD, *Highlights form a Symposium* May 8, 2007.

Use of Low-Dose Hormone Therapy in Menopause: Changing Perspectives, Pinkerton MD et. al., *Contemporary OB/GYN,* December, 2008.

The Evolution of Estrogen Therapy: A Modern-Day Management Option for Menopause, Simon MD, *PV Update Publishing,* 2007.

The Long and Winding Road of Hormone Therapy: Where Are We Today? Goldstein MD, Stencil MD, *Women's Health Update,* Special Supplement, March, 2008.

Breast Cancer Risk Reduction: SERMS, Surgery, and Beyond, Dronca MD, et al, *Menopause Management,* Vol 18, Number 2, 2009.

Management of Hot Flashes: Alternatives to Estrogen Therapy, Shifren MD, *Menopause Management,* Vol 18, Number 2, 2009.

Clinical Perspectives on the Role of Hormone Therapy in Menopausal Management, Shoppe MD, Goldstein MD, *Ob.*

Gyn. News, Supplement, 2007.

In Perspective: Estrogen Therapy Safely and Effectively Reduces Total Mortality and Coronary Heart Disease in Recently Menopausal Women, Hodis MD, Mack MD, *Menopause Management,* March, 2008.

Understanding the Controversy: Hormone Testing and Bioidentical Hormones, Simon MD, et al, *Monograph Postgraduate Course North American Menopause Society,* March 2008.

Vitamin D: Essential for Lifelong Health in Women, Pizza MD, *The Female Patient,* Vol 34 No. 5, May 2009.

Investigation, Treatment, and Monitoring of Late-Onset Hypogonadism in Males, Wang MD, et al, *International Journal of Impotence Research,* Vol 20, No. 5, October 2008.

Vaginal pH, Estrogen and Genital Atrophy, Freedman MD, *Menopause Management,* Vol 19. No. 4, August 2008.

Testosterone Therapy in Adult Men with Androgen Deficiency Syndrome, An Endocrine Society Clinical Practice Guideline, *The Endocrine Society's Clinical Guidelines,* 2006.

Diagnosing Hypoactive Sexual Desire Disorder in Peri- and Postmenopausal Women, Labium PhD, *Supplement to Menopause Management* 19th Annual Meeting NAMS, Vol 18 Suppl. 1, 2009.

Women's Sexual Health Issues: Practical Management Strategies, Update 2009, Goldstein MD, Parish MD, Schwenkhagen MD, *ISSWSH Annual Pre-Course Conference,* February, 2009.

Testosterone Improves Sexual Function in Women Not Taking Estrogen, Davis MD, et al, *New England Journal of Medicine,* 359, 2008.

Nurses' Health Study: Health Lifestyle Lowers Mortality in Middle-aged Women, Van Dam et al, *British Medical Journal,* 2009.

Menopause and the Metabolic Syndrome, Janssen MD, et al, *Archives of Internal Medicine,* 168, 2008.

Health related Quality of Life After Combined Hormone Replacement Therapy, Walton MD, et al, *British Medical Journal*, 2008.

Hormone Therapy Update, Carr MD, *Contemporary OB/GYN*, August, 2007.

Postmenopausal Hormone Therapy and Risk of Cardiovascular Disease by Age and Years Since Menopause, Rossouw MD, et al, *JAMA*, 297, 2007.

The Beneficial Effect of Hormone Therapy on the Mortality and Coronary Heart Disease in Younger verses Older Postmenopausal Women, Hodis MD, Mack MD, *Medscape OB/Gyn & Women's Health*, March, 2008.

Feminine Forever, Round 2: the Bioidentical Cult, Utian MD, *Menopause*, January, 2008.

Postmenopausal systemic Hormone therapy: Putting Risks Into Perspective, Utian MD, *Medscape* sponsored by NAMS and National Association of Nurse Practitioners in Women's Health. April, 2008.

Postmenopausal Hormone Therapy in Clinical Perspective, Hodis MD, *Menopause*, 14, 2007.

Change in health related quality of life over the menopausal transition, Avis MD, Colvin MD, *Menopause*16; *2009*; 860-869.

Microdose transdermal estrogen therapy for the relief of vulvo-vaginal symptoms in postmenopausal women, Bachman, GA, Schaefers, M, Uddin A, Utian WH. *Menopause* 16; 2009; 877-882.

Topical estrogen therapy in the management of postmenopausal vaginal atrophy, Al-Baghdall O, Ewies AA. *Climacteric* 12; 2009; 91-105.

Non-hormonal therapies for menopausal hot flashes: systematic review and meta-analysis. Nelson HD, Vesco KK, Haney F. *JAMA* 295; 2006; 2057-2071.

Vasomotor symptoms and mortality: the Rancho Bernardo Study. Svartberg J, von Muhlen D, *Menopause* 16; 2009; 888-891.

Postmenopausal testosterone: time for a reappraisal?. Buster J. *Female Patient* 32; 2007; 22-36.

Menopausal hot flushes revisited. Andrikoula M, Prelevic G. *Climacteric* 12; 2009; 3-15.

Vasomotor symptoms and cardiovascular risk. Gambacciani M, Pepe A. *Climacteric* 12; 2009; 32-35.

Quality of life and sexuality issues in aging women. Birkhaser M. Climacteric 12; 2009; 52-57.

Temporal association of hot flashes and depression in the transition to menopause. Freeman EW, Sammel MD, *Menopause* 16; 2009; 728-734.

Hippocampal volumes are larger in postmenopausal women using estrogen compared to past users, never users, and men; a possible window of opportunity effect. Lord C, Buss C, Lupien SJ, Pruessner JC. *Neurobiol Aging* 29; 2008; 95-101.

Depression during the menopause transition: window of opportunity. Soares CN. *Menopause* 15; 2008; 207-209.

Depression and cardiovascular sequelae in postmenopausal women. Wasser-Hall S, Shumaker S, Ockene J. *Arch Intern Med* 164; 2004; 289-298.

Risk for new onset depression during the menopause transition. Cohen LS, Soares CN, Vitonis AF, Otto ML, Harlow BL. *Arch Gen Psychiatry* 63; 2006; 385-390.

The interface of depression, sleep, and vasomotor symptoms. Shaver JL *Menopause* 16; 2009;626-629.

Coronary heart disease and depression: a review of recent mechanistic research. Skala JA, Freedland KE. *Can J Psychiatry* 51; 2006; 738-745.

Estrogen, menopause, and the aging brain: How basic science can inform hormone therapy in women. Morrison JH, Brinton RD. *J Neurosci* 26; 2006; 10332-10348.

Hormone therapy in menopausal women with cognitive complaints: a randomized, double-blind trial. Maki PM, Gast MJ, Vieweg AJ *Neurology* 69; 2007; 1322-1330.

Hormone therapy and cognitive function. Maki PM, Sunderman E. *Hum Reprod Update* 2009 May 25.

Effects of the menopause transition and hormone use on cognitive performance in midlife women. Greendale GA, Huang MH, Wright RG. *Neurology* 72; 2009; 1850-1857.

Menopause, cognitive ageing, and dementia: practical implications. Henderson VW. *Menopause International* 15; 2009; 41-44.

Lipoprotein management in patients with cardiometabolic risk. Brunzell JD, Davidson M. *Diabetes Care* 31; 2008; 811-822.

Estrogen in the prevention of atherosclerosis. Hodis HN. Lobo RA, Mack WJ. *Ann Intern Med* 135; 2001; 939-953.

Gender differences in osteoarthritis. Price MD, Herndon JH. *Menopause* 16; 2009; 624-625.

Postmenopausal hormone therapy and risk of cardiovascular disease by age and years since menopause. Rossouw JE, Prentice RL, Manson JE. *JAMA* 297; 2007; 1465-1477.

Skin: impact of menopause, aging, and hormones. Utian WH. *Menopause Management* 18; 2009; 11-25.

Diagnosis and treatment of the metabolic syndrome in menopausal women. Pokrywka G. *Menopause Management* 6;2007; 16-28.

Authors' Biography

Lovera Wolf Miller, M.D. and David C. Miller, M.D. are wife and husband physicians living in their hometown: LaPorte, Indiana. They met at a piano recital in the fifth grade. The fact that they are best friends and do everything together is a happy accident because their attraction was purely physical. They have two exceptional and beautiful semi-adult daughters: Sasha, married to Kash Franger, and Brienna Miller, a free agent.

Lovera graduated with honors in Biology from Andrews University in Berrien Springs, Michigan and obtained her medical degree from Loma Linda University School of Medicine in Loma Linda, California. She completed a residency in Obstetrics and Gynecology at Glendale Adventist Medical Center in Glendale, California and is a Board Certified OBGyn and a Fellow in the American College of Obstetrics and Gynecology. Lovera is a NAMS Certified Menopause Practitioner. She is President of health 4 her in Michigan City, Indiana and limits her practice to gynecology and the treatment of perimenopause, menopause, and postmenopause.

David graduated from Purdue University with a degree in English and obtained a Masters degree in physiology from The University of California in Riverside, California. He studied neurophysiology for a PhD at the Brain research Institute at UCLA in Los Angeles, California before obtaining a medical degree from Loma Linda University in Loma Linda, California. David completed a residency in Anesthesiology at the University of Iowa in Iowa City, Iowa and completed fellowship requirements for the specialty of pain management. He is Board Certified in Anesthesiology (American Board of Anesthesiology) and Pain (American Board of Pain Medicine, Fellow of Interventional Pain Practice, American Board of Interventional Pain Physicians). He is also a NAMS Certified Menopause

Practitioner. David is President of Woodland Pain Center in Michigan City, Indiana and limits his practice to the evaluation and treatment of chronic pain.

Lovera and David are a lot more fun than the dry details of their education. They love to travel, hike, kayak, ski, read, garden, and write. They are active in Haitian Support Ministries (haitiansupportministries.org) and have been doing medical trips to Jacmel, Haiti twice a year for many years and were in Haiti for medical relief the week after the earthquake. They both play the harp (one of them much better than the other).

The authors would love to hear from you!

Web page: womenopausebook.com

Email: womenopausebook@mac.com

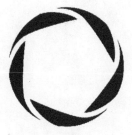

BOOKS

O is a symbol of the world, of oneness and unity. In different cultures it also means the "eye," symbolizing knowledge and insight. We aim to publish books that are accessible, constructive and that challenge accepted opinion, both that of academia and the "moral majority."

Our books are available in all good English language bookstores worldwide. If you don't see the book on the shelves ask the bookstore to order it for you, quoting the ISBN number and title. Alternatively you can order online (all major online retail sites carry our titles) or contact the distributor in the relevant country, listed on the copyright page.

See our website **www.o-books.net** for a full list of over 500 titles, growing by 100 a year.

And tune in to myspiritradio.com for our book review radio show, hosted by June-Elleni Laine, where you can listen to the authors discussing their books.

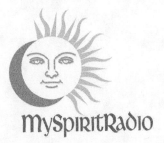

mySpiritRadio